Good Clinical Practice Guide

Compiled by the Medicines and Healthcare products Regulatory Agency

CW00952670

First published 2012

ISBN 978 0 11 708107 9

Printed in the United Kingdom for The Stationery Office

22567 09/12

Contents

Foreword

This guide is the result of eight years' experience of working under the remit of the Clinical Trials Directive 2001/20/EC. The Clinical Trials Directive came into force in May 2004 and was greeted with some trepidation by parts of the clinical trial community. The Directive was put into place to provide a consistent set of rules for clinical trials, applied across the European Union (EU), to ensure that the rights, well-being and safety of clinical trial subjects are not jeopardised, and that the results produced from trials are credible so that sound marketing and prescribing decisions can be made. Ultimately, the intention is to safeguard both current trial subjects and future patients.

Despite inherent flexibilities in the regulations and guidance, over the years it has become apparent that a 'one size fits all' philosophy has developed and this does not work successfully across the wide range of trials conducted in the UK. A contributing factor to this is the lack of authoritative and comprehensive guidance on how the regulations, and in particular Good Clinical Practice (GCP) principles, should be implemented in practice. Depending on the investigational medicinal product, and the indication and subject population in which it is to be used, it is clear that different approaches can be taken with regard to management of the conduct of the trial, using a risk-based proportionate approach. In the UK, a risk-adapted approach has been promoted since April 2011, with guidance being published on the MHRA website at that time. The assessment and management of risk is a theme which runs throughout this guide. The GCP Forum was launched on the MHRA website in October 2011, and allows researchers and organisations to discuss practical issues relating to clinical trials. Both the GCP Forum and this guide are a result of requests from stakeholders for additional guidance on conducting trials.

It is hoped that this guide will provide some insight into a more proportionate way to manage clinical trials within the regulatory framework.

Rebecca Stanbrook
Group Manager, Inspections (GCP, GPvP and GLP)
Dr Martyn Ward
Manager, Clinical Trials Unit (CTU)

Foreword continues

This guide has been driven by the Good Clinical Practice (GCP) Inspectorate at the MHRA, with collaboration from the Health Research Authority (HRA) through the National Research Ethics Service (NRES), and the Clinical Trials Unit and Statistics Unit of the MHRA Licensing Division.

It was recognised that there was a need to provide additional information to the various stakeholder communities in the GCP arena, and therefore this guide has been produced. While this guide does not replace existing documents on the subject, it does offer valuable practical guidance on GCP and how it is possible to comply within the existing legal framework.

I commend this useful reference to you, as the MHRA, sponsors and others involved in clinical trials of investigational medicinal products work together to further benefit public health by safeguarding trial subjects and future patients.

Gerald Heddell
Director, Inspection, Enforcement and Standards Division

Acknowledgements

With regard to the writing of this guide, prepared under the auspices of the MHRA, particular thanks should go to the Good Clinical Practice (GCP) Inspectorate of the MHRA Inspection, Enforcement and Standards Division, who devised and reviewed the guide as well as authoring the majority of the chapters. Thanks must also be given to the authors and reviewers within the Clinical Trials Unit and Statistics Unit of the MHRA Licensing Division, the other MHRA Inspectorates, and the Health Research Authority, as well as to our stakeholders for their review and contributions. Without all these individuals and groups, this guide would not have been possible.

Feedback

Questions or comments on the content or presentation of this guide are encouraged and will be used to develop further editions. Your views are valued and both the MHRA and The Stationery Office (TSO) would appreciate you taking the time to contact us by post, telephone, fax or email.

Good Clinical Practice (GCP) Inspectorate
Inspection, Enforcement and Standards Division
Medicines and Healthcare products Regulatory Agency
151 Buckingham Palace Road
London SW1W 9SZ
www.mhra.gov.uk (Home/How we regulate/Medicines/Inspection and standards/Good Clinical Practice)
Email: info@mhra.gsi.gov.uk
Phone: 020 3080 6000
Fax: 0203 118 9803

For general queries about clinical trials:
Clinical Trial Helpline
Email: clintrialhelpline@mhra.gsi.gov.uk
Phone: 020 3080 6456

For queries relating to clinical trial submissions:
Regulatory Information Service
Email: RIS.CT@mhra.gsi.gov.uk
Phone: 020 3080 7400

For general enquiries about the MHRA:
Central Enquiry Point
Email: info@mhra.gsi.gov.uk
Phone: 020 3080 6000

Abbreviations

AAPEC   Appointing Authority for Phase I Ethics Committees
ABPI   Association of the British Pharmaceutical Industry
AE   adverse event
ALS   advanced life support
API   active pharmaceutical ingredient
AR   adverse reaction
ARSAC   Administration of Radioactive Substances Advisory Committee
ASCII   American Standard Code for Information Interchange
ASR   annual safety report
ATIMP   advanced therapy investigational medicinal product
ATMP   advanced therapy medicinal product
BEMA   Benchmarking of European Medicines Agencies
CAPA   corrective and preventative action
CHM   Commission on Human Medicines
CHMP   Committee for Medicinal Products for Human Use
CIOMS   Council for International Organizations of Medical Sciences
CMDh   Co-ordination Group for Mutual Recognition and Decentralised
           Procedures – Human
CMO   contract manufacturing organisation
CoA   certificate of analysis
CPA   Clinical Pathology Accreditation
CPMP   Committee for Proprietary Medicinal Products
CPRD   Clinical Practice Research Datalink
CRA   clinical research associate
CRF   case report form
CRN   Clinical Research Network
CRO   contract research organisation
CSR   clinical study report
CSV   computer system validation

CTA	clinical trial authorisation
CTEAG	Clinical Trials Expert Advisory Group
CTFG	Clinical Trials Facilitation Group
CTU	MHRA Clinical Trials Unit
DCF	data clarification form
DH	Department of Health
DIBD	development international birth date
DLP	data lock point
DMC	data monitoring committee
DMP	data management plan
DSMB	data safety monitoring board
DSUR	development safety update report
eCRF	electronic case report form
EDC	electronic data capture
EEA	European Economic Area
EHR	electronic health records
EMA	European Medicines Agency
eSUSAR	electronic SUSAR online reporting tool
eTMF	electronic trial master file
EU	European Union
EudraCT	European Union Drug Regulating Authorities Clinical Trials
EVCTM	EudraVigilance Clinical Trial Module
FIH	first in human
GAMP	Good Automated Manufacturing Practice
GCP	Good Clinical Practice
GDP	Good Distribution Practice
GLP	Good Laboratory Practice
GMP	Good Manufacturing Practice
GNA	grounds for non-acceptance
GP	general practitioner
GPvP	Good Pharmacovigilance Practice
GTAC	Gene Therapy Advisory Committee
GxP	good practice standards
HFEA	Human Fertilisation and Embryology Authority

HMA	Heads of Medicines Agencies
HRA	Health Research Authority
HTA	Human Tissue Authority
IB	investigator's brochure
IBD	international birth date
ICH	International Conference on Harmonisation
ILS	immediate life support
IMP	investigational medicinal product
IMPD	investigational medicinal product dossier
IRAS	Integrated Research Application System
IRT	interactive response technologies
ISF	investigator site file
ISO	International Organization for Standardization
ITT	intention to treat
MA	marketing authorisation
MAA	marketing authorisation application
MAH	marketing authorisation holder
mCTA	model clinical trial agreement
MedDRA®	Medical Dictionary for Regulatory Activities
MHRA	Medicines and Healthcare products Regulatory Agency
MIA	manufacturer's/importer's authorisation
MIA(IMP)	manufacturer's authorisation for investigational medicinal products
MRC	Medical Research Council
NCR	no carbon required
NHS	National Health Service
NIHR	National Institute for Health Research
nIMP	non-investigational medicinal product
NRES	National Research Ethics Service
OCR	optical character recognition
pCRF	paper case report form
PD	pharmacodynamic
PDCO	Paediatric Committee
PDF	portable document format

PI	principal investigator
PIC	subject or patient identification centre
PIP	paediatric investigation plan
PK	pharmacokinetic
PSF	product specification file
PSUR	periodic safety update report
QA	quality assurance
QC	quality control
QMS	quality management system
QP	Qualified Person
R&D	research and development
REC	research ethics committee
RSI	reference safety information
SAE	serious adverse event
SAP	statistical analysis plan
SAR	serious adverse reaction
SDV	source data verification
SMO	site management organisation
SOC	system organ class
SOP	standard operating procedure
SPC	summary of product characteristics
SQL	structured query language
SSA	site-specific assessment
SSI	site-specific information
SUSAR	suspected unexpected serious adverse reaction
TMF	trial master file
TSC	trial steering committee
UAT	user acceptance testing
UKECA	United Kingdom Ethics Committee Authority
URS	user requirements specification
VAS	visual analogue scale
VHP	Voluntary Harmonisation Procedure
WHO	World Health Organization
XML	extensible markup language

Preface

There are a large number of legislative documents that govern clinical trials, at a European and national level. At the European level, these are also supported by a number of guidance documents that explain how organisations may comply with the required legislation. In general, guidelines are not legally binding, but as they effectively spell out how legal obligations may be met in a harmonised manner, organisations are expected to comply with them, unless they have appropriate justification for not doing so. Guidelines are also intended to further harmonise European procedures; therefore, compliance with these guidelines should facilitate assessment, approval and control of clinical trials. However, it should be noted that not all guidelines have the same legal status and some may be 'quasi-binding' when they are referenced in the legislation. This means that Good Clinical Practice (GCP) is not always black and white; 'grey' areas exist.

The European Medicines Agency (EMA) has published a document that explains the legislative framework, EMEA/P/24143/2004 'Procedure for European Union guidelines and related documents within the pharmaceutical legislative framework', which can be found on the EMA website.

The EMA also publishes question and answer documents and reflection papers; these are not legally binding and inspectors do not inspect against them. The purpose of these documents is to provide responses to frequently asked questions and to give comment on the current thoughts of European regulators on particular topics.

The International Conference on Harmonisation's Topic E6 (R1) – 'Guideline for Good Clinical Practice' (hereinafter 'ICH GCP') merits a specific reference in relation to guidance for clinical trials. ICH GCP is not explicitly mentioned in the UK legislation; although some Member States have incorporated ICH GCP directly into national legislation, the UK has not. Therefore, ICH GCP is not (in its totality) legally binding in the UK. However, the UK legislation includes the requirements to comply with the conditions and principles of GCP, as outlined in Directive 2005/28/EC. ICH GCP (as adopted by the Committee for Medicinal Products for Human Use (CHMP)) is part of European guidance, as an element of EudraLex Volume 10, and as such should be taken into consideration, as appropriate, as an established standard for GCP. In particular, if a study is to be included as part of a marketing authorisation application, it is an expectation that ICH GCP should be complied with, and this is referred to in the annexes to the Notice to Applicants (Volume 2B) for the Common Technical Document.

However, if organisations claim compliance with ICH GCP as a quality standard, or cite compliance with ICH GCP within protocols or study reports, then it is expected that ICH GCP is followed, and this may be reviewed on inspection.

We are often asked to distinguish between what is a requirement, what is in guidance and what is simply good practice, and which of these must be followed. It is an absolute requirement that the legislation, that is European Regulations, Directives and UK Statutory Instruments, is followed. The guidance contained in EudraLex Volume 10 is largely there to support the legislation and instructs organisations how to comply with the law.

This guide covers legislation, guidance and good practice. Therefore to distinguish between these in the text, the words 'must' and 'required' or 'requirement' refer to legislative requirements, the word 'should' refers to guidance-related practices, and 'recommended' or 'suggested' refers to good practice. To avoid confusion it should be noted that the legislation often uses the word 'shall'; this terminology is interpreted as a requirement and will appear as 'must' in this guide. The following examples are provided to illustrate this approach:

- The word 'should' is used in relation to the production of standard written procedures; although it is a requirement that *'necessary procedures to secure the quality of every aspect of the trial should be complied with'* (Part 2 (4) of Schedule 1 to SI 2004/1031)) this does not always necessitate the need for written procedures for each and every aspect of the trial. Procedures could be contained elsewhere (for example, the protocol), where appropriate, and therefore quality systems need to be proportionate. However, the procedures, whatever they are, 'must' be complied with.
- The words 'must' and 'should' are also both used in relation to the trial master file (TMF). For example, there are some documents that are required as part of the TMF, such as protocols, whereas other documents (for example, 'relevant communications') are referred to in guidance such as ICH GCP. However, those documents that are required to demonstrate whether a trial has been conducted according to the legislation are a requirement of Regulation 31 A(4b) of SI 2004/1031. These documents could also be 'relevant

communications', such as decisions regarding substantiality of an amendment, or communicating the sponsor release of investigational medicinal product (IMP), and therefore 'must' be retained in the TMF.

Throughout this guide, the terms 'must' and 'required'/'requirement' are, for ease of reference, number-coded in the text where used and the corresponding references in the legislation are found at the end of each chapter and annex.

Introduction

The MHRA has identified the need for creating and publishing a guide to Good Clinical Practice (GCP). Similar guidance documents exist for other areas of good practice (GxP): *The Good Pharmacovigilance Practice Guide*; *Rules and Guidance for Pharmaceutical Manufacturers and Distributors*; and the *Guide to UK GLP Regulations*. This guide relates to the conduct of clinical trials of medicinal products for human use in the UK. It is intended that this guide will complement currently available legislation and guidance and provide practical advice to stakeholders about implementing the principles of GCP for the various types of clinical trials in a risk-proportionate way, within the context of the clinical trial regulatory framework in the European Union (EU).

The guide is aimed at any individual and/or organisation involved in conducting clinical trials with medicines in the UK (for example, both commercial and non-commercial sponsors and hosts of clinical trials), as well as contract research organisations, clinical research consultants and other niche providers. However, many of the principles and much of the advice that the guide contains are also relevant to clinical research more generally and may also be useful for organisations conducting trials in other countries.

GCP is a set of internationally recognised ethical and scientific quality requirements that must be observed for designing, conducting, recording and reporting clinical trials that involve the participation of human subjects. Compliance with this good practice provides assurance that the rights, safety and well-being of trial subjects are protected, and that the results of the clinical trials are credible and accurate. Following the implementation of the Clinical Trials Directive 2001/20/EC on 1 May 2004, compliance with the principles of GCP became a legal requirement for everyone in the EU involved in the conduct of a clinical trial with an investigational medicinal product and was transposed into national law in each Member State. This was further developed by the publication and implementation of the GCP Directive 2005/28/EC in 2005. The Clinical Trials Directive 2001/20/EC applies to all interventional clinical trials of medicinal products in Europe, from 'first in human' trials to pragmatic comparisons of commonly used medicines.

The purpose of Directive 2001/20/EC was to develop an increasingly harmonised approach to the approval and conduct of all clinical trials carried out within the EU. The EU Member States were required to adopt and publish national legislation and administrative provisions necessary to comply with Directive 2001/20/EC before 1 May 2003, and had to apply these provisions at the latest with effect from 1 May 2004.

In the UK, these requirements were achieved through The Medicines for Human Use (Clinical Trials) Regulations 2004, Statutory Instrument No. 1031 (SI 2004/1031). SI 2004/1031 sets out the processes for both regulatory and ethical review of all interventional trials of medicinal products in humans in order to gain a clinical trial authorisation (CTA) and favourable research ethics committee (REC) opinion. In addition, the Statutory Instrument sets out requirements by which these trials must be conducted (GCP) and provides the basis for powers to regulate clinical trials, such as inspection and enforcement. This Statutory Instrument has been amended a number of times since 2004 to accommodate new legislation (for example, the GCP Directive 2005/28/EC), but SI 2004/1031 is the commonly used reference for the legislation underpinning clinical trials in the UK. Clinical trials using advanced therapy medicinal products or conducted in the paediatric population are performed under the same regulations; however, these trials also need to take into account the additional regulations specific to these areas.

Additional legislation and guidance documents are detailed in Annex 2. It is important to note that this guide is not intended to replace the existing legislation and guidance and therefore it does not act as a single reference document for all requirements.

This guide is the result of collaboration between different groups within the MHRA, including the Inspectorates (GCP, GMP, GDP, GPvP and GLP) and the Clinical Trials Unit (CTU) as well as external bodies such as the Health Research Authority (HRA). With a combined experience of performing over 700 inspections, the MHRA GCP Inspectorate has encountered many models for conducting clinical trials and also many examples of both good and poor practice. The MHRA GCP Inspectorate also plays an active role within Europe, as does the MHRA CTU, working with European colleagues to develop regulatory requirements and guidance for clinical trials. For example, the MHRA GCP Inspectorate is part of the European Medicines Agency (EMA) Inspectors Working Group, while the MHRA CTU is represented at the Clinical Trials Facilitation Group (CTFG), a working group of the Heads of Medicines Agencies

(HMA), which acts as a forum for agreeing common principles and processes to be applied throughout the European medicines regulatory network. In addition, together with the HRA, the MHRA CTU and GCP Inspectorate provide UK input on the development of guidance at the European Commission Expert Working Group on Clinical Trials.

It is recognised that there are differences in terms of structure, organisation, resources, experience and approach between all those involved in conducting clinical trials and therefore the way in which organisations can achieve compliance varies immensely; what is appropriate for one may be hugely unrealistic or unnecessary for another. It is not possible to address all scenarios within this guide or to provide information that will satisfy the requirements of all individual organisations, but it is hoped that by highlighting the areas in which issues with compliance are commonly found and providing specific examples of good and poor practice this guide can assist organisations in developing effective systems to manage and conduct clinical trials of medicinal products in a risk-proportionate and compliant way.

With the ever-changing regulatory environment, it is inevitable that aspects of this guide will not remain current, although the general principles of GCP will always be relevant. The MHRA intends to revise and update the guide at appropriate time points and, in particular, after experience is gained on the new legislation, following any revisions to EU clinical trial legislation.

The MHRA's mission is to enhance and safeguard the health of the public by ensuring that medicines and medical devices work, and are acceptably safe. We aim to protect, promote and improve public health, and it is hoped that the information provided within this guide will contribute to these aims, by assisting organisations in developing and maintaining appropriate and effective systems for conducting trials in the UK.

The content of external websites referenced in this guide is not the responsibility of the MHRA.

Information given is general guidance and is not an authoritative statement of the law.

CHAPTER 1

Sponsor oversight

Editor's note

Any legal entity that is established in the European Economic Area (EEA), or has an established legal representative within the EEA, can sponsor a clinical trial of an investigational medicinal product (IMP) in the UK. The sponsor may be a single person or organisation or two or more persons or organisations (joint/co-sponsorship). The types of clinical trial sponsors seen in the UK are wide-ranging and come from both the commercial and non-commercial sectors.

In the Medicines for Human Use (Clinical Trials) Regulations 2004 (SI 2004/1031), the sponsor has specific responsibilities with regard to the authorisation for clinical trials and ethics committee opinion, Good Clinical Practice (GCP) and the conduct of clinical trials, pharmacovigilance, and the manufacture, importation and labelling of IMP. Although the sponsor can formally delegate one or more of these functions of sponsorship, ultimately the sponsor remains responsible. Therefore, the sponsor is required to implement sufficient processes to maintain oversight of the clinical trial so that it can ensure that the legislation is complied with and that the sponsor's legal responsibilities are met.

This chapter describes what any organisation needs to consider when sponsoring, managing and overseeing a clinical trial (Figure 1.1), the legal responsibilities of a sponsor, and the ways in which sponsor oversight of the trial can be achieved by different types of organisations and various sponsorship models. Aspects of this chapter may therefore also be applicable to those organisations or individuals who have been delegated all or some of the functions of sponsorship.

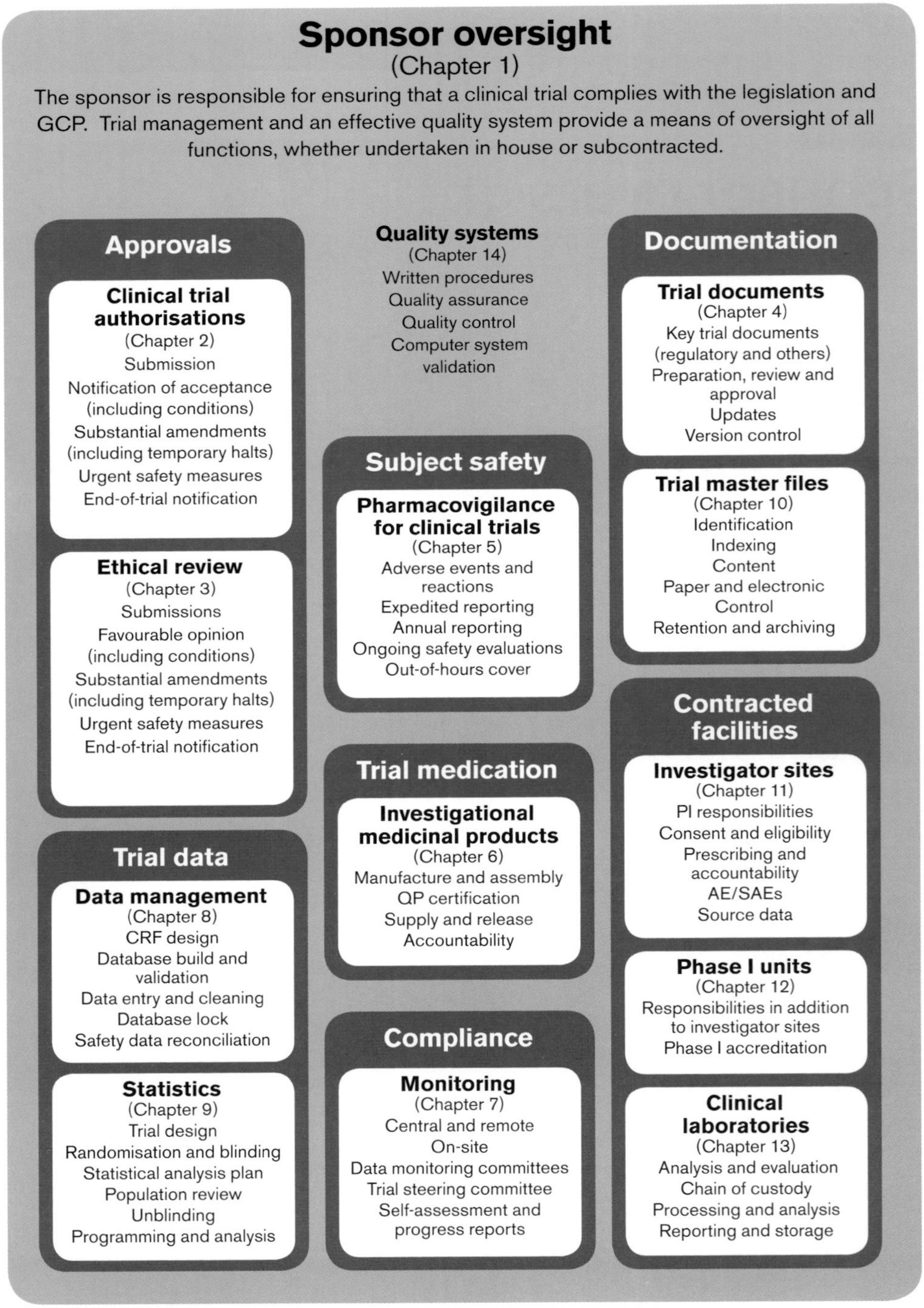

Sponsor oversight
(Chapter 1)

The sponsor is responsible for ensuring that a clinical trial complies with the legislation and GCP. Trial management and an effective quality system provide a means of oversight of all functions, whether undertaken in house or subcontracted.

Approvals

Clinical trial authorisations
(Chapter 2)
Submission
Notification of acceptance
(including conditions)
Substantial amendments
(including temporary halts)
Urgent safety measures
End-of-trial notification

Ethical review
(Chapter 3)
Submissions
Favourable opinion
(including conditions)
Substantial amendments
(including temporary halts)
Urgent safety measures
End-of-trial notification

Quality systems
(Chapter 14)
Written procedures
Quality assurance
Quality control
Computer system
validation

Subject safety

Pharmacovigilance for clinical trials
(Chapter 5)
Adverse events and reactions
Expedited reporting
Annual reporting
Ongoing safety evaluations
Out-of-hours cover

Documentation

Trial documents
(Chapter 4)
Key trial documents
(regulatory and others)
Preparation, review and approval
Updates
Version control

Trial master files
(Chapter 10)
Identification
Indexing
Content
Paper and electronic
Control
Retention and archiving

Contracted facilities

Investigator sites
(Chapter 11)
PI responsibilities
Consent and eligibility
Prescribing and accountability
AE/SAEs
Source data

Trial data

Data management
(Chapter 8)
CRF design
Database build and validation
Data entry and cleaning
Database lock
Safety data reconciliation

Statistics
(Chapter 9)
Trial design
Randomisation and blinding
Statistical analysis plan
Population review
Unblinding
Programming and analysis

Trial medication

Investigational medicinal products
(Chapter 6)
Manufacture and assembly
QP certification
Supply and release
Accountability

Compliance

Monitoring
(Chapter 7)
Central and remote
On-site
Data monitoring committees
Trial steering committee
Self-assessment and progress reports

Phase I units
(Chapter 12)
Responsibilities in addition to investigator sites
Phase I accreditation

Clinical laboratories
(Chapter 13)
Analysis and evaluation
Chain of custody
Processing and analysis
Reporting and storage

Figure 1.1 Aspects of sponsor oversight

1.1 Sponsors

1.1.1 Who can be a sponsor?

Regulation 3 (1) of SI 2004/1031 defines the sponsor, as:

'(in relation to a clinical trial) the person who takes responsibility for the initiation, management and financing (or arranging the financing) of that trial.'

The sponsor must[1] be established in the EEA or have a legal representative who is so established (see section 1.1.6). Any organisation that is a legal entity can sponsor a clinical trial. The legislation does allow for a single individual to become a sponsor (although many organisations do not permit their staff to take personal responsibility for sponsoring a clinical trial due to the risks and legal liabilities involved) or for two or more persons or organisations to sponsor a clinical trial together. The latter is referred to as joint or co-sponsorship (see section 1.1.5).

The types of clinical trial sponsors seen in the UK include commercial pharmaceutical companies (from small or virtual companies to global organisations), research councils, medical charities and other non-commercial bodies, such as the employer of an investigator undertaking a clinical trial (for example, NHS Trusts and universities).

1.1.2 Approach to sponsorship

Firstly, the sponsor must identify whether the proposed research falls under the clinical trial legislation; if it does, it is recommended that the sponsor then determines the categorisation of the trial to Type A, B or C, in line with the MRC/DH/MHRA paper 'Risk-adapted approaches to the management of clinical trials of investigational medicinal products' (hereinafter 'risk-adapted approach guidance') (Chapter 2). For each clinical trial it is strongly recommended that a risk assessment be undertaken at the protocol development stage; this then allows the sponsor to decide on whether to proceed with the sponsorship and assists in identifying and mitigating any potential risks associated with the trial. The risk to those participating in clinical trials and the risk to the integrity of the data vary considerably, depending on a number of factors. As part of the risk assessment, sponsors should consider assessing the risks posed by the knowledge and clinical experience of the IMP in the population under trial and any other interventions in the trial design, as well as considering the financial and legal risks to the organisation.

Performing a risk assessment allows the sponsor to identify areas of higher risk and put in place plans to mitigate them. The risk assessment is also useful for planning the overall approach to the trial's management and establishing how the sponsor's responsibilities can be met, and how elements can be adapted in line with the risk-adapted approach guidance. The risk assessment can also form the basis for determining the extent of monitoring activities for overseeing vendors and investigator sites involved in the clinical trial. However, the risk assessment or risk mitigation plan is considered a living document and therefore the sponsor should refer to it throughout the trial to ensure that it is being complied with and that it is kept updated as required to reflect any changes or new information.

The development of a risk assessment or risk mitigation plan is further discussed in section 4.7.1, with additional considerations for the Voluntary MHRA Phase I Accreditation Scheme included in Chapter 12.

1.1.3   What are the responsibilities of a sponsor?

The sponsor has specific legal responsibilities defined in SI 2004/1031. These relate to obtaining and maintaining the authorisation for clinical trials and research ethics committee (REC) opinion, GCP and trial conduct, pharmacovigilance and IMP manufacture and labelling. These responsibilities are summarised in Table 1.1.

The sponsor can formally delegate one or more of the functions of sponsorship; for example, a commercial pharmaceutical company may employ a contract research organisation (CRO) to perform monitoring activities or an NHS Trust may delegate certain functions to the chief investigator of the clinical trial. (Note: the term 'vendors' will be used to refer to all the various types of providers to which a sponsor may delegate its functions, such as CROs, contract manufacturing organisations (CMOs), laboratories, consultants, freelancers/ contractors and niche providers.)

Table 1.1 Summary of the sponsor's functions and responsibilities

Sponsor's functions and responsibilities	UK SI 2004/1031 reference
A. Authorisation for clinical trials and research ethics committee opinion	
Obtain required authorisations to commence the trial (clinical trial authorisation and favourable research ethics committee opinion)	Part 3, Regulations 12, 13, 17, 18, 19 and 20. Schedules 3, 4 and 5
Keep records of all amendments to the authorisations and obtain approval where approvals are required	Part 3, Regulations 22, 24, 25 and 26
Produce undertaking to allow inspection of premises in third countries if required	Part 3, Regulation 21
Notify all relevant bodies of the conclusion or termination of the trial within the specified timeframes	Part 3, Regulation 27
B. GCP and the conduct of clinical trials	
Ensure that the conditions and principles of Good Clinical Practice are satisfied or adhered to	Part 4, Regulation 28 Schedule 1
Ensure that the trial is conducted in accordance with the protocol and subsequent amendments	Part 4, Regulation 29
Notify any serious breaches of Good Clinical Practice or the protocol, or any urgent safety measures taken to the appropriate authorities	Part 4, Regulations 29A and 30
Ensure investigational medicinal products and relevant devices are available to subjects free of charge	Part 4, Regulation 28
Keep a trial master file to hold all documents relating to that trial	Part 4, Regulation 31A
Appoint named individuals responsible for archiving the trial essential documents	Part 4, Regulation 31A
C. Pharmacovigilance	
Ensure an investigator's brochure exists and is validated and updated at least annually	Part 1, Regulation 3A
Keep records of all adverse events relating to that trial which are reported by investigators	Part 5, Regulation 32
Recording and reporting suspected unexpected serious adverse reactions to appropriate authorities within specified timelines	Part 5, Regulation 33
Ensure investigators are informed of suspected unexpected serious adverse reactions	Part 5, Regulation 33

Table continues

Table 1.1 *continued*

Sponsor's functions and responsibilities	UK SI 2004/1031 reference
Ensure all suspected unexpected serious adverse reactions including those in third countries are entered into the European database	Part 5, Regulation 34
Provide annual list of suspected serious adverse reactions and a safety report to the appropriate authorities	Part 5, Regulation 35
D. Manufacture and labelling of investigational medicinal products	
Meet requirements for the authorisation to manufacture and import investigational medicinal product (including the use of hospital exemptions)	Part 6, Regulations 36 and 37 Schedules 6, 7 and 8
Certification of the investigational medicinal product by a Qualified Person	Part 6, Regulation 43
Two-step release process of investigational medicinal product ('technical release' and 'regulatory release')	Part 6, Regulation 43
Ensure investigational medicinal product is labelled in accordance with Article 15 of Commission Directive 2003/94/EC	Part 7, Regulation 46

Ultimately, the sponsor remains accountable for all functions of sponsorship, whether delegated or not. This is stated in Regulation 3 (12) of SI 2004/10/31:

'A person who is a sponsor of a clinical trial in accordance with this regulation may delegate any or all of his functions under these Regulations to any person but any such arrangement shall not affect the responsibility of the sponsor.'

Regulation 28 (2) of SI 2004/1031 states that the *'sponsor of a clinical trial shall put and keep in place arrangements for the purpose of ensuring that with regard to that trial the conditions and principles of GCP are satisfied or adhered to'*. Therefore, the sponsor is required to implement sufficient processes to maintain oversight of the clinical trial so that it can ensure that the legislation is complied with and that the sponsor's legal responsibilities are met. This in turn helps to ensure the safety and well-being of clinical trial subjects, and the integrity of the data and results generated.

How sponsors manage their oversight of clinical trials may vary significantly, depending on the nature and size of the organisation. For example, responsibility may lie with the research and development (R&D) office or chief investigator or clinical trials unit/facility in a non-commercial organisation or with the project management function in commercial organisations. Examples of how non-commercial and commercial organisations may be set up are provided in Figure 1.2. The sponsor's responsibilities and the methods by which these responsibilities can be met by various organisations are discussed in more detail in this chapter.

1.1.4 Non-commercial sponsorship

Although the concepts discussed in this chapter are applicable to both commercial and non-commercial sponsors, there are some additional points that are particularly relevant to non-commercial sponsors and these are discussed below.

It is recommended that sponsors should assess the risk of the trial at the protocol development stage to assist them in making their decision as to whether it is a trial that falls under the Clinical Trials Regulations and then whether they wish to sponsor the trial or not. These processes are of particular relevance to non-commercial organisations, where the decision to sponsor a clinical trial is made on a case-by-case basis in response to either a request from the organisation's employees (for example, a researcher asking their employer, an NHS Trust, to act as sponsor) or from someone external to the organisation (for example, a researcher asking a university, of which they are not an employee, to act as sponsor). Therefore, non-commercial organisations should develop written procedures to describe how the clinical trial and sponsorship decision will be made and documented. The lack of such procedures can lead to trials being misclassified and trials that come under the Clinical Trials Regulations not being conducted according to those regulations. It is recommended that the procedures include what requirements need to be met by the requester in order for the organisation to agree to sponsor the clinical trial, as well as any terms and conditions that need to be adhered to and how sponsorship can be withdrawn in the event of non-compliance. The decision on sponsorship by non-commercial sponsors can form part of the risk assessment. Where sponsorship is a new undertaking for an organisation, the organisation may wish to begin work in clinical trials by sponsoring small (that is, at a few sites or a single site) or lower-risk trials. With more experience, the sponsorship could then be expanded to include different types of trials, thus ensuring that sponsorship of trials falls within the sponsor's capabilities.

Once a decision has been made to sponsor a clinical trial, the sponsor's functions, as described in the legislation, must[2] be formally delegated and agreed

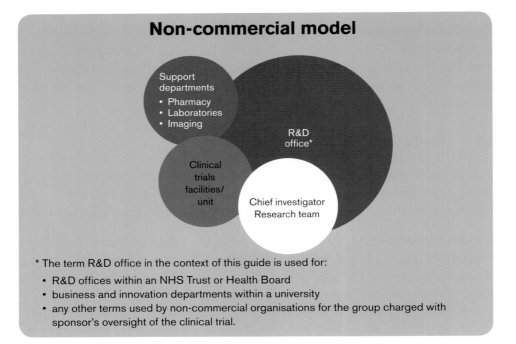

Non-commercial model

Support departments
• Pharmacy
• Laboratories
• Imaging

R&D office*

Clinical trials facilities/ unit

Chief investigator Research team

* The term R&D office in the context of this guide is used for:
• R&D offices within an NHS Trust or Health Board
• business and innovation departments within a university
• any other terms used by non-commercial organisations for the group charged with sponsor's oversight of the clinical trial.

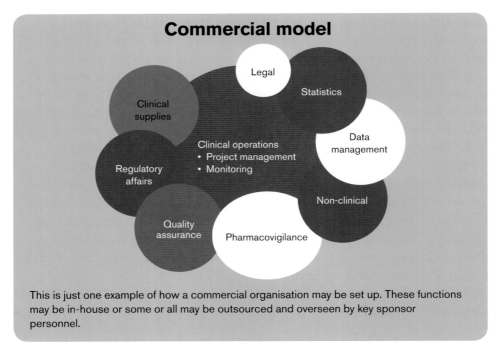

Commercial model

Legal

Statistics

Clinical supplies

Data management

Clinical operations
• Project management
• Monitoring

Regulatory affairs

Non-clinical

Quality assurance

Pharmacovigilance

This is just one example of how a commercial organisation may be set up. These functions may be in-house or some or all may be outsourced and overseen by key sponsor personnel.

Figure 1.2 Example models of organisation set-up

between the relevant parties. For example, with non-commercial sponsors, a number of functions are often delegated to the chief investigator and other host sites (if multi-centred), such as another NHS Trust. Therefore, formal arrangements should be put in place between the sponsor and the chief investigator and host sites to ensure that all parties are aware of their delegated sponsor functions. The sponsor must[3, 4] also have assurance that the chief investigator and host organisation(s) are competent and that they are able to manage and conduct the clinical trials and perform their delegated sponsor functions. This may involve the following:

- performing a pre-assessment of the capabilities of the investigator and/or host site, and arranging for appropriate training in research methods and GCP for the chief investigator and members of the research team as required

- assessing any quality system at the investigator and/or host site to ensure that it meets expectations and suitable standards.

If these functions are not adequately delegated, this can lead to sponsors failing to meet their responsibilities outlined in the legislation (for example, if the function of safety reporting has been delegated to a chief investigator who has not been adequately trained or if the chief investigator is unaware of what has been delegated to them, this can result in safety reports not being submitted in the required timelines).

In addition, sponsors should ensure that there are formal processes in place to allow them to maintain oversight of delegated functions. This usually consists of some form of audit and monitoring activities to detect and rectify poor compliance. The risk assessment performed before the clinical trial begins can be used to plan these details as well as the overall approach for managing the clinical trial.

1.1.5 Joint or co-sponsorship

A sponsor is often a single organisation, which is usually the case for clinical trials being sponsored by commercial pharmaceutical companies. Clinical trials can also be sponsored by two or more persons or organisations. This is referred to as joint or co-sponsorship and is more common in clinical trials being sponsored by non-commercial organisations where a group of partners may make collaborative arrangements to initiate, manage and fund a trial.

Regulation 3 (2) of SI 2004/1031 allows joint or co-sponsors of a trial to take joint responsibility for carrying out the functions of the sponsor of that trial or to allocate among themselves responsibility for carrying out those functions.

1.1.5.1 Joint responsibility

If the partners choose to take joint responsibility, all of them would accept joint liability for all of the sponsor's responsibilities. In this case, each partner organisation is required[4] to have suitably qualified and trained staff to perform or oversee all of the sponsor's responsibilities, should maintain clear documented evidence of this oversight and must[5] ensure that appropriate insurance arrangements are in place (see section 1.3.8).

1.1.5.2 Allocated responsibility

If the partners each choose to take on a set of sponsorship responsibilities, these must[6] be detailed in the clinical trial authorisation (CTA) submitted to the competent authority and would be grouped by function into the following: authorisation for clinical trials and REC opinion, GCP and the conduct of clinical trials, pharmacovigilance, and IMP manufacture, assembly and labelling. In this case, the partners would collaboratively cover all of the sponsor's functions with each responsibility performed by the named organisation/person.

1.1.5.3 Decision process and agreements

Before a decision can be made as to whether sponsorship will be a joint or allocated responsibility (and, if it is to be an allocated responsibility, who will take responsibility for the specific functions), a formal assessment should be carried out of each individual co-sponsor's capabilities to ensure that responsibilities are allocated appropriately. This could be, for example, via an audit, review of CVs or assessment of the co-sponsor's quality system.

In addition, the division of regulatory responsibilities (that is, Parts 3, 4, 5, 6 and 7 of SI 2004/1031) between the partners must[6] be agreed before the trial starts. For example, this can be documented using a contract or memorandum of understanding either issued per clinical trial or as an overarching master agreement for all clinical trials associated with a particular project or programme of work. It is recommended that this document also describes the process for the transfer of obligations between parties for specific activities.

There should be a process in place to allow for adequate oversight by each partner of tasks being conducted by another partner. This can be achieved using a variety of different methods, such as regular meetings (to discuss trial progress, any key trial-related issues and to document agreement with any key decisions taken), producing progress reports and developing formal escalation processes, as well as monitoring and auditing. Further suggestions are noted below:

- meeting minutes from discussions with internal functions and external vendors
- progress reports
- documenting key decisions taken
- documenting review of regular progress reports from vendors/partners
- documenting review of self-assessment reports from investigator sites
- documenting review of key trial documents and checklists
- defined processes for the escalation and resolution of issues
- documenting review of monitoring visit reports and follow-up letters
- performing co-monitoring visits and documenting the outcome of these visits
- a defined plan for the ongoing review of a vendor's/partner's performance.

Joint sponsorship can work well when responsibilities are clear. However, problems can arise when there is no, or inadequate, documentation of delegation of the joint sponsor responsibilities between the parties. When this occurs it can become unclear who is responsible for what, or if both parties were jointly responsible. This can result in functions either not being performed or being duplicated unnecessarily. Oversight can also be problematic if it is not clearly defined such that there is no, or inadequate, oversight of sponsor responsibilities that have been contracted to the joint sponsor. An example is where a university takes responsibility for obtaining authorisation and REC opinion, but the actual activity is undertaken by the NHS Trust R&D office, with no oversight by the university that this is performed satisfactorily.

1.1.6   Legal representative

If the sponsor is not based in the EEA, it is a statutory requirement[1] to appoint a legal representative who is established and contactable at an address in the EEA.

The legal representative may be an individual person or a representative of a corporate entity. They do not have to be a legally qualified person; however, they must be willing to act as the agent of the sponsor in the event of any legal proceedings instituted in the European Community (for example, the service of legal documents).

The legal representative does not assume any of the legal liabilities of the sponsor(s) for the clinical trial as part of their role as legal representative. However, in some cases legal representatives enter into specific contractual arrangements to undertake some or all of the statutory duties of the sponsor in relation to the trial, in which case the legal representative would also be regarded as a co-sponsor, and would also require insurance/indemnity.

1.2   Clinical trial authorisations and research ethics committee opinion

The sponsor's responsibilities regarding obtaining and maintaining authorisation by the competent authority and a favourable REC opinion for a clinical trial are summarised in Table 1.1 (Part A) and in the following sections. The detail of these activities and requirements is described in Chapter 2 and Chapter 3.

1.2.1   Obtaining and maintaining clinical trial authorisations

In order to obtain and maintain the required regulatory authorisations, the sponsor should consider implementing formal written procedures that describe the steps to be taken. In preparing these written procedures, the sponsor may find it useful to refer to the MHRA website, the Health Research Authority (HRA) website and any relevant European Commission guidance.

For all clinical trials, it is necessary to obtain initial approval from the competent authority, which in the UK is the MHRA, in the form of a clinical trial authorisation (CTA). Any subsequent substantial amendments to the CTA are also subject to approval by the competent authority (and/or the REC). In large commercial organisations, these activities are usually performed by the regulatory affairs department, while in smaller commercial organisations, these may be delegated to the trial manager and/or assistant(s). Once the initial authorisation is obtained (and any necessary subsequent authorisations for amendments) this information should be disseminated to the rest of the trial team as necessary, so that there is appropriate awareness that the competent authority approval has been obtained. It is recommended that this dissemination of information is documented in the trial master file (TMF) and this could take the form of emails or records of updates provided at project team meetings.

If the sponsor has delegated the function of obtaining competent authority approval to an external vendor, then it is necessary for the sponsor to have processes in place to ensure that the vendor provides the sponsor with information about the approval status of the clinical trial (and any conditions associated with the approval) in order for the sponsor to conduct or delegate any further tasks upon which these depend. This may be achieved in a number of ways, for example:

- the vendor copying the sponsor in on any correspondence to and from the competent authority and sending the sponsor copies of the approvals once received
- the vendor submitting status reports to the sponsor
- other documented means of communication between the parties (such as emails, meeting/teleconference minutes).

In the case of non-commercial sponsors, the task of obtaining and maintaining the CTA may be performed by the sponsor's R&D office or delegated to either a clinical trial facility/unit or the chief investigator. If this task is delegated to the chief investigator, then the non-commercial sponsor will need to have a mechanism in place for reviewing the CTA and obtaining input from other supporting departments (for example, the pharmacy department) to ensure that there is consistency between the documents produced and that there has been input from those with the relevant expertise. Any reviews and comments should be documented and retained in the TMF as evidence. The sponsor should ensure that there are processes in place for it to be informed of the trial authorisation and any subsequent updates to the authorisation (this information is usually a prerequisite for obtaining the local R&D approval).

1.2.2 Obtaining and maintaining favourable research ethics committee opinion

The sponsor of a clinical trial is also required[7] to obtain a favourable REC opinion prior to starting the trial. Regardless of whether the sponsor is commercial or non-commercial, the application must[8] be made by the chief investigator for the trial, but usually with assistance from the sponsor or delegated external vendor to assist with the completion of the application form. Further guidance on completing the REC application can be found in Chapter 3 and within the Integrated Research Application System (IRAS). The sponsor should ensure that sufficient processes are in place for it to be informed of the initial and subsequent (as relevant) favourable REC opinion status of the clinical trial. The sponsor needs to receive all relevant information in a timely manner to ensure that this is communicated to other involved parties so that they are aware of changes and are able to implement them appropriately (or to prevent their implementation prior to approval). This may be achieved in the same ways as those examples provided for the CTA (see section 1.2.1).

1.2.3 Additional considerations for authorisations and research ethics committee opinion

During the process of obtaining the required authorisation and favourable REC opinion, there may be a request to change the protocol by either the competent authority or the REC. Should this occur, the authorisation and favourable REC opinion may be for different versions of the protocol. Therefore, the sponsor needs to consider whether the requested change should be submitted to the other party or not. Any decision and its justification must[9, 10] be documented as evidence, as this would constitute an amendment (see section 1.2.5) and therefore must be assessed for substantiality.

Authorisations and/or favourable REC opinions may be granted subject to conditions. The sponsor must[11] ensure that there is evidence that these conditions have been reviewed and met.

Lastly, the sponsor should review the authorisation and favourable REC opinion to ensure that it accurately reflects the documentation submitted and to seek clarification should it contain errors (for example, REC letters listing the incorrect version of the protocol and/or subject information sheet). It is also important to ensure that the correct authorisation or approval letter is used to implement a change. For example, two substantial amendments were made simultaneously to the MHRA for the same trial, one for an expiry date extension and one for a protocol amendment. An authorisation letter was subsequently received; however, the letter was not adequately reviewed and, as a result, the authorisation for the expiry date was incorrectly used to implement the protocol amendment (which was still being assessed by the MHRA).

1.2.4 Other required approvals

It may also be necessary to obtain advice and other approvals in addition to the competent authority approval and favourable REC opinion. For example, depending on the IMP under investigation, it may be necessary to obtain advice on the IMP-associated risk factors from the Clinical Trials Expert Advisory Group (CTEAG) (see section 2.5).

In addition, it will be necessary to apply for site-specific assessments or NHS management permission, depending on the type of site (see section 3.2.4). Other applications may also be needed – for example, Administration of Radioactive Substances Advisory Committee (ARSAC) certification. Further guidance on the approvals required for a particular trial is available within IRAS and described in Chapter 3. These additional approvals depend on the location of the investigator sites (commercial units or NHS sites), the type of IMP under investigation, internal host organisation processes, and the assessments or procedures being undertaken in the clinical trial. The sponsor should consider what additional approvals are required in the planning stages of the clinical trial (this can be incorporated into the risk assessment process) and put in place processes to ensure that these approvals are obtained prior to the trial commencing.

1.2.5   Implementation of amendments

Sponsors should implement a formalised process for the management of amendments. This will include their identification, assessment and approval in addition to the control and implementation (at sponsor and investigator sites) of any updated trial-related documents that are associated with such amendments (for example, changes to the protocol and subject information sheets). A formal implementation process will provide clear documented evidence of when updated documents were implemented and will reduce the likelihood of superseded documents being used.

It has been a common finding on inspections that the implementation of amendments has been inadequately overseen, such that it was not possible to verify the date that the new protocol and any associated documentation started to be used, or it was found that superseded subject information sheets and consent forms continued to be used.

The sponsor must[9] assess whether amendments to the documents submitted to the competent authority and the REC are substantial and therefore whether they are required to be submitted to the competent authority, the REC or both. (General guidance is provided in section 2.3.6.1 to assist the sponsor in deciding whether a substantial amendment requires authorisation, or an ethical opinion, or both.) The substantiality assessment and subsequent submission requirements (including the justification) must[10] be documented and retained in the TMF. This is especially important if the amendment is considered non-substantial, as there is no requirement to submit this to either the competent authority or the REC; therefore, this is the only method to verify that a submission was not required. It is

ysisPro output.

sisProoutput.

not acceptable to only be able to identify non-substantial amendments by making an assumption that the change is non-substantial if there is no corresponding submission and competent authority authorisation or favourable REC opinion. It is also important to ensure that where an NHS Trust is the sponsor and has delegated the responsibility for amendments to the chief investigator, the R&D office is aware of any changes to ensure continued sponsorship agreement and management permission.

1.2.6 Notifying relevant bodies of the conclusion or early termination of a trial

As part of the sponsor's responsibilities, the sponsor is required[12] to inform the competent authority and the REC of the conclusion or early termination of the clinical trial. The sponsor must[10] retain sufficient documentation to demonstrate that this was performed within the required timeframes.

The sponsor may make use of electronic trackers and spreadsheets to record key trial events, such as the last subject last visit or other protocol-defined definition of end of trial, to help track the date by which the end-of-trial or early termination notification is to be submitted. Some sponsors may delegate this task to an external vendor or the chief investigator, but the sponsors should have mechanisms in place to maintain oversight of these activities to ensure that they are being performed. For example, sponsors may expect to be copied in on relevant correspondence, and to be sent status reports detailing key trial events or receive confirmation by email that the necessary notifications have been sent.

1.3 Good Clinical Practice and conduct of clinical trials

The sponsor's responsibilities relating to GCP and the conduct of the trial are summarised in Table 1.1 (Part B).

1.3.1 Oversight of internal functions and external vendors

In order to ensure that the clinical trial is conducted in accordance with the legislation, protocol and GCP, the sponsor must[13, 14] implement a suitable quality system for the functions it undertakes (Chapter 14), and then should develop processes to assess internal compliance with that system. Also, throughout the clinical trial, the sponsor must[2] maintain oversight of internal functions, which can be achieved by, for example, holding regular project team meetings, documenting key decisions and following predefined escalation processes for the reporting and resolution of significant trial-related issues. These methods are further described in section 1.6.

Other mechanisms to maintain oversight and assess compliance can include monitoring or auditing; these are two very separate activities and the terms should not be used interchangeably. The term 'monitoring' is used for the activity of overseeing the progress of a clinical trial and of ensuring that it is conducted, recorded and reported in accordance with the protocol, written procedures, GCP and applicable regulatory requirements (Chapter 7). Monitoring is conducted by someone who is part of the trial team, who is familiar with and has been trained in the trial and therefore can perform a quality control (QC) check of the trial activities, usually at the investigator sites. On the other hand, the term 'auditing' is used for a quality assurance (QA) activity where there is an independent examination of trial-related activities in accordance with the protocol, written procedures, GCP and applicable regulatory requirements. Auditing is conducted by someone independent of the trial team (Chapter 14).

In today's evolving clinical trials environment, not all sponsors perform all of the clinical trial activities in-house and often a variety of different service models are used to conduct clinical trials, which use CROs, external vendors or consultants/freelancers to varying degrees. The sponsor may delegate a significant proportion of the functions (for example, project management and monitoring) or may only delegate discrete activities (for example, laboratory analysis, data management and statistics). In some cases, the sponsor may delegate all of its functions to vendors and act as a 'virtual' sponsor. The model used often depends on the sponsor's R&D strategy, in-house expertise and resource capacity, and the location of the sponsor in relation to the investigator sites to be used. Regardless of the model used, the sponsor retains ultimate responsibility for the clinical trial.

It is important to ensure that oversight is maintained of all vendors; this includes contract consultants or freelancers contracted by the sponsor to undertake functions as if they were part of the organisation. These activities can be easily overlooked and a lack of oversight may potentially lead to the sponsor inadvertently breaching the legislation or GCP. For example, a small virtual organisation contracted a consultant medical advisor to make pharmacovigilance assessments on its behalf; however, the contractor was not adequately trained to perform those functions and was unfamiliar with the legislation. This resulted in late expedited reporting of suspected unexpected serious adverse reactions

(SUSARs) by the sponsor and also in poor documentation of the sponsor's assessment of these events in the TMF.

Some non-commercial sponsors arrange to have IMP supplied by a pharmaceutical organisation or by the marketing authorisation holder (MAH) free of charge for use in a clinical trial. In these circumstances, the IMP supplier would also be considered a vendor. On occasions, the supplier may specify a particular distributor to be used, although the contract is held between the sponsor and distributor. When this occurs the sponsor must[14] satisfy itself that this distributor is acceptable and follow its own vendor selection process before signing any agreement with them.

It should be noted that, although the sponsor retains ultimate responsibility for all functions, all vendors must[3, 15] show due diligence when performing any functions they have been delegated as all persons involved in the conduct of a clinical trial have a legal responsibility to comply with GCP, the protocol and the terms of the competent authority authorisation and favourable REC opinion.

1.3.2   Selection of vendors

The process of vendor oversight begins with the selection of a suitable vendor. As such, the sponsor should implement processes for assessing the suitability of any vendors to be used, prior to the signing of contracts. A variety of assessment methods can be considered when assessing the suitability of a vendor and some examples are given below:

- pre-qualification questionnaires
- assessment of CVs and previous experience
- obtaining suitable references
- referring to prior knowledge of the vendor from use in other clinical trials
- assessing quality system/written procedures
- conducting audits.

The process for assessing the suitability of a vendor will vary depending on the risk associated with the tasks being delegated and what is previously known about the vendor. For example, for critical activities such as manufacture and cold-chain supply of IMP by a vendor not previously used by the sponsor, it may be appropriate to conduct an audit prior to signing the contract and allowing the vendor to perform these activities. For other tasks, such as shipping trial documents to various locations, it may be more suitable to review the vendor's

> **Examples of inadequate assessment of the vendor's suitability by a sponsor, leading to issues with the activity the vendor has been contracted to perform**
>
> *Example 1*
>
> IMP is manufactured by an external CMO; however, neither the chief investigator nor the R&D office (as the sponsor representative) has assessed the vendor's suitability; the CMO has been selected based on informal recommendation only. As a result, the IMP is not labelled according to the CTA, nor is it Annex 13 compliant.
>
> *Example 2*
>
> The R&D office is unaware that the investigator has organised an external laboratory to analyse samples and neither party assesses whether the laboratory could perform this activity in compliance with GCP. As a result, samples are analysed using a non-validated method and the results are unreliable (that is, they are not reproducible) and cannot be used.
>
> *Example 3*
>
> A sponsor conducts an audit of a CMO and identifies that it has a number of issues related to randomisation activities; however, the sponsor fails to follow up on these issues before contracting the CMO. As a result, the CMO assembles subject kits in such a way that the randomisation allocation of the kits is incorrect.

previous experience, obtain references and ask pertinent questions. The information obtained from these assessments will then be used to make a decision about the suitability of the vendor. Sponsors should ensure that an adequate assessment of the vendor has been performed (including adequate responses to audit findings, if applicable) prior to confirming vendor selection. It is recommended that the decision to select a particular vendor is documented and that the rationale for selection is clear.

Some sponsors may develop 'preferred providers' lists, which detail vendors that have been pre-qualified for use by the sponsor and, as such, individuals within the sponsor's organisation will be instructed to select vendors from this list.

After the selection of a vendor, appropriate contracts should be put in place prior to the commencement of work. Contracts should clearly detail the delegated tasks, duties and functions between the parties, the required standards of service and the process for further subcontracting by the vendor (to ensure that subcontracting does not occur without sponsor approval). Processes should also be implemented to ensure that these contracts are kept current. Section 1.3.7 describes the process of preparing and maintaining contracts and agreements.

1.3.3 Maintaining oversight of vendors

Once the vendor has been selected, the sponsor will need to consider how it will maintain continuing oversight of the vendor's clinical trial-related activities. This oversight can be achieved through a variety of different methods, but often relies on clear and well-defined communication channels. Sponsors often rely on regular communication with vendors to be made aware of how the trial is progressing and to discuss any issues that arise. This can be achieved through regular teleconferences or face-to-face meetings, or review of specific activities (for example, regulatory green-light checks (see section 1.5.2.3), and review or audit of the TMF). However, whatever the process chosen, this must[10] be clearly documented (including the outcome of any discussions) and retained in the TMF.

In addition to this, some sponsors request regular written update reports, which detail how the trial is progressing and highlight any significant issues (for example, status or progress reports). In this situation, there should be a process to define what review and assessment these reports undergo once received by the sponsor and how this is documented. Depending on the activities delegated to vendors, sponsors may also consider reviewing and being one of the authorisation signatories on key trial documents such as:

- trial-specific instruction manuals and guidelines (for example, pharmacy, laboratory and safety)
- case report form (CRF) design approvals
- data management and statistical analysis plans
- communication plan (especially if multiple vendors are being used).

In order to maintain effective oversight, sponsors may also consider defining an escalation process for any significant issues, so that these are reported and addressed in a timely manner. A significant issue could be, for example, a major GCP compliance issue at an investigator site identified through the vendor's monitoring of the trial that the monitor is unable to resolve. An example was seen on inspection where, although the monitor had identified issues and recorded them in the monitoring report, these issues were not dealt with and this led to further non-compliances, such that the site was eventually closed following a serious breach. Early escalation and management at both the sponsor and investigator site (for example, by the sponsor contacting the investigator or the investigator's R&D office) may well have resulted in a more positive outcome.

The sponsor is also responsible for ensuring that it provides vendors with all the appropriate documentation to enable them to perform their delegated functions (for example, copies of the protocol and investigator's brochure (IB)). This must[4] also include providing any written procedures (and relevant training if the vendor is to use the sponsor's written procedures) and include a mechanism to ensure that the vendor receives any updates to these documents. It is a common finding during inspection that vendors are not provided with adequate access to the sponsor's written procedures (in particular where there are updates) during the course of their activities.

As part of the sponsor's overall quality assurance programme, consideration also needs to be given to how often vendors undergo a formal assessment (for example, in the form of an audit) once they have been selected for use. This assessment helps to ensure the ongoing suitability of the use of the vendor and the vendor's compliance with the regulations, protocol, GCP standards and contracts. A formal assessment is particularly important if the vendor is a 'preferred provider' and being used for numerous trials, as non-compliance could then impact on not just one trial but multiple trials, resulting in systemic non-compliance. This may impact on subject safety or data integrity and cause delays to the trial. On inspection it was observed that a laboratory was not performing the safety assessment analysis as per the validated method and, as a result, incorrect values were provided to the investigators to assess the subjects' eligibility across all the trials for which the vendor was contracted to provide analysis. Consequently, ineligible subjects were recruited, putting these subjects at risk and invalidating the results to such an extent that the trials had to be repeated, incurring additional costs to the sponsor.

Regardless of the oversight methods to be used, these methods should be clearly defined prior to the commencement of clinical trial activities, either in the sponsor's quality system or any relevant trial-specific documents (for example, the trial contract, vendor oversight plans or manuals). This will result in a well-defined vendor oversight programme, which will assist the sponsor in assessing and ensuring the vendor's compliance with the legislation.

1.3.4   Oversight of investigator sites

Prior to selecting an investigator site, the sponsor should perform a suitability assessment or evaluation. This may occur in the form of a pre-qualification questionnaire or a visit to the site to assess the site facilities and capacity as well as the experience and qualifications of the trial team. Sponsors may also rely on their previous knowledge and experience of working with a particular investigator site, or on recommendations from other researchers and investigators. After this initial assessment, investigator sites will undergo some form of site initiation process to ensure that the site is suitably prepared for conducting the clinical trial.

Throughout the active phase of the trial, the sponsor's main method of investigator site oversight will be through monitoring. The frequency, scope, detail and type of monitoring should be identified prior to the start of the clinical trial (this should ideally form part of the risk assessment plan) and the details should be defined in a trial-specific monitoring plan or within the sponsor's quality system. However, these monitoring parameters will vary depending on the risk, purpose, design and complexity of the clinical trial. For example, some clinical trials may require frequent on-site monitoring visits, while other clinical trials may be suitable for central monitoring, or a combination of the two approaches. These concepts are discussed further in Chapter 7.

Regardless of the type and extent of monitoring performed, staff performing monitoring activities must[4] be appropriately trained for their role and have sufficient guidance from the sponsor on what is expected from the investigator site. In addition, the information gathered through monitoring should be appropriately reviewed and escalated (as necessary) within the sponsor's organisation. This could be achieved by the review of monitoring visit reports by designated individuals within the sponsor organisation and a clearly defined issue escalation process.

In situations where the monitoring activities are delegated to an external vendor, the sponsor will still need to implement processes to maintain oversight of the investigator sites. Examples of methods through which this can be achieved are regular meetings with the vendor, reviewing the monitoring visit reports (or a sample of the reports) produced by the vendor, conducting co-monitoring visits with the vendor (in accordance with a frequency determined by the sponsor), and establishing a clearly defined issue escalation process. In addition, sponsors may want to consider how monitors are assigned (for example, defining minimum standards for monitors' experience and training) and what handover processes are in place when those monitors change (that is, for continuity of site management) to ensure a focus on quality is maintained.

1.3.5 Protocol compliance and serious breaches

A sponsor of a clinical trial should list all significant protocol non-compliances/ deviations in the clinical study report (CSR) or publication, and must[16] assess whether any of these non-compliances should be reported to the MHRA as a serious breach of GCP and the protocol. In order to ensure that the sponsor meets these requirements, appropriate processes should be in place for identifying, capturing, assessing and reporting protocol and GCP non-compliance. These processes may include:

- definition of non-compliances for a trial, including classification (such as major or minor; this is usually part of the statistical analysis plan)
- identification and capture of the non-compliances
- management and escalation of non-compliances, including corrective and preventative actions
- how non-compliances will be consolidated from the various sources (for example, those identified at site by the trial team or by monitoring activities, or identified during analysis of samples by clinical laboratories)
- circulation to appropriate functions in order to assess:
  » seriousness for those required to be reported to the MHRA
  » impact on the population for inclusion in the analysis
  » inclusion in the CSR.

1.3.5.1 Protocol waivers

Protocol waivers are prospective deviations or waivers to the protocol. These types of non-compliances are not acceptable as they constitute a deliberate breach of Regulation 29 of SI 2004/1031:

> 'Subject to regulation 30, no person shall conduct a clinical trial otherwise than in accordance with – (a) the protocol relating to that trial, as may be amended from time to time in accordance with regulations 22 to 25'

For example, it is not acceptable for the sponsor (or the chief investigator on behalf of the sponsor) to allow subjects to be included in a trial when the subjects do not meet one or more of the eligibility criteria or restrictions defined in the protocol. If there are difficulties in subject recruitment related to eligibility criteria or restrictions, it is instead expected that these are addressed via a substantial amendment to change the inclusion/exclusion criteria and/or restrictions defined in the protocol. Review of screening logs will assist in identifying if there are any of these issues.

1.3.5.2 Protocol non-compliances

Protocol non-compliances are departures from the protocol that have been identified retrospectively – for example, a missed visit window because the subject did not turn up for the appointment. These types of non-compliances are impossible to predict and therefore it is almost inevitable that some protocol non-compliances will occur.

It is a common misconception that the protocol non-compliances will all be identified via the CRF. However, the CRF will only identify non-compliances in relation to the data collected (for example, time/visit windows outside that defined in the protocol or laboratory/vital signs outside the protocol-defined limits for continued dosing/dose reductions). The CRF will not identify other potentially important non-compliances (for example, incorrectly consented subjects, a malfunctioning piece of equipment, incorrect sample handling/processing) that may equally have an impact on the analysis of trial results and should also be discussed in the CSR (see sections 4.7.6 and 9.7.1).

If the process for capturing non-compliances is not formally defined, they may be easily overlooked and, as a result, the sponsor may include subjects in the analysis that could bias the results or produce a clinical study report that does not reflect the actual conduct of the trial. For example, a sponsor 'waived' numerous subjects into a clinical trial; these subjects were then incorrectly described as meeting the eligibility criteria in the CRF and subsequently in the clinical trial summary report. This report was submitted as part of the marketing authorisation application for the product and the sponsor was required to re-analyse the data, after correcting the eligibility status, before the data were accepted by the regulators.

There are many ways to capture protocol and GCP non-compliance; however, it is recommended that consideration is given to ensuring that the data captured are structured for ease of assessment, for example:

- documenting and collating in the monitoring visit reports
- creating a non-compliance log with category fields such as eligibility, missed windows, consent and IMP issues
- collation of any IMP issues – for example, issues with temperature monitoring or dosing errors.

1.3.5.3   Serious breaches

In order to ensure that the sponsor meets the requirement[16] for reporting any serious breaches of GCP and the protocol within 7 days of becoming aware of the breach, there should be a formal process for identifying, assessing and reporting non-compliances. The process should include a clear audit trail of when the non-compliance was received, assessed as serious and then when it was submitted to the MHRA (and REC, if applicable). It should also clearly document the rationale for the decisions taken.

The relevant staff must[4] be suitably trained in these processes. Investigator site staff should also be aware of these reporting requirements as it may facilitate the timely identification of such issues. In situations where external vendors are to be used, sponsors should be clear with regard to who will be delegated the function for reporting serious breaches. If the sponsor delegates the reporting responsibilities to an external vendor, then it is recommended that this is detailed in the agreement between the sponsor and external vendor.

It is acknowledged that some serious breaches may be identified and reported by vendors and/or investigator sites to the sponsor, who may disagree with the serious breach assessment. Alternatively, the vendor may become aware that the sponsor has committed a serious breach. In these cases, vendors will need to consider what actions to take; this may include direct reporting to the MHRA. It is expected that organisations exercise due diligence and as such make every effort to ensure that both themselves and the sponsor comply with the legislation, and retain documentation as evidence of this attempt.

More detailed guidance for reporting serious breaches can be found on the MHRA website.

1.3.6   Trial master file and archiving

The sponsor is responsible for keeping a TMF for a clinical trial that must[17] be readily available at all reasonable times for inspection by the competent authority or any person appointed by the sponsor to audit the clinical trial. The TMF must[10] contain all documents that enable both the conduct of the clinical trial and the quality of the data produced to be evaluated and show that the trial is, or has been, conducted in accordance with the legislation. The legislation also states that the clinical trial information must[18] be stored in such a way that it can be accurately reported, interpreted and verified.

The sponsor and the chief investigator must[19] ensure that the essential documents and medical files of trial subjects are retained for at least 5 years after the conclusion of the trial and that, during this period, the essential documents are readily available to the competent authority on request, and are complete and legible. It should be noted that some sponsors may have to retain essential documents for longer periods of time if the data are to be used to support a marketing authorisation application.

In order to ensure compliance with the legislation, the sponsor organisation should implement processes for the maintenance and archiving of essential documents and must[20] appoint a named individual(s) responsible for archiving. Access to the archived documents must[20] be restricted to these appointed individuals. These processes should also consider the arrangements when the task of TMF maintenance is delegated to a vendor, including how the sponsor will maintain oversight. The sponsor can consider providing the vendor with a copy of its own TMF maintenance procedure (or review the vendor's procedure), visiting the vendor to perform TMF checks or requesting copies of key documents from the vendor for the sponsor's own files. In this situation, it is recommended that the sponsor also considers implementing processes to describe how the external vendor TMF and sponsor files are to be consolidated and reconciled at the end of the trial, including how this process will be performed without losing evidence of what records the sponsor held (and when) during the active phase of the trial. If this evidence is lost, it may not be possible to verify on inspection how the sponsor maintained oversight during the trial.

If the sponsor is using an external vendor for archiving, then as part of vendor oversight the sponsor will need to ensure that the vendor's facilities are appropriate for the storage of the essential documents (via some form of pre-contract assessment). The sponsor should also ensure that appropriate contracts are in place and may consider including a clause to prevent documents being moved to locations that are not approved by the sponsor. The sponsor should also consider implementing processes for the ongoing assessment of the vendor and the ongoing integrity of the documents.

Sponsors should discuss archiving arrangements with the investigator site for the investigator site file (ISF) during the preparation stage of the clinical trial (for example, at the site initiation), to ensure that appropriate arrangements can be made in time for the end of the trial.

The requirements for TMF and archiving, and associated legislation, are discussed further in Chapter 10.

1.3.7   Preparation and oversight of contracts and agreements

In addition to there being many types of contracts/agreements (for example, service level agreements, master service agreements with associated work or task orders and investigator site agreements), sponsors and vendors may each have their own templates and agreement requirements. Therefore, in order to ensure the needs of each party are met, a process for the development and execution of a contract should be formalised.

1.3.7.1   Vendor contracts

It is acknowledged that, in order to minimise delays, trial set-up activities may be undertaken by vendors prior to a fully executed contract being in place. If this is the case it is important that a formal agreement, sometimes known as a 'letter of intent', is in place which, as a minimum, clearly identifies what activities are to be undertaken, the standards to be adhered to and a time limit or expiry of the agreement. However, it should be clearly documented either in the letter of intent or the organisation's quality system that IMP should not be shipped and no subjects screened (that is, trial-specific screening) or dosed prior to the full (main) contract being in place, as this could invalidate the insurance and thus affect the subjects' rights.

There should be written procedures in place for the preparation, review and execution of contracts, which may include:

* who is responsible for preparing, reviewing and signing contracts
* the requirement for clear delegated tasks, duties and functions between the parties
* the required standards of service (that is, which applicable laws and guidance, and procedures are to be adhered to)
* clear instructions that the contract should not take precedence over the protocol
* the process for subcontracting by the vendor (to ensure that subcontracting does not occur without the sponsor's knowledge or approval)
* how relevant safety information will be provided (for example, from IMP suppliers to the sponsor or the sponsor to investigators)
* quality control checks of the contract against relevant documents (for example, the protocol).

Once a contract is executed, processes should ensure that these contracts remain current and that the requirements of the contract are being met by all parties. It is also important that everyone with contractual obligations is aware of and has access to the contract. Insufficient contract oversight can result in:

* no contract in place with a vendor
* a contract in place a significant time after the activities have begun
* an organisation not being aware of and therefore not fulfilling its contractual obligations
* tasks continuing under an expired contract
* additional tasks being undertaken without a contract extension/amendment.

Oversight of contracts could be achieved by planning periodic reviews of the contracts or by defining specific triggers for the review, such as protocol amendments, updates to relevant legislation or changes to the quality system.

1.3.7.2   Investigator site agreements

There should be fully signed investigator agreements in place prior to authorising the shipment of IMP to the investigator sites and informing investigators that they can start recruitment. The content of these agreements may vary; however, there are standard templates ('model agreements') available on the Association of the British Pharmaceutical Industry (ABPI) website (www.abpi.org.uk) for both commercial and non-commercial investigator site agreements. These are recognised by the UK Department of Health as well as industry and used as a basis for agreements for trials in the UK.

As with vendor contracts, it is recommended that these agreements are regularly checked to ensure that the terms are being met; for example, there may be changes to the principal investigator and changes to the number of subjects to be recruited during the trial that may require the agreements to be updated.

1.3.8   Clinical trials insurance

In accordance with Part 2 (14) of Schedule 1 to SI 2004/1031, the following condition applies to all clinical trials:

'Provision has been made for insurance or indemnity to cover the liability of the investigator and sponsor which may arise in relation to the clinical trial.'

Therefore, the sponsor and relevant parties must[5] ensure that appropriate provisions are in place for the duration of the trial and that the insurance policies being used to provide cover are appropriate for the clinical trial (for example, that they contain no exclusions that could impact on cover for clinical trial subjects).

As per Regulation 15 (5j) of SI 2004/1031, it is also the responsibility of the REC to consider any insurance or indemnity to cover the liability of the investigator or sponsor when giving its opinion on a REC application.

During inspections, several examples have been identified where the insurance cover has not been adequate as a result of the exclusions listed on the insurance policy. For example, an insurance policy excluded cover in relation to:

- certain subject populations
  - » subjects with HIV in an HIV trial
  - » subjects with Hepatitis B in a trial of the disease
  - » children in a paediatric trial
  - » pregnant women in an obstetrics trial
- regulatory issues
  - » excluding a trial without correct competent authority authorisation or favourable REC opinion
  - » excluding subjects that were not appropriately consented.

While the insurance may still be acceptable, depending on the exclusion, it is important that the sponsor is aware of the insurance policy exclusions, so that provisions can be considered. For example:

- applying for a waiver or additional premium for a subject population for a particular trial
- having a robust mechanism for ensuring initial approvals and any subsequent amendments are submitted to the competent authority and the REC, and that any specified conditions have been met.

There should be a process in place for the sponsor to check the insurance for each individual trial; it is recommended that this check is documented and filed in the TMF.

It is also recommended that vendors providing clinical trials services (for example, Phase I units and trial management) have insurance in place to meet claims arising from their negligence, whether from subjects directly or (in the case of

Phase I trials) from sponsors seeking reimbursement of their costs in meeting claims from subjects. Vendors are expected to have a mechanism in place for ensuring that there are no exclusions within the sponsor policy that affect the cover for the trial. This may be documented in a number of ways; for example, a copy of the policy could be included with the certificate, the certificate could clearly list the exclusions or there could be some form of formal sign-off to verify that someone from the sponsor or vendor has checked that the exclusions are acceptable.

The regulations state that provision must[5] be made for insurance or indemnity; therefore it is not acceptable in the UK for commercial organisations to self-insure, unless the sponsor can clearly demonstrate that a separate and adequate fund has been established by the organisation to meet its insurance obligations, which would provide compensation to subjects even if the sponsor ceases to trade. In this case, variations of 'self-insurance' may be acceptable, and this should be clear in the REC application.

For collaborative academic clinical trials (that is, non-commercial trials) public bodies (for example, Department of Health, Ministry of Defence, Medical Research Council and NHS bodies) do not require specific insurance as a named sponsor for a clinical trial. They must, however, ensure that the research (and any consequent interaction with patient care) is covered by NHS indemnity in respect of negligent harm. This is achieved as part of the process for giving management permission for research to go ahead. Specific checks are undertaken, and agreements are made, to ensure that the appropriate indemnity arrangements are in place. This process formalises the NHS body's duty of care towards the subject who consents to participate in research undertaken within the NHS. It is also important for the sponsor to be aware of the position on product liability in academic trials. For example, it has been observed that where an IMP supplier is providing the IMP free of charge, the contract may state that there is no product liability if it is not used within the terms of the marketing authorisation. The sponsor needs to be aware of this and the impact in relation to the risks of the trial.

Universities already have insurance cover for negligent harm; therefore, there will be no need for them to take non-negligent cover unless the REC identifies a specific need for such cover. It is acknowledged that some universities may already have non-negligent cover; however, universities should still check their insurance arrangements to ensure that the population to be studied is not excluded in the insurance policy.

Where a trial has joint sponsorship between a public body and non-public body, adequate checks should be made by each party that their sponsor responsibilities have adequate insurance cover.

1.4 Pharmacovigilance

The sponsor has defined legal responsibilities in relation to pharmacovigilance in clinical trials (Table 1.1, Part C). The sponsor should have robust processes in place to cover the various aspects relating to these responsibilities. These may include:

- identifying, collecting and reporting adverse events and serious adverse events (SAEs)/SUSARs
- provision of a safety section in the protocol
- assessing the need for a safety plan (for example, where the reporting mechanism is complex or involving various vendors)
- assessing and taking action in relation to safety signals (both clinical and non-clinical)
- use of independent data monitoring committees (DMCs)
- urgent safety measures
- production of development safety update reports (DSURs).

Detailed requirements for pharmacovigilance activities are described in Chapter 5.

1.4.1 Investigator's brochure

The sponsor is required[21] to produce an investigator's brochure (IB) and review the IB at least annually. Production of this document (see section 4.7.3) may be completed in-house or contracted out to a vendor; in either case, it should be clear who has been assigned this function. The TMF must[10] contain clear evidence not only that the IB has been reviewed even when the review concludes that no update is required, but also that this has been communicated to all relevant parties involved in the trial.

To ensure that this annual review is conducted, the sponsor can consider making use of the following tools:

- reminders in calendars

- manual spreadsheets
- electronic trackers with electronic alerts.

In the case of non-commercial sponsors, the requirement to produce and update the IB may be delegated to the chief investigator or the IB may be provided by the IMP supplier (usually a pharmaceutical company). In either case the sponsor must[21] ensure that the IB is reviewed on at least an annual basis. To ensure this, the sponsor can consider making use of the tools listed above, as well as the following:

- request this information to be included in self-assessment reports completed by the chief investigator
- verify compliance with this requirement through monitoring and audit activities
- request to be copied into the relevant correspondence (confirming review and/or submission of these documents to the competent authority and REC).

If there is a marketing authorisation and summary of product characteristics (SPC) for the IMP, and an IB is being used for trials, the sponsor should also ensure that the reference safety information (RSI) in the IB is consistent with that in the SPC, or have documented justification for any significant differences. If the IMP has a marketing authorisation and it is being used within its authorisation in the specified population, there may be no need to make use of an IB as an SPC may suffice as the RSI.

1.4.2 Urgent safety measures

Where the sponsor or an investigator takes urgent safety measures in order to protect the subjects of a trial against any immediate hazard to their health or safety, the competent authority and REC must[22] be notified immediately and in any event within 3 days that such measures have been taken and the reasons why they have been taken (see section 2.3.7 for further details on reporting urgent safety measures).

1.4.3 Safety reporting

1.4.3.1 Deciding on what safety data to record and report

As part of the risk assessment the sponsor could consider the following before initiating a clinical trial:

- What are the specific requirements for recording and notifying adverse events in the trial?
- Which events should be recorded and where?
- Which events should be notified to the sponsor and what are the timelines for notification?
- Is a DMC required?

The risk associated with the clinical trial in relation to safety will depend on:

- the authorisation status of the IMP(s)
- the extent of knowledge of the risk–benefit profile of the IMP(s)
- the population to be studied in the clinical trial
- the clinical trial objectives
- the assessments and procedures associated with the clinical trial design.

The proposed procedures for assessing, recording, notifying and reporting adverse events should then be detailed in the trial protocol and the sponsor's quality system.

1.4.3.2 Oversight of adverse events

As part of the site initiation process and pre-trial communications (for example, face-to-face, webinar or online training), investigators are instructed to report adverse events to the sponsor (as per the process specified in the protocol). These are usually reported via the CRF and can be verified through source data verification (SDV) during monitoring of the investigator site, where trial records are reviewed to ensure that all necessary adverse events have been reported.

1.4.3.3 Oversight of serious adverse events

If an investigator determines that an adverse event fulfils one of the seriousness criteria (as defined in the protocol) then they must[23] report this event as an SAE to the sponsor or its delegated external vendor immediately and this should be within 24 hours of becoming aware of the event. The event is then assessed and a decision is made as to whether the event is reportable to the competent authority and the REC as a SUSAR and in what required timeframe (7 or 15 days depending on the seriousness criteria; see section 5.5).

The identification and reporting of SAEs can be verified through SDV during monitoring of the investigator site. In addition, the sponsor should ensure that sufficient processes are in place to verify that all necessary reports are being

Table 1.2 Example tracker for documenting the serious adverse event assessment process

Subject ID	Event	Dates						
		Event occurred	Notified to PI	Reported to sponsor	Received by sponsor	Assessed	Reported to CA	Reported to REC
AB/01	Stroke	01/Oct/11	02/Oct/11	02/Oct/11	02/Oct/11	03/Oct/11	05/Oct/11	06/Oct/11

CA, competent authority; ID, identification; PI, principal investigator; REC, research ethics committee

submitted within the required timeframes. This can be achieved by tracking and documenting key steps of the SAE process to ensure that the timelines are complied with, as illustrated in Table 1.2.

Using tools, such as trackers and spreadsheets, to document each step of the SAE process can assist in collation and oversight of this information in a meaningful way for both large clinical trials (with multiple sites in multiple countries with differing requirements) and small clinical trials with a single site and low reporting rate of SAEs. If an external vendor is being used for this service, then reports summarising this information can be requested from the vendor to assess compliance with the legislation. For blinded clinical trials it is important to consider who will oversee this information in order to ensure that the blinded status of the trial is not compromised.

1.4.3.4 Informing investigators of SUSARs

The sponsor is required[24] to ensure that the investigators responsible for the conduct of a trial are informed of any SUSARs that occur in relation to an IMP used in the trials it is involved with. This is the case whether that SUSAR occurs in the trial that the investigator is involved in, or another trial using the same IMP for which the sponsor is responsible. No timelines are specified in the regulations for reporting to investigators; however, this should be done in a timely manner to ensure that investigators are kept fully informed of all safety information.

This requirement is usually met by sending the investigators periodic listings of SUSARs or individual CIOMS I forms as each event occurs. It should be clear who within the sponsor organisation has responsibility for this activity and processes should be implemented to ensure that this requirement is met. The sponsor could consider adding another column to Table 1.2 to track the submission of SUSARs to investigators. Monitoring of investigator sites can also be used to verify that investigators have received and read this information (see section 5.5 for further information).

In the case of multi-centre clinical trials with a non-commercial sponsor, this responsibility is usually delegated to the chief investigator, who would be responsible for collating safety information and periodically sending it to the other investigators. In order to maintain oversight, the sponsor can consider requesting that this information is included in self-assessment reports completed by the chief investigator and verifying compliance through monitoring and audit activities.

1.4.3.5 Development safety update reports

The sponsor must[25] provide the competent authority and REC with an annual report on the safety of subjects in all clinical trials of the product for which the sponsor is responsible, whether in the UK or elsewhere. All annual safety reports (ASRs) should be in the format of DSURs (see section 5.15 for further details of the requirements for DSURs, including format and content). In the case of non-commercial sponsors, the requirement to provide an annual list of suspected serious adverse reactions and a safety report is often delegated to the chief investigator.

In order to ensure that DSURs are being produced and submitted on time, the sponsor can consider using the same tools as those examples provided for the IB (see section 1.4.1).

1.5 Manufacture, assembly, importation and labelling of IMP

The sponsor's responsibilities relating to manufacture, assembly, importation and labelling of IMP are summarised in Table 1.1 (Part D).

1.5.1 Requirements for the authorisation to manufacture and import IMP

The sponsor has a number of responsibilities relating to the manufacture, assembly, importation and labelling of IMP. The legislation states that these activities must[26] occur in accordance with the manufacturing authorisation granted by the competent authority. (In the UK this is a specific manufacturer's authorisation for investigational medicinal products (MIA(IMP)), with appropriate authorisations. In other EU countries this may be authorised and identified differently by the competent authority; however, throughout this guide the term 'MIA(IMP)' will be used to describe the manufacturing authorisation.) Therefore, the sponsor must[26] ensure that the requirements for authorisation to manufacture, assemble and import the IMP are met (see Chapter 6 for further detail on these requirements).

The sponsor must[26] assess whether the activities it intends to perform require an MIA(IMP). If so, the sponsor should obtain the necessary authorisation or ensure a suitable CMO is contracted to undertake these activities on behalf of the sponsor. The sponsor is responsible for assessing that the CMO is suitable to undertake these activities (for example, by using appropriate vendor selection tools, as described in section 1.3.2). If the sponsor is using an external vendor for all or part of these activities, then as part of vendor oversight it must[26] ensure that the vendor is authorised to perform these activities.

The sponsor should ensure that responsibilities relating to IMP activities are not delegated to individuals who are inappropriately trained and qualified (for example, delegation to a chief investigator or pharmacy not trained in Annex 13 of the EU Guidelines to GMP), as this may lead to failures to comply with the legislation (for example, manufacturing IMP or investigator sites receiving IMP directly from outside the EEA without an MIA(IMP)).

1.5.2 Authorisation to start the trial

It is a legislative requirement[7] that a trial does not start until an authorisation has been granted and favourable REC opinion has been received – 'regulatory release', and that IMP must[27] not be sold or supplied until an authorisation has been granted and it has been certified by a Qualified Person (QP) where required – 'technical release'. Both these steps must[10] be recorded and retained in the relevant trial files held by or on behalf of the sponsor.

The sponsor's authorisation to start the trial is usually marked by the shipment of IMP to the investigator sites. However, there are occasions where this may vary. For example:

- Where off-the-shelf authorised products are the IMP, this would be the authorisation to start recruitment, as no technical release may be required (see section 6.3.3). However, the sponsor should still perform some type of formally documented 'regulatory green-light' check (see section 1.5.2.3) to ensure that all the necessary regulatory approvals are in place.

- IMP may be shipped under quarantine, prior to technical release. This may only occur where the IMP is being shipped to a department controlling release of the IMP to the investigator (for example, a pharmacy in a Phase I unit). However, this should only be undertaken provided the receiving site has a regulatory green-light check to ensure QP certification is received to remove the IMP from quarantine for release to the investigator. Therefore, the site must[14] comply with robust quarantine procedures.

1.5.2.1 Step 1: Qualified Person certification (or 'technical release')

The sponsor must[28] ensure that a QP certifies that the IMP has been manufactured to EU Good Manufacturing Practice (GMP) standards and in accordance with the CTA and product specification file. The circumstances where QP certification is not required (for example, when unaltered licensed products are used for a clinical trial) are covered in section 6.3.3.

QP certification may be performed by the sponsor or contracted out; however, the sponsor must[29] assure itself that there is appropriate access to a named QP. There should be written procedures to describe the certification process and relevant staff must[4] be appropriately trained. In addition, if this function is to be performed by an external vendor, then the sponsor should ensure that the responsibilities are clearly described (for example, in the contract and/or a technical agreement with the external vendor). The sponsor should also ensure that the vendor is supplied with all the relevant paperwork to perform QP certification (for example, the entire CTA as approved by the competent authority, including any conditions of approval and subsequent amendments).

Further requirements for QP certification can be found in section 6.3.3.

1.5.2.2 Step 2: Regulatory checks (or 'regulatory release')

The sponsor must[7] not start a clinical trial until clinical trial authorisation has been granted for the trial (and all conditions of that authorisation have been met) and a favourable REC opinion has been granted (and any conditions have been met). This is referred to as 'regulatory release'.

Note that, although it is possible to advertise and recruit a subject provided a favourable REC opinion has been granted, if there is no competent authority authorisation, then no trial-specific activities must[7] be conducted. Any recruitment (for example, generic screening) should only be undertaken where there are robust quarantine procedures in place to ensure that IMP is not administered.

1.5.2.3   Regulatory green light

In addition to the requirements for technical and regulatory release, it is also expected that the sponsor verifies that other aspects required to comply with the Clinical Trials Regulations are in place prior to authorising the start of the trial. These will vary between organisations and trials, but may include checking that the contracts with the investigator site(s) and any vendors have been finalised and signed, that insurance is in place and adequate, or that any other approvals have been granted (for example, ARSAC).

There should be clear documentation to verify that all the necessary documents have been received and checked by the sponsor prior to the authorisation to start the trial; that is, there should be clear evidence of what documents have been checked (including versions), who has checked each document and when, and who has authorised the start of the trial at each site and when. This documented check is commonly referred to as the 'regulatory green light' and usually marks the sponsor's authorisation to ship the IMP to the investigator sites. There should be a written procedure to cover this process.

Examples of inadequate regulatory green-light processes include those where:

- there was no documented process to verify that all the required documents were received prior to shipping the IMP
- the regulatory green light did not cover all the key checks required; for example, it did not ensure that there was 'technical release' as there was no requirement to check that there was a QP certification where required
- a regulatory green-light checklist was produced which only contained ticks next to the documents and, as there was no signature or date to verify who made the checks and when, it could not be verified that authorisation was given after all the relevant checks had been made
- the regulatory green-light procedure consisted of a document that was signed and dated to state that all required documents and approvals were in place; however, this document was simply filed in the TMF and not related to any trigger to ship the IMP to investigator sites and, therefore, there was no procedure in place to prevent shipment of the IMP to site without relevant approvals.

It is recommended that the sponsor considers who is responsible for performing this check and authorisation, so it is not repeated by numerous staff. For example:

- Non-commercial organisations often have both R&D and pharmacy making the same checks; therefore consideration should be given to who is best placed to give the final 'authorisation'.
- For multi-centre trials, this regulatory green-light check can be separated into two parts, where the trial or country-level documents are checked once for the whole trial (for example, the CTA and favourable REC opinion) and then the investigator site-level documents are checked for each site (for example, the site-specific approvals), prior to authorising the start of the clinical trial at that investigator site.

If the sponsor is reliant on an external vendor for obtaining the required approvals then the regulatory green-light check may also be delegated. As a result, the sponsor should implement processes for maintaining oversight of this activity prior to the commencement of the clinical trial. For example, the sponsor may:

- review the external vendor's regulatory green-light procedure and/or checklist to ensure that the external vendor has an appropriate process in place for performing this function
- approve or review the regulatory green-light checks for the first few investigator sites initiated, and then occasionally perform spot checks of any further regulatory green-light checks completed
- request that it is sent copies of all the documented regulatory green-light checks as they are completed
- organise a joint regulatory green-light check with the vendor (that is, the checklist may initially be completed by the external vendor and then checked and approved by the sponsor).

1.5.3 Labelling of IMP

The sponsor should implement processes to ensure that the IMP is appropriately labelled. The requirements of labelling are described in section 6.7.

1.5.4 Oversight of IMP activities at investigator sites

The sponsor should ensure that it has sufficient oversight of the IMP while it is at the investigator site. This can be achieved through monitoring activities (which check that the IMP is appropriately stored, dispensed and accounted for) or update reports from suppliers of interactive response technologies (IRT), if being used.

The sponsor also should ensure that investigator sites are sufficiently supplied (and re-supplied) with IMP. In order to do so, an initial calculation needs to be made to determine what quantity of IMP is required. This quantity will depend on the number of subjects the investigator site plans on recruiting and the site's storage capacity. The information obtained from monitoring and IRT suppliers (if used) can then be used to determine how often re-supplies are required to ensure that the site is sufficiently supplied with IMP.

1.6   Trial/project management

Clinical trial or project management refers to a process that is initiated and followed to successfully manage and coordinate all activities involved in the conduct of clinical trials. Without good project management, a clinical trial can be rendered worthless, subjects will have been exposed to IMP unnecessarily and many thousands of pounds can be lost. Project management ensures that the trial runs smoothly and that vital resources are used as optimally as possible. The practicalities of maintaining sponsor oversight also often fall to the project management function of an organisation. Project management is therefore a key part of clinical research.

For a new commercial product there will usually be a development programme in place and project or programme management activities will start before the first trial commences and continue until the development programme for a compound is completed or curtailed. Project managers may be involved in the clinical programme, of which one trial may form only a small part of the programme (Figure 1.3).

In non-commercial trials, many small trials do not have a project manager as this is often the role of the chief investigator or principal investigator; however, larger trials may have trial managers or trial coordinators who take on many of the project management activities of the trial.

This section will discuss the role project management has to play in relation to a single trial and how sponsor oversight can be achieved by making use of good project management skills.

Some of the key project management considerations before, during and after the trial are detailed in Table 1.3.

Development programme

Programme project manager

Responsible for oversight of multiple clinical trials and ensuring that information from each trial and non-clinical activities is assessed and circulated to all other relevant teams

Clinical

Phase I trials
- Early phase trials, usually involving healthy volunteers (but may be patients)
- Main focus is on safety, tolerability and pharmacokinetics

Phase II trials
- Larger trials in patients for continuing safety and efficacy
- Project management is key to managing the oversight of multiple sites and multiple countries

Phase III trials
- Large trials in many patients and sites for continuing safety and efficacy
- May be pivotal trials being used in MAA submissions
- Project management is key to managing the oversight of multiple sites and multiple countries (there may be multiple project managers, depending on the size of the trial)

Marketing/Post-marketing

Phase IV trials
- Trials to ascertain more information on safety and efficacy in the general population
- May be run by the pharmaceutical organisation's affiliate or R&D group
- Project management is key to oversight of these trials (there may be multiple project managers depending on the size of the trial)

Non-interventional trials
- Not within the remit of the clinical trials legislation

Related aspects

Non-clinical data
- Liaison with non-clinical/translational science regarding non-clinical data

Investigational medicinal product manufacture
- Liaison with clinical supplies group/pharmacy

Pharmacovigilance
- Liaison with pharmacovigilance group regarding clinical safety

Figure 1.3 Example of a clinical development programme

Table 1.3 Key trial/project management considerations

Project/trial management		
Before	**During**	**End/After**
Communication		
Project team set-up	Project meetings and telephone/video conferences	Trial debrief
Project plan/milestones	Progress/status reports	
Communication plan	Dissemination of key information/minutes etc.	
	Changes to trial team	
Documentation		
Prepare trial master file	Maintain trial master file	Complete and archive trial master file
Risk assessment	Review/update/circulate risk assessment	Clinical study report
Key trial documents (for example, protocol, investigator's brochure, subject information sheet/consent forms, accountability records)	Review/update/circulate key trial documents, trial plans, written procedures etc.	
Regulatory green-light check	Amendments (including substantiality decision and implementation)	
Trial manuals/plans (for example, pharmacy, laboratory manuals)	Document and circulate any actions and decisions	
Written procedures		
Regulatory and ethical correspondence		
Competent authority authorisation	Substantial amendments	End-of-trial notification
Favourable research ethics committee opinion	Annual progress reports to research ethics committee	Clinical trial summary report
	Serious breaches	
	Urgent safety measures	
	Development safety update reports	

Project/trial management		
Before	**During**	**End/After**
Vendors		
Vendor selection	Oversight	Vendor performance assessment
Contracts and insurance	Review of contracts	
Provision of required documentation	Ensure obligations of all parties being met	
Training	Status updates	
	Visits/audits	
	Management and escalation of issues	
Investigational medicinal product		
Manufacture, packaging and labelling	Ongoing supply	Complete accountability
Qualified person certification	Ongoing accountability	Return/destruction
Randomisation and blinding	Maintenance of blinding	
Release and distribution	Temperature excursions	
Investigational medicinal product dossier/summary of product characteristics	Shelf-life changes	
Investigator site		
Monitoring plan	Routine on-site/central monitoring	Notification of end of recruitment
Monitors assigned	Recruitment updates	Close-out
Site selection	Issue identification and escalation	Complete and archive Investigator site file
Initiation and training	Collection of case report form data	
	Data query answering	
	Additional investigator sites initiation and training	
Pharmacovigilance		
Safety plan	Adverse event collection, assessment and reporting	Final reconciliation of safety and clinical databases
	Ongoing safety updates	
	Safety signal detection	

Table continues

Table 1.3 *continued*

Project/trial management		
Before	**During**	**End/After**
Pharmacovigilance *continued*		
	Data monitoring committee/ data safety monitoring board	
	Investigator's brochure update/validation	
	Development safety update reports preparation	
	Reconciliation of safety and clinical databases	
Data management and analysis		
Case report form design and preparation	Data entry	Final electronic data transfer
Define major non-compliances	Protocol non-compliance collection and circulation	Protocol non-compliance review for analysis
Database build	Data queries	Final analysis (for example, statistical and pharmacokinetic)
Computer system validation and validation of application builds	Electronic data transfer	
Data management plan	Interim analyses (including dose escalation)	
Statistical analysis plan		

1.6.1   Project team

A project manager is not expected to be an expert in all areas of clinical research; instead they are the key communicator and coordinator for the trial to ensure that key decisions are made by relevant and well-informed staff in a timely manner and that these decisions are documented and retained. Therefore, the project manager is responsible for producing a realistic and agreed project plan for the trial, tracking progress of the trial against the plan's timelines and milestones, and generally maintaining oversight of the trial as a whole. How this oversight is managed depends on what resources or tools the project manager has available; tools can range from simple spreadsheets to more complex Gantt charts, project plans or bespoke clinical trials management systems.

To perform project management effectively, one of the first tasks is to assign a project/trial team and clearly define the roles and responsibilities within the project team, in line with the agreed project plan and timeline. Doing this upfront will avoid duplication of effort and ensure that all team members take ownership of the functions and tasks assigned. Where this is not done, it could result in important decisions not being actioned and followed up for completion. For example, in a large global trial involving a sponsor and two CROs, the pharmacovigilance group identified a safety concern relating to how the IMP was packaged that increased the potential for overdose. Although the issue was identified and actions were agreed to mitigate this, the project team failed to adequately document the issue to ensure that responsibility for the action was assigned and implemented. As a result there was a significant delay in an alert being issued to the investigator sites, in which time further overdoses occurred, one leading to the death of a subject. This issue is a clear demonstration of how serious issues can arise, simply by the lack of documentation and communication.

In some organisations (for example, non-commercial or virtual organisations), a number of the functions undertaken by the project team may be undertaken by the same person (that is, R&D personnel, chief investigator, research nurse). Also there may be circumstances where these functions are undertaken by an external party/vendor (for example, a CRO or consultant). Both of these scenarios are acceptable, so long as the responsibilities are clearly defined and they are included as part of the trial team.

Throughout the trial the project manager would usually liaise with the various members of the project team and convene meetings as required (these may be face-to-face or using teleconferences or videoconferences) to discuss the progress of the trial (in line with any risk management plan) and any potential barriers to the trial proceeding in the expected timeframes. The attendance at these meetings may vary throughout the trial depending on the expertise required at each stage of the trial.

Where the project management activities are contracted out to a vendor, the vendor's project manager may be required to provide the sponsor with regular status/progress reports.

1.6.2 Communication and tracking

Whether it is a single-centre or multi-centre trial or a series of clinical trials being run as part of a programme, communication is critical as there will potentially be a variety of groups involved, both internally and externally (such as vendors, contractors and investigator sites). Therefore it is recommended that the project manager ensures that the lines of communication are clear. Depending on the complexity of the trial, and the number of different parties involved, it is sometimes useful to have an agreed communication plan in place so that all involved parties are clear who needs to communicate what to whom and when.

If a trial is simple, and there are only a few groups or a small local team of people working together throughout the trial, it may only be necessary to meet as required to discuss progress.

Any meetings (and any other important communications collected or disseminated) must[10] be adequately documented and retained in the TMF as well as documentation of key decisions relating to the trial (including details of who made the decision and when it was made). Documentation can be in the form of emails, meeting minutes or other activity-specific or trial-specific documents. For example:

- forms tracking trial items such as CRF pages, IMP and laboratory samples
- approval forms for various trial-specific documents
- checklists such as those used for regulatory green-light or quality control processes
- spreadsheets to track amendments and their approvals
- logs for the collection of protocol deviations, SAEs or site contact details.

It is acknowledged that where there is a small team discussion may happen 'across the desk'; however, no matter what the size and location of the team, all key decisions must[10] be documented so that the trial can be reconstructed without the need for the team to be available (for example, team members may not remember events, may leave or may be unavailable during an inspection).

1.7   Chapter legislative references

Throughout this chapter, specific terminology – 'must', 'required' or 'requirement' – has been used to interpret activities that are legislative requirements. These terms have been number-coded in the text where used, and the corresponding reference in the legislation can be found below.

1. Regulation 3 (11) of SI 2004/1031
2. Regulation 3 (12) of SI 2004/1031
3. Regulation 28 (1) of SI 2004/1031
4. Schedule 1, Part 2 (2) of SI 2004/1031
5. Schedule 1, Part 2 (14) of SI 2004/1031
6. Regulation 3 (2) and (5) of SI 2004/1031
7. Regulation 12 of SI 2004/1031
8. Regulation 14 (1) of SI 2004/1031
9. Regulation 24 of SI 2004/1031
10. Regulation 31A (4) of SI 2004/1031
11. Regulation 18 (4) of SI 2004/1031
12. Regulation 27 of SI 2004/1031
13. Regulation 28 (2) of SI 2004/1031
14. Schedule 1, Part 2 (4) of SI 2004/1031
15. Regulation 29 of SI 2004/1031
16. Regulation 29A of SI 2004/1031
17. Regulation 31A (2) of SI 2004/1031
18. Schedule 1, Part 2 (9) of SI 2004/1031
19. Regulation 31A (7) of SI 2004/1031
20. Regulation 31A (9) of SI 2004/1031
21. Regulation 3A of SI 2004/1031
22. Regulation 30 of SI 2004/1031
23. Regulation 32 (1) of SI 2004/1031
24. Regulation 33 (5) of SI 2004/1031
25. Regulation 35 of SI 2004/1031
26. Regulation 36 of SI 2004/1031
27. Regulation 13 of SI 2004/1031
28. Article 13 (3) of Directive 2001/20/EC
29. Regulation 43 of SI 2004/1031

1

CHAPTER 2

Clinical trial authorisations

2

Editor's note

According to the Clinical Trials Directive 2001/20/EC, clinical trials of medicinal products in human subjects require authorisation by the competent authority (the MHRA in the UK) and a favourable opinion by an ethics committee. This competent authority authorisation is granted in the form of a clinical trial authorisation (CTA).

Clinical trials involving only medical devices, food supplements or other non-medicinal therapies (such as surgical interventions) as well as non-interventional trials are not covered by Directive 2001/20/EC and, as such, a CTA would not be required. The assessments of applications from sponsors to conduct clinical trials with medicinal products are carried out by the MHRA Clinical Trials Unit (CTU). The types of trials assessed range from 'first in human' studies for new compounds to trials with products which already have marketing authorisations. In addition to assessment activities, the MHRA CTU carries out many different functions in relation to the regulation of clinical trials including the review of evolving safety data, provision of advice on clinical trials, and meeting with organisations to provide scientific or regulatory advice.

This chapter provides an overview of clinical trials which are covered by Directive 2001/20/EC. The format and content of CTA applications and the assessment thereof is described in detail; common issues with deficient applications are also discussed to help applicants with future applications. Risk-adapted approaches to the management of clinical trials are reviewed, including the Notification Scheme for lower-risk investigational medicinal products (IMPs) and applications for higher-risk trials requiring expert advice. Lastly, the Voluntary Harmonisation Procedure (VHP) for EU multinational clinical trials is described.

2.1 Legal definition of a clinical trial

The Medicines for Human Use (Clinical Trials) Regulations 2004 (SI 2004/1031) only apply to trials of medicinal products. Medicinal products are substances, or combinations of substances, which either prevent or treat disease in humans or are administered to humans with a view to making a medical diagnosis or to restore, correct or modify physiological functions (Article 1 of Directive 2001/83/EC).

Consequently, a clinical trial is an investigation in human subjects which is intended to *'discover or verify the clinical, pharmacological or other pharmacodynamic effects of one or more medicinal products, to identify any adverse reactions to one or more such products, or to study absorption, distribution, metabolism and excretion of one or more such products, with the object of ascertaining the safety or efficacy of those products'* (Regulation 2 of SI 2004/1031). This definition includes pharmacokinetic studies.

An IMP is defined in Regulation 2 of SI 2004/1031 as a pharmaceutical form of an active substance or placebo being tested or used as a reference product in a clinical trial. IMPs can include authorised products used in their approved form, either within or outside their licensed indication, or manufactured and assembled (formulated or packaged) in a way that is different from the authorised form. For example, a tablet product of active substance X may be authorised for use as an anti-hypertensive. A clinical researcher has found evidence that X may have anti-microbial activity and wants to carry out a clinical trial in patients with severe chest infections with X administered as an injection. In this case, X solution for injection would be an IMP for the proposed clinical trial as an active substance authorised as a different form for a different indication. Alternatively, the authorised product (X in tablet form) could be used as the IMP in a clinical trial to investigate the long-term safety of X when used to treat hypertension. In this case, the purpose of the proposed clinical trial is to gain further information on the use of X tablets in an authorised indication.

To find out whether a clinical trial is covered by the Clinical Trials Directive 2001/20/EC, an algorithm 'Is it a clinical trial of a medicinal product?' has been developed. This algorithm is provided in the annex to the 'Question & Answers' document in EudraLex Volume 10, Chapter V, and is also available on the MHRA website.

2

If, after working through the algorithm, there is still uncertainty about whether or not the clinical trial is covered by Directive 2001/20/EC, an email can be sent to the MHRA's Clinical Trial Helpline (clintrialhelpline@mhra.gsi.gov.uk) marked 'Scope – protocol review' followed by the trial title (short) in the subject line requesting an opinion on the status of the trial. A copy of the protocol or protocol proposal should be provided with the request. Where possible, responses to such 'scope' queries will be sent within 7 days.

Clinical trials involving only medical devices or other non-medicinal therapies (such as surgical interventions) are not covered by Directive 2001/20/EC. Clinical trials involving a medicine and a medical device will be subject to clinical trials regulations and may also be subject to medical device regulations depending on the purpose of the clinical trial. In such cases, the applicant can check the regulatory position with the MHRA if in any doubt. Advice from the MHRA Devices Division should be sought for clinical trials involving non-CE marked devices or CE marked devices used outside the conditions of the CE marking. The applicant should refer to any correspondence with the Devices Division in the cover letter of the CTA application. The regulations do not apply to non-interventional trials (as defined in Regulation 2 of SI 2004/1031 and Article 2 (c) of Directive 2001/20/EC). Epidemiological methods should be used for the data analysis of such trials. Clinical trials with food supplements are also not covered by Directive 2001/20/EC; however, where a food supplement (for example, a vitamin) is presented as a pharmaceutical form (for example, a tablet), and is being evaluated for a medicinal purpose, then it will be considered as a medicine and the requirements of Directive 2001/20/EC will apply.

Some clinical trials also involve medicinal products which are classified as non-investigational medicinal products (nIMPs). For example, an active substance may be used as a probe to investigate the role of a certain liver enzyme on the metabolism of an IMP. Standard-of-care medicines that are already being administered to a subject, but are continued during the clinical trial, are generally considered to be nIMPs. Additional examples of clinical trials involving nIMPs are available on the MHRA website to assist organisations in making the decision as to whether a product is an IMP or a nIMP. Further information on nIMPs is provided in Chapter 6.

2.1.1 European Union Drug Regulating Authorities Clinical Trials database

The European Union Drug Regulating Authorities Clinical Trials (EudraCT) database provides competent authorities with a common set of information on clinical trials taking place in the European Union (EU) that commenced from 1 May 2004 onwards. The EudraCT system comprises a website (http://eudract.eudra.org) available to clinical trial sponsors and a secure database available only to the competent authorities, the European Commission and the European Medicines Agency (EMA). Each clinical trial is provided with a unique identifier known as the EudraCT number. Competent authorities enter information into EudraCT on the authorisation of the clinical trial, the research ethics committee (REC) opinion, amendments, the end of the trial and inspections. Public access to the EudraCT database is possible, allowing members of the public to access certain information on EU-approved clinical trials and data following the end of trials through the EU Clinical Trial Register (https://www.clinicaltrialsregister.eu).

2.2 Format and content of a clinical trial authorisation application

Details of the documentation required to support a CTA application (as per Regulation 17, and Part 2 of Schedule 3 to SI 2004/1031) are available in the European Commission 'Detailed guidance on the request to the competent authorities for authorisation of a clinical trial on a medicinal product for human use, the notification of substantial amendments and the declaration of the end of the trial' (hereinafter 'detailed guidance CT-1').

In order for an application to be considered as valid, a submission should contain a file for each of the following documents:

- cover letter
- CTA application form and valid XML
- protocol
- investigator's brochure (IB) or equivalent document (for example, the summary of product characteristics (SPC))
- investigational medicinal product dossier (IMPD)
- nIMP dossier (if required)
- scientific advice
- EMA decision

- trial-specific labelling of the IMP (or justification for its absence)
- proof of payment
- manufacturer's authorisation or importer's authorisation together with a Qualified Person (QP) declaration on compliance with Good Manufacturing Practice (GMP) for each manufacturing site.

Further details of these documents are provided in the following sections.

2.2.1   Cover letter

A signed cover letter should be submitted with all other documentation. Typically it will list the documentation that is being submitted, details of the trial (including EudraCT number and protocol number) and the contact details of the person submitting the application. It should be in an MS Word® format or Adobe Acrobat® optical character recognition (OCR) format so it is readily readable. The cover letter should also include identification of the reference safety information (RSI) that will be used to determine expectedness in the trial and make it clear whether the trial involves vulnerable populations, whether it is a 'first in human' (FIH) trial or part of a paediatric investigation plan (PIP), or if scientific advice has been sought from the EMA or competent authority.

2.2.2   Clinical trial authorisation application form and valid XML

An XML file is the data format of the saved CTA application form information. It is created via the Integrated Research Application System (IRAS) or the EudraCT database. The XML file of the completed CTA application form is required to enable the entry of the details of the trial into the EudraCT database, a role the competent authority is obliged to fulfil by Directive 2001/20/EC.

2.2.3   Protocol

The content and format of the protocol should comply with the ICH Topic E6 (R1) – 'Guideline for Good Clinical Practice'. Information on the production of the protocol is detailed in Chapter 4. The version of protocol submitted should include all currently authorised amendments and a definition of the end of the trial (see section 2.3.10 for further information on the definition of the end of the trial). The protocol should be identified by the title, a sponsor's reference code (applicable to all versions), a version number and date (that will be updated when it is amended) and by any short title or name assigned to it. It should be signed by the sponsor and principal investigator (or coordinating investigator for multi-centre trials).

2.2.4   Investigator's brochure or equivalent document

The IB should be prepared from all available information and evidence that supports the rationale for the proposed clinical trial and the safe use of the IMP in the trial. It should be presented in the format of summaries rather than the full trial reports and it should be made clear whether this information is from final or draft data. Information on the production of this document is detailed in Chapter 4. The SPC will replace the IB if the IMP is authorised in any EU Member State and it is being used in accordance with the terms of the marketing authorisation. When the conditions of use in the clinical trial differ from those authorised, the SPC should be supplemented with a summary of relevant data that support the use of the IMP in the clinical trial. This can be provided in the form of an IB or, in some cases, may be incorporated into the protocol. The section of the IB that refers to, and clearly allows the assessment of, the expectedness of adverse reactions should be clear and also identified in the cover letter.

2.2.5   Investigational medicinal product dossier

An IMPD must[1] accompany each application. However, on a case-by-case basis, this may be a full dossier or a simplified dossier, which may be the SPC for an EU-authorised product. The content of the IMPD (for drug substances other than those produced by biotechnology) is described in the EMA 'Guideline on the requirements to the chemical and pharmaceutical quality documentation concerning investigational medicinal products in clinical trials' (CHMP/QWP/185401/2004) and that for biological products is described in the EMA 'Guideline on the requirements for quality documentation concerning biological investigational medicinal products in clinical trials' (CHMP/BWP/534898/2008) in EudraLex Volume 10, Chapter III. These guidelines are available on the European Commission website. Information on the production of this document is detailed in Chapter 4.

For an additional protocol with the same IMP or a cross-referral submission (that is, where one sponsor uses an IMP and cross-refers to another application, with permission), no new IMPD or IB data should be provided; however, copies of the relevant manufacturer's authorisation(s) and QP declaration (if applicable) must[1] still be provided since these are trial-specific. In the case of a cross-referral submission, this should be addressed in the cover letter.

2.2.6 Non-investigational medicinal product dossier

In general, the documentation requirements[1] in the CTA application dossier for IMPs also apply to nIMPs. However, there are possibilities for simplified documentation requirements (that is, a 'simplified dossier') depending on the extent of knowledge of the nIMP. Annex 2 of the 'Guidance on investigational medicinal products (IMPs) and non-investigational medicinal products (nIMPs)' in EudraLex Volume 10, Chapter III, sets out those simplified documentation requirements.

2.2.7 Scientific advice

If it is available, a copy of the summary of scientific advice received from any Member State or the EMA with regard to the clinical trial should be provided in the CTA application.

2.2.8 Decision of the European Medicines Agency

If the clinical trial is part of an agreed PIP, a copy of the EMA's decision on the agreement on the PIP, as well as the opinion of the Paediatric Committee (PDCO) should be provided, unless these documents are fully accessible via the internet. If this is the case, the link to this documentation in the cover letter is sufficient.

2.2.9 Labelling of the investigational medicinal product

The detailed guidance CT-1 requires the submission of the content of trial labelling as part of the application for a CTA. Where a sponsor wishes to claim an exemption from the need for trial-specific labelling under the provisions of Regulation 46 (2) of SI 2004/1031, a statement to this effect should be included in the application. Labelling requirements for a clinical trial are covered in section 6.7.

2.2.10 Proof of payment

Proof of payment must[2] be submitted at the same time as all the other documentation; it can be included in the cover letter and/or as a separate document. This can take the form of a banker's draft or other proof of payment (for example, a photocopy of a cheque or confirmation of bank transfer).

Documentation should be in MS Word format or Adobe Acrobat OCR. If proof of payment is not received then this would constitute an invalid application and it would be rejected at the validation stage.

The requirement to pay fees at the time of submission of a CTA application is a legal requirement specified in The Medicines (Products for Human Use) (Fees) Regulations, as amended. Payment at a different time is not acceptable.

The fee depends on the type of clinical trial: Phase I/II/III trials with an unknown product, and Phase II/III trials with a known product, cost significantly more than Phase IV trials, additional protocols (same sponsor and same product(s)) and cross-referral applications. Further information on fees for clinical trials can be found on the MHRA website.

2.2.11 Manufacturer's or importer's authorisation and QP declaration

The manufacture and/or assembly (packaging and labelling) of an IMP must[3] be undertaken by the holder of an authorisation for the manufacture of IMP (that is, a manufacturer's authorisation for investigational medical products (MIA(IMP)), except in those situations described below. A copy of the manufacturer's authorisation must[1] be provided for each EU site undertaking any manufacturing step in the preparation of the test product or any comparator (including placebos). Blinding of a comparator product by over-encapsulation is also considered to be manufacturing (see section 6.8). Copies of relevant manufacturer's authorisations, including those issued by the MHRA GMP Inspectorate, must[1] be provided otherwise the CTA application is invalid. Also, their inclusion demonstrates that the sponsor has satisfied itself that the proposed sites of manufacture have appropriate authorisations (for example, for sterile product manufacture).

However, the requirement to hold a manufacturer's authorisation for IMP does not apply in the following situations:

* the manufacture or assembly is in accordance with the terms and conditions of a marketing authorisation relating to that product (Regulation 36 (2) of SI 2004/1031)

- the assembly is carried out in a hospital or health centre by a doctor, a pharmacist or a person acting under the supervision of a pharmacist and the IMPs are assembled exclusively for use in that hospital or health centre, or any other hospital or health centre which is a trial site for the clinical trial in which the product is to be used (Regulation 37 of SI 2004/1031).

Where manufacture and/or assembly occurs outside the EEA, the product has to be imported by the holder of a manufacturer's authorisation covering the activity of importation of IMP. In addition, a copy of the QP declaration on GMP equivalence to EU GMP must[1] be provided. The QP declaration is usually signed by a QP named on the manufacturer's authorisation of the importer but may be signed by a QP at the batch release site (if this is different). In such cases, a copy of the manufacturer's authorisation for the batch release site is also required[1]. The QP declaration is trial-specific and product-specific (including placebos). The details to be included on the batch release certificate should be in accordance with the harmonised format found in Attachment 3 to Annex 13, EudraLex Volume 4; this facilitates the free movement of IMP between Member States. Refer to section 6.3 for further details on the required authorisations and QP declaration.

In cases where a document is not required in support of an application, such as when the type of submission does not require details of the content of the labelling, the file should still be provided; however, it should contain an explanation for why the document has not been supplied.

2.2.12 Failure to submit a valid application

Approximately 15% of applications fail at the validation step. The most frequent causes of an application being considered as invalid are listed below:

- failure to supply a EudraCT XML file of the completed CTA application form
- failure to complete section C1 of the CTA application form or section D1 of the notification of amendment form – these sections provide information on the person authorised by the sponsor to correspond with the competent authority on behalf of the sponsor; this information is required in order to be able to communicate with the sponsor
- failure to provide proof of payment
- failure to provide the correct product name in section D3.1 of the CTA application form – the product name provided in this section should be the trade name for the product or the name routinely used by the sponsor to identify the IMP in the clinical trial documentation.

2.3 Clinical trial authorisation applications – assessment and amendments

2.3.1 Assessment process

Three assessors are usually involved in the assessment of a CTA application – a non-clinical, medical and pharmaceutical assessor. However, where there is no new non-clinical information to assess, the CTA application will be assessed by a medical assessor and a pharmaceutical assessor only. Each assessor reviews and evaluates the relevant supporting data for the CTA application and prepares an assessment report. For example, the pharmaceutical assessor assesses the quality section of the IMPD, manufacturer's authorisations and labelling. The authorisation of the CTA application is dependent on an agreement from all three (or two, as applicable) disciplines. Sponsors should note that the approval applies to the CTA application and that the associated documents are not approved as such as they only support the approved CTA.

FIH clinical trials (that is, the first-ever trial in a human using the drug substance) and first time in UK (FTUK) clinical trials (that is, the first trial in the UK using the drug substance) are discussed at a weekly meeting of MHRA CTU assessors. The multi-disciplinary nature of the meeting ensures that there is a consensus on the outcome of the assessment. For certain higher-risk FIH clinical trials, expert advice is sought (see section 2.5).

The decision on whether to accept the request for a CTA, to request further information or to reject the application is made based on safety considerations, that is, the risk–benefit analysis of the proposed clinical trial. The fundamental question that is asked is: 'Do the data supplied support the use of this product, administered in this way, in the proposed dose for the proposed duration, to this "type" of subject?' Approval of a CTA application is contingent on risk mitigation making the risk–benefit acceptable. For example, this may mean that the proposed dose is lowered to reduce the incidence and severity of side effects, or the safety measures in the proposed clinical trial are enhanced.

2.3.2 Common issues found during assessment

Following an MHRA CTU evaluation of deficiencies with CTA applications, issues have been commonly identified in the following areas and applicants are recommended to ensure that these points are addressed in future CTA applications:

- appropriateness of dose rationale in terms of both the dose and duration
- adequacy of safety monitoring
- adequacy of safety reporting
- adequacy of contraceptive advice
- justification for the inclusion of lactating women and/or women of child-bearing potential
- adequacy of follow-up provisions (for example, in terms of duration)
- inclusion of appropriate manufacturer's authorisations and trial- and product-specific QP declarations
- inclusion and accuracy of labelling
- accuracy of the application form and its consistency with other information provided (for example, the IMPD)
- inclusion of information on placebo products.

Further details of these points are provided in the following sections.

2.3.2.1 Appropriateness of dose rationale (dose and duration)

Dose and duration need to be addressed on both a non-clinical and a clinical basis. The sponsor needs to justify the starting dose and the maximum dose to be administered. For later stage clinical trials, the doses are generally based on Phase I or Phase II clinical data. For earlier stage trials, both the starting dose and the maximum dose should be based on non-clinical data (see Jones and McBlane (2011); *Regulatory Rapporteur* 8 (10): 24–26). The sponsor also needs to be able to justify that the duration of dosing is sufficient to meet the trial objectives. From a non-clinical point of view, in principle, the duration of the animal toxicity studies conducted in two mammalian species (one non-rodent) should be equal to or exceed the duration of the human clinical trials up to the maximum recommended duration of the repeated-dose toxicity studies (see ICH Topic M3 (R2) – 'Non-clinical safety studies for the conduct of human clinical trials and marketing authorization for pharmaceuticals'; ICH Topic S6 (R1) – 'Preclinical safety evaluation of biotechnology-derived pharmaceuticals'; ICH Topic S9 – 'Non-clinical evaluation for anticancer pharmaceuticals'). In circumstances where significant therapeutic gain has been shown, trials can be extended beyond the duration of supportive repeated-dose toxicity studies on a case-by-case basis.

2.3.2.2   Adequacy of safety monitoring

The protocol should include adequate safety monitoring requirements for the trial. For example:

- If the SPC requires liver function to be monitored every four weeks, this requirement should be followed in the trial and included in the protocol, unless alternative arrangements can be justified
- If the IMP is cardiotoxic, and if QTc interval increases are a withdrawal criterion, then the permitted QTc interval should be defined and conform to the recommendation for QT interval assessment, which can be found on the MHRA website.

2.3.2.3   Adequacy of safety reporting

The statement 'All adverse events will be reported' in a protocol is not sufficient. There are specific requirements[4] for safety reporting in the legislation. Therefore, the protocol should include a safety section that clearly defines the responsibilities of the sponsor and investigator in terms of safety reporting. The protocol should indicate which adverse events will or will not be reported immediately. Further advice on safety reporting is included in Chapter 5 and is also available on the MHRA website.

2.3.2.4   Adequacy of contraceptive advice

Contraceptive advice for fertile male and/or female subjects should be provided based upon the availability and results of reproductive toxicity data. Highly effective methods of birth control are defined as those, alone or in combination, that result in a low failure rate (that is, less than 1% per year) when used consistently and correctly. For subjects using a hormonal contraceptive method, information regarding the product under evaluation and its potential effect on the contraceptive should be addressed. In addition, the contraception requirements should extend to a suitable period after the last dose of trial medication (for example, a whole spermatogenic cycle plus five drug half-lives). Further information is available on the MHRA website.

2.3.2.5   Justification for the inclusion of lactating women and/or women of child-bearing potential

Clinical trials in pregnant women are extremely rare due to potential adverse effects on the foetus. In extremely rare cases, trials may be carried out (for example, drugs to delay labour in pre-term pregnancy).

2.3.2.6 Adequacy of follow-up provisions

For some trials, such as those trials using advanced therapy investigational medicinal products (ATIMPs), it will be appropriate to include longer follow-up for subjects in the trial (see section 5.13 and Annex 3). Some trials, depending on the nature of the IMP and pharmacokinetic properties, may need longer follow-up in terms of safety reporting and monitoring.

2.3.2.7 Inclusion of appropriate manufacturer's authorisations and QP declarations

Manufacturer's authorisations are regularly omitted from CTA applications. Also, occasionally, copies of manufacturer's authorisations for sites which are not mentioned in the IMPD are included, resulting in the need for clarification, or QP declarations are provided that are neither trial- nor product-specific.

2.3.2.8 Inclusion and accuracy of labelling

Labelling is often omitted, particularly for non-commercial clinical trials. Sometimes, labelling is provided for the IMP, but not for the comparator product. Other common problems are inconsistency of storage instructions (for example, storage temperature with respect to those stated in the IMPD), unclear dosing instructions and lack of justification for non-compliance with labelling requirements.

The submitted IMP label should match the one that is formally approved by the sponsor, and filed in the trial master file (TMF). Examples have been seen on inspection where the label used in the trial was different from that submitted and approved by the MHRA as part of the CTA.

2.3.2.9 Accuracy of the application form and consistency with other information provided

The application form needs to be consistent with other supporting documentation, such as the protocol, IB and IMPD. For example, comparator products may appear to be licensed products on the application form, but may have been modified resulting in the submission of an IMPD. Additional examples where incorrect or inconsistent information has been provided in the CTA application include those where:

* the application for a trial stated that the IMP had a marketing authorisation within the UK; however, it did not

- the IMP, which was an authorised product, had been re-packaged and labelled for trial use, but this information on re-packaging had not been detailed in the CTA application
- for a Phase I trial, the labels and manufacturing information provided in the CTA application related only to the bulk supply, and did not reflect the final, finished IMP.

2.3.2.10 Inclusion of information on placebo products

Incomplete information is sometimes provided on placebo products; for example, the application form may only state that the placebo product is the same composition as the IMP except for the absence of the drug substance, and may not provide the other necessary information in terms of the manufacturing, testing and stability.

2.3.3 Timelines of assessment

All timelines for CTA applications are measured in terms of calendar days. The initial assessment of a CTA application must[5] be performed within 30 days. The only exception is for trials using ATIMPs. If the competent authority consults with a relevant committee for advice, a further 90 days[6] is added. For the purposes of this calculation, the day of receipt of the valid application by the MHRA CTU is day 0. Applications for Phase I trials will be assessed and processed within an average of 14 days or less.

If, as a result of the initial assessment, the sponsor has to amend the CTA application, the amended application must[7] be assessed by the competent authority within 60 days from the date on which the original CTA application was received. However, for this to apply, the sponsor must[8] provide the amended application to the competent authority within 14 days from the date on which the result of the initial assessment was received. The only exception is again for trials using ATIMPs, where the time limit is 90 days, or 180 days[9] if advice from a relevant committee is sought, from the date on which the original CTA application was received.

2.3.4 Outcomes of the clinical trial authorisation application assessment

There are three possible outcomes following the initial assessment of the CTA application (Regulations 18, 19 and 20 of SI 2004/1031):

61

(i)   The application may be accepted without the need for any further information or amendment. In this case, the acceptance letter states that the CTA is effective from the date of the letter and includes a reminder that a favourable opinion from the REC is also required before the clinical trial can proceed.

(ii) The application may be accepted without the need for any further information or amendment, but with certain conditions applied. In such cases, the acceptance letter for the CTA will include the following statements, together with the specific conditions:

'Authorisation of your clinical trial is subject to the following condition(s):

<<Description of the specific conditions>>

If these conditions are met, the trial is authorised and you do not need to respond to this letter. If your trial does not meet these conditions, your trial does not have authorisation and therefore you cannot proceed with the trial. You must inform the MHRA immediately if the trial does not meet the above conditions. All changes to the terms and conditions of this trial must be made as a request for a substantial amendment to this clinical trial authorisation.'

It is important to note that without satisfying the conditions of approval stated in the CTA acceptance letter, the authorisation is not valid and proceeding with the trial would be illegal.[10] For example, as part of the conditions of approval of a particular trial, the MHRA CTU could request that a valid MIA(IMP) be submitted to it (as it did not form part of the original application) and if the MIA(IMP) is subsequently not supplied to the MHRA, the trial does not have approval and the sponsor cannot initiate the trial. Other examples of conditions or remarks on acceptance letters could be a request for provisions for safety reporting to be confirmed before the trial commences or a requirement for acceptable methods of contraception to be listed in the protocol before the trial can go ahead.

(iii) The sponsor may be sent a letter requesting further information and/or changes to be made to the supporting documentation (for example, the protocol). This request is sent as a 'grounds for non-acceptance' (GNA) letter which is not a rejection of the CTA application. The sponsor may respond to the grounds identified in this letter within 14 days, or 30 days for trials of ATIMPs, otherwise the application will be deemed to have been refused. The response to the GNA letter should cover all the issues raised, but nothing additional. In the vast majority of cases, the provision of the additional information and/or revision of the supporting documentation results in the acceptance of the CTA application.

All documentation from the initial CTA submission to authorisation must[11] be present in the TMF in order to be able to reconstruct the events of the trial; this includes any initial GNA letter.

2.3.5   What makes a good clinical trial authorisation application?

A good CTA application is likely to be approved by the MHRA CTU without the need for providing further information and is also more likely to be approved without the need for conditions. It is recommended that applicants focus on the following areas:

- Providing an informative cover letter, including an explanation of what has been included in the CTA application and a justification for omitting any documents. It is very useful if the applicant provides references (EudraCT numbers) of previous clinical trials approved in the UK with the same drug substance and/ or drug product and what changes, if any, have been made to the IMPD. This can save time re-assessing the same information.

- Submitting an application form detailing exactly what is to be used as an IMP in the proposed clinical trial and, if appropriate, who is certifying the finished IMP(s).

- Providing clear and concise information on the IMP(s) to be used in the proposed clinical trial. This information may simply be the SPC for a marketed product or a full or simplified IMPD for a new drug substance and drug product.

- Submitting a protocol providing information on the objective(s), design, methodology, dose rationale, statistical considerations, safety reporting and organisation of the proposed clinical trial.

- Providing an IB (or SPC) summarising relevant non-clinical and clinical data for the IMP(s) with clear sections for the assessment of the expectedness of adverse reactions.

- Supplying either labelling which complies with Annex 13, EudraLex Volume 4, or a justification for the absence of trial-specific labelling.

- Providing authorisations for all EU sites of manufacture and assembly. In the case of non-EU sites, copies of the authorisations for the importer and the site certifying the finished IMP (if different) should be provided, together with a QP declaration on GMP equivalence to EU GMP.

- Submitting any scientific advice that has been requested from EMA or any competent authority.
- Providing the opinion of the REC, if available.
- Ensuring consistency of submitted documents.

2.3.6   Amendments

2.3.6.1   Substantial or non-substantial, authorisation or ethical opinion?

There are two types of changes to clinical trials and their associated documentation – substantial and non-substantial amendments. Except when taking urgent safety measures (see section 2.3.7), the sponsor of a clinical trial is required[12, 13] to obtain authorisation from the competent authority and/or a favourable opinion from the REC before implementing any amendment that is considered to be substantial. Non-substantial amendments do not require prior authorisation, but such changes must[12] be recorded by the sponsor (ideally including the sponsor's rationale as to why the amendment is non-substantial) and must[12] be made available upon request.

The definition of a substantial amendment, together with examples, is provided in the detailed guidance CT-1. A substantial amendment is a change that is likely to have a significant impact on the safety or physical or mental integrity of the clinical trial subjects, or the scientific value of the clinical trial. Examples of these include changes to the primary objective of the trial, addition of a trial arm or placebo group and changes to the RSI. However, it is up to the sponsor of the clinical trial to assess whether an amendment is to be regarded as substantial or not. It is also the responsibility of the sponsor to decide whether a substantial amendment requires authorisation, or an ethical opinion, or both (such decisions and rationale may be reviewed during a Good Clinical Practice (GCP) inspection). The general guidance on amendments provided in Table 2.1 has been agreed between the MHRA and the National Research Ethics Service (NRES) (as part of the Health Research Authority (HRA)), taking account of guidance from the European Commission. (Note that the list in Table 2.1 is not exhaustive.)

There is no need to inform the competent authority if the substantial amendment is only an amendment requiring REC favourable opinion and, similarly, there is no need to inform the REC of substantial amendments only requiring competent authority approval.

Table 2.1 General guidance on amendments

Amendments
Amendments normally requiring authorisation only
New toxicological or pharmacological data or new interpretation of toxicological or pharmacological data of relevance for the investigator
Changes to the reference safety information for the development safety update report (DSUR)
Changes to the investigational medicinal product dossier
Reduction in the sponsor's planned level of monitoring for the trial
Amendments normally requiring a favourable research ethics committee (REC) opinion only
Significant changes to information provided to subjects – for example, subject information sheets, consent forms, diaries, letters to GPs or other clinicians, letters to relatives/carers (whether generic to the whole trial or specific to a particular trial site)
Significant changes to recruitment and consent procedures, including the inclusion of adults lacking capacity in the trial
Significant increase to the radiation exposures to subjects from the protocol
Change of insurance or indemnity arrangements for the trial
Change to the payments, benefits or incentives to be received by subjects or researchers in connection with taking part in the trial, or any other change giving rise to a possible conflict of interest on the part of any investigator/collaborator
Change of the chief investigator
Change of principal investigator at a trial site
Addition of new trial sites not listed with the original request for authorisation and REC application
Change to the definition of a trial site
Any other significant change to the conduct or management of the trial at particular trial sites
Early closure or withdrawal of a site
Any other significant changes to the terms of the REC application
Amendments normally requiring both authorisation and a favourable REC opinion
Change of the main objective of the trial
Change of primary or secondary end-points likely to have a significant impact on the safety or scientific value of the trial
Use of a new measurement for the primary end-point
New toxicological or pharmacological data or new interpretation of toxicological or pharmacological data which is likely to impact on the risk–benefit assessment
Addition of a trial arm or placebo group

Table continues

Table 2.1 *continued*

Amendments
Amendments normally requiring both authorisation and a favourable REC opinion *continued*
Significant change of inclusion or exclusion criteria (for example, age range) likely to have a significant impact on the safety or scientific value of the trial
Change of a diagnostic or medical monitoring procedure likely to have a significant impact on the safety or scientific value of the trial
Withdrawal of an independent data monitoring committee
Change of investigational medicinal product(s)
Change of dosing/mode of administration of investigational medicinal product(s)
Any other change of trial design likely to have a significant impact on primary or major secondary statistical analysis or on the risk–benefit assessment
Change of the sponsor or sponsor's legal representative
Temporary halt of the trial or temporary halt at a trial site, and re-start of the trial following a temporary halt
Change of the definition of the end of the trial
Amendments not normally requiring notification
Changes to the identification of the trial (for example, change of title)
Increase in duration of the trial, provided that the exposure to treatment is not extended, the definition of the end of trial is unchanged and there is no change to monitoring arrangements
Changes to the numbers of subjects planned in the UK as a whole or at individual trial sites, provided that there is no change to the total number of subjects in the trial or the increase/decrease is insignificant in relation to the overall sample size
Change in the documentation used by the research team to record trial data (for example, case report form or data collection form)
Additional safety monitoring which is not part of an urgent safety measure but is taken on a precautionary basis
Changes to the research team other than to chief or principal investigators
Changes to contact details
Changes to the internal organisation of the sponsor or persons to whom tasks have been delegated
Changes to the logistical arrangements for transporting or storing samples
Changes to technical equipment
Inclusion or withdrawal of another Member State or third country
Minor clarifications to the protocol
Minor clarifications or updates of subject information documentation
Corrections of typographical errors

2

2.3.6.2 Submitting a substantial amendment to the MHRA

When submitting a substantial amendment to the MHRA CTU, the applicant must[12] provide the following key documents:

- a signed notification of amendment (Annex 2) form in PDF format available on the EudraCT section of the EMA website
- an updated XML and PDF file of the CTA form (Annex 1) with changes highlighted, if the amendment impacts on the information previously submitted
- description of the amendment
- reasons for the proposed amendment
- a copy of the proposed changes to the protocol or any other documents (such as the IMPD), showing previous and new wording, where applicable
- supporting data for the amendment, including, as applicable, summaries of data, updated overall risk–benefit assessment, possible consequences for subjects already in the trial and possible consequences for the evaluation of results
- proof of payment.

The assessment of a substantial amendment must[12] be performed within 35 days. For the purposes of this calculation, the day of receipt of the valid application by the MHRA CTU is day 0. Amendments for Phase I trials will be assessed within 35 days, with an average of 14 days or less. When the amendment has been assessed, the applicant may be sent a letter informing them of one of the following:

(i) acceptance of the amendment

(ii) acceptance of the amendment subject to conditions

(iii) grounds for non-acceptance of the amendment (usually requiring a re-submission of the amendment).

See section 2.3.4 for further details on these three possible outcomes.

2.3.7 Urgent safety measures

An urgent safety measure is an action that the sponsor and investigator may take in order to protect the subjects of a trial against any immediate hazard to their health or safety (for example, an organisation identifies that there is a significantly higher incidence of death at one UK site, and as a result suspends recruitment at that site as an urgent safety measure). The MHRA (and REC, see section 3.5.1) must[13] be notified immediately and, in any event, within 3 days that such a measure has been taken and the reasons why it has been taken. The initial notification to the MHRA should be by telephone. A notice in writing must[13] be sent within 3 days. The notice should set out the reasons for the urgent safety measure and the plan for further action.

If the process in place for implementing and reporting urgent safety measures is not robust, or if responsibilities for the process are not clearly defined (for example, in contracts, especially when third-party vendors are used to manage investigator sites and trials), this may lead to issues. Timelines for reporting may not be met (for example, if urgent safety measures are implemented at investigator sites, but are not submitted to the MHRA until some time later as an amendment), or there may be inappropriate use of the term 'urgent safety measure' when classifying protocol amendments (for example, protocol amendments being submitted to the MHRA as urgent safety measures when no investigator sites have yet been opened in the UK and there is therefore no immediate hazard to subjects).

2.3.8   Temporary halt of a trial

When a sponsor halts a trial temporarily, it should notify the MHRA (and REC; see section 3.6.2) immediately and at the latest within 15 days from when the trial is temporarily halted. This includes trials where the stoppage was not envisaged in the approved protocol and where there is an intention to resume it. It does not include trials where recruitment may be temporarily halted for logistical reasons, such as trial team unavailability. The notification should be made as a substantial amendment and clearly explain what has been halted (for example, stopping recruitment and/or interrupting treatment of subjects already included) and the reasons for the temporary halt. To restart a trial that has been temporarily halted, the sponsor should make the request as a substantial amendment providing evidence that it is safe to restart the trial. If a sponsor decides not to recommence a temporarily halted trial, the MHRA and REC must[14] be notified in writing within 15 days of the decision, using the end-of-trial declaration form and including a brief explanation of the reasons for ending the trial prematurely.

2.3.9   Early termination of a trial

In the case of early termination, the sponsor must[14] notify the end of the trial to the competent authority (and REC, see section 3.6.3) immediately and at the latest within 15 days after the trial is halted, clearly explaining the reasons and describing follow-up measures, if any, to be taken for safety reasons. This does not include trials that complete early because full recruitment has been achieved. Early termination of a trial may be due to reasons other than safety concerns, such as financial or business difficulties of the sponsor or related to slow recruitment. For whatever reason, both the competent authority and REC must[14] be notified.

2.3.10   End of the trial

The sponsor must[14] notify the competent authorities of the Member States concerned as well as the REC that the clinical trial has ended within 90 days of the end of the trial as it is defined in the trial protocol.

The formal process for notifying the competent authority of the end of the trial is the completion of the declaration in EudraCT. Once the declaration of the end of a clinical trial form has been received by the competent authority, only the clinical trial summary report will be accepted (that is, no further amendments can be submitted). Note that the MHRA can be informed separately by email of the end of the trial in the UK when other non-UK sites remain active, in order to terminate the annual service fee (see section 2.3.11); however, this is a separate process from the formal notification of end of trial. Further details are available on the MHRA website.

The sponsor should provide the clinical trial summary report within one year of the end of the complete trial for non-paediatric clinical trials. For paediatric clinical trials of IMPs with an authorisation and sponsored by the marketing authorisation holder, the timelines are set out in the European Commission Communication 2009/C28/01 ('Guidance on the information concerning paediatric clinical trials to be entered into the EU Database on Clinical Trials (EudraCT) and on the information to be made public by the European Medicines Agency (EMEA), in accordance with Article 41 of Regulation (EC) No. 1901/2006'), that is, the timelines to submit this report are 6 months after the end of the trial, but could be extended to 12 months if the submitting party has demonstrated that it is not possible to submit within the timeline for objective scientific reasons. Further details on the clinical trial summary report can be found in the detailed guidance CT-1.

2.3.11 Annual service fees

In line with the periodic fees for marketing authorisations and licensing regulations (The Medicines (Products for Human Use) (Fees) Regulations), all sponsors who hold open CTAs on 1 April receive an invoice for an annual service fee. Annual service fees apply to all trials which have been approved by the MHRA and for which an end-of-trial declaration has not been received by the MHRA. This may include approved trials that have not yet started or that have been temporarily halted. The definition of the end of the trial should be provided in the protocol and any change to this definition, for whatever reason, should be notified as a substantial amendment (see section 2.3.6). In most cases it will be the date of the last visit of the last subject undergoing the trial. The end of the recruitment period does not automatically signify the end of the trial. Further information on the end of the trial is provided in section 2.3.10.

To advise the MHRA that a trial is no longer active at any UK site (when other non-UK sites remain active), and therefore that the trial is no longer subject to an annual service fee, an email should be sent to the MHRA email address (ct.submission@mhra.gsi.gov.uk). This is a separate process from the formal notification of end of trial. Once the MHRA CTU has received a confirmation that a clinical trial has been completed at all UK sites, the notification will be processed and an acknowledgement will be sent to confirm that the details have been updated. Following submission of this email, the MHRA CTU does not expect to receive any further trial amendments since such amendments will not be applicable to UK sites as they are no longer actively participating in the clinical trial.

2.4 Risk-adapted approach to the management of clinical trials

The regulatory framework in the UK provides for a range of risk-adapted approaches that simplify the processes involved in initiating and managing a clinical trial. This is particularly useful, for example, in clinical trials in authorised products, where there is some potential for adverse event monitoring, record keeping, IMP storage, and documentation requirements to be adapted based on a risk assessment. Further information on this approach can be found in the MRC/DH/MHRA paper 'Risk-adapted approaches to the management of clinical trials of investigational medicinal products' (hereinafter 'risk-adapted approach guidance').

2.4.1   Assessment of risk in clinical trials

Risk in a clinical trial can be defined as the likelihood of a potential hazard occurring and causing harm to the trial subject/participant and/or an organisation, or detrimentally affecting the reliability of the trial results. A clinical trial commonly involves several different organisations and each should consider its specific responsibilities and duties with respect to the trial and the level of risk in relation to these. For every clinical trial, there is a core set of risks inherent to the protocol that relate to the safety and rights of the subjects and to the credibility of the results.

Risk assessment is essentially a process of identifying the potential hazards associated with that trial, and assessing the likelihood of those hazards occurring and resulting in harm.

Within a particular clinical trial, risks to subject safety in relation to the IMP can be categorised in relation to how much is known about the IMP being investigated. These potential risks should be assessed relative to the standard of care for the relevant clinical condition and the level of clinical experience with the intervention rather than the subjects' underlying illness or the recognised adverse effects of the intervention.

The potential risks should be balanced against the level of risk that a trial subject would be exposed to outside the trial as follows:

- Type A = no higher than the risk of standard medical care
- Type B = somewhat higher than the risk of standard medical care
- Type C = markedly higher than the risk of standard medical care.

The risk-adapted approach guidance provides a pragmatic approach to achieving this categorisation by using the marketing authorisation status of the IMP as shown in Table 2.2. This simple method for categorising the risk associated with the IMP and its use allows for elements of clinical trial management to be adapted within the scope of the Directive 2001/20/EC. For lower-risk category trials, this may simplify the requirements for both obtaining regulatory approvals and conducting the trial. However, although the IMP has implications for the level of risk, it does not fully determine it. Therefore, it is recommended that a full bespoke risk assessment is completed for all trials. Phase I trials or trials applying the risk-adapted approach should, however, conduct a risk assessment. See section 4.7.1 for details on how to perform and document this assessment.

Table 2.2 Categorisation of clinical trials based on potential risk associated with the investigational medicinal product and its use

Trial categories based upon the potential risk associated with the investigational medicinal product	Examples of types of clinical trials
Type A: no higher than that of standard medical care	Trials involving IMPs authorised in any EU Member State if: • they relate to the authorised range of indications, dosage and form, or • they involve off-label use (such as in paediatrics and in oncology etc.) if this off-label use is established practice and supported by sufficient published evidence and/or guidelines.
Type B: somewhat higher than that of standard medical care	Trials involving IMPs authorised in any EU Member State if: • such products are used for a new indication (different patient population/ disease group), or • substantial dosage modifications are made for the licensed indication, or • if they are used in combinations for which interactions are suspected. Trials involving medicinal products not authorised in any EU Member State if the drug substance is part of a medicinal product authorised in the EU. (A grading of *Type A* may be justified if there is extensive clinical experience with the product and no reason to suspect a different safety profile in the trial population.)[a]
Type C: markedly higher than that of standard medical care	Trials involving IMPs not authorised in any EU Member State. (A grading other than *Type C* may be justified if there are extensive class data or non-clinical and clinical evidence.)[a]

[a] If a grading other than those indicated is felt to be justified, the rationale and evidence should be presented in the CTA application.

EU, European Union; IMP, investigational medicinal product

2.4.2 Notification Scheme

As part of the risk-adapted approach, notifications may be submitted to the MHRA CTU for the majority of Type A trials (as defined in the risk-adapted approach guidance) conducted in the UK. This 'Notification Scheme' came into operation in April 2011. The process of notification involves the applicant sending the standard EudraCT application form and accompanying documents in the usual way. The notification is then acknowledged by the MHRA CTU with an accompanying statement to say that the clinical trial may go ahead after 14 days from receipt of notification, if the MHRA CTU has not raised any objections. This means that the acknowledgement letter acts as the authorisation. If the MHRA CTU raises objections to the notification, then the submission will be assessed as for a standard request for authorisation. In this case, the initial assessment will be performed within 30 days. For the purposes of this calculation, the day of receipt of the valid notification by the MHRA CTU is day 0. All interventional clinical trials with an IMP conducted in the UK will continue to require a favourable opinion from a REC before the start of the clinical trial.

2.4.2.1 What trials can be submitted under the Notification Scheme?

The Notification Scheme is open to clinical trials meeting the criteria for Type A category trials (see Table 2.2), and may include randomisation of subjects to different authorised products or re-packaging and/or re-labelling of the marketed product(s). Placebo-controlled trials in subjects will not be open to the Notification Scheme, nor will clinical trials in which the authorised product has been modified (for example, by over-encapsulation), even if they otherwise meet the criteria for categorisation to Type A. In addition, trials that have been categorised as Type A, but involve an IMP outside its authorisation (although supported by data of its use in standard clinical practice), will not qualify for the Notification Scheme. Consequently, while all notifications will be for Type A clinical trials, not all Type A clinical trials can be submitted under the Notification Scheme.

2.4.2.2 Documents to send in a submission under the Notification Scheme

In order for an application to be considered as valid, a submission should contain a file for each of the following documents:

- cover letter, which includes the statement that it is a submission under the Notification Scheme
- CTA application form and valid XML

2

> **Examples of trials where it would be appropriate to submit notifications under the Notification Scheme**
>
> *A comparison of subject-controlled analgesia and routine care (nurse-titrated analgesia) in an accident and emergency setting*
>
> The IMP to be used is morphine sulphate 1 mg/ml solution for injection, which is licensed in the UK. The indication, subject population, dose, trial duration and inclusion/exclusion criteria are in line with the SPC for the IMP. Safety monitoring and the provisions for safety reporting are also acceptable, therefore the notification may be authorised.
>
> *A trial on the effect of prednisolone as a glucocorticoid replacement therapy on hypoglycaemia frequency in people with Type 1 diabetes and adrenal insufficiency*
>
> The IMPs (prednisolone, 1 mg or 5 mg gastro-resistant tablets) are licensed in the UK. The indication, subject population, dose, trial duration and inclusion/exclusion criteria are in line with the SPC for the IMP. Safety monitoring and the provisions for safety reporting are also acceptable, therefore the notification may be authorised.
>
> *A trial in the use of propofol as an anaesthetic during electroconvulsive therapy (ECT) for depression*
>
> The IMP (propofol, 10 mg/ml emulsion for infusion) is licensed in the UK. The indication, subject population, dose, trial duration and inclusion/exclusion criteria are in line with the SPC for the IMP. Safety monitoring and the provisions for safety reporting are also acceptable, therefore the notification may be authorised.

- protocol including:
  - » an evaluation of the anticipated benefits and risks
  - » a justification for including subjects who are incapable of giving informed consent, or other special populations if applicable
  - » a rationale/justification for the use of the product in the trial where it is not being used strictly within the terms of its SPC
  - » procedures for eliciting and recording adverse event reports, as well as the investigator's responsibilities for reporting both serious adverse reactions (SARs) and suspected unexpected serious adverse reactions (SUSARs) to the sponsor
- SPC (if this document is originally in a language other than English, an English translation should be provided)
- proof of payment
- justification for absence of trial-specific labelling (or the content of trial-specific labelling if this will be used)

> **Examples of trials where it would not be appropriate to submit notifications under the Notification Scheme; any submitted notifications would be invalid and these trials would be subsequently assessed as a standard CTA application**
>
> *An exploratory trial of intravitreal pegaptanib in diabetic macular oedema*
>
> The IMP (pegaptanib solution for injection) is licensed in the UK. The subject population and inclusion/exclusion criteria are in line with the SPC for the IMP. Safety monitoring and the provisions for safety reporting are also acceptable. However, the indication (diabetic macular oedema), dose (0.3 mg every four weeks) and trial duration are not in line with the SPC, so the notification would be invalid.
>
> *A trial of testosterone replacement for young male cancer patients*
>
> The IMP (testosterone 2% gel) is licensed in the UK. The indication, subject population, dose, trial duration and inclusion/exclusion criteria are in line with the SPC for the IMP. Safety monitoring and the provisions for safety reporting are also acceptable. However, the applicant wants to use a placebo arm in the clinical trial as a control, therefore the notification would be invalid.
>
> *A pilot trial of simvastatin dose and cholesterol control in older subjects*
>
> The IMPs (simvastatin 10/20/40/80 mg tablets) are licensed in the UK. For blinding purposes, the tablets will be over-encapsulated in size 00 Swedish orange hard gelatin capsules and back-filled with lactose monohydrate. The indication, subject population, dose, trial duration and inclusion/exclusion criteria are in line with the SPC for the IMP. Safety monitoring and the provisions for safety reporting are also acceptable. However, the use of a modified licensed product, namely over-encapsulated tablets, in the clinical trial is unacceptable in a notification.

2

- justification for the absence of a manufacturer's authorisation (or a copy of the authorisation for each manufacturing site involved in re-packaging of the marketed product, where this site is not a hospital or health centre).

It is suggested that the chief investigator's/sponsor's assessment of the IMP risk category and a safety monitoring plan are also included with the notification, either as an appendix to the protocol, or incorporated into the body of the protocol or the cover letter. These documents would be reviewed by the MHRA assessor and agreed as acceptable (or not).

When the MHRA CTU receives a notification of a clinical trial, the notification will be validated. If the notification is not valid (for example, incomplete information is supplied) then the person making the application will be contacted and told that there are deficiencies. If the deficiencies are minor, the applicant may be asked to provide the missing information. The submission will not be progressed until the missing components are provided, although once the submission is complete it will be processed as normal. If the deficiencies are major, the applicant may be required to re-submit a complete application.

Once the notification is valid (that is, complete) the review period will begin and an acknowledgement letter will be sent to the person submitting the notification by post. The acknowledgement letter provides authorisation of the trial unless an objection is raised by the MHRA CTU within 14 days. If an objection is raised, this will be sent by email and by post.

If modifications are subsequently made to the use of the IMP in the trial, but these modifications are still within the terms of the SPC (that is, with regards to the indication, subject population, dosage) and they do not affect the risk category, then the MHRA does not need to be notified. However, if modifications go beyond the terms of the SPC or result in the risk category increasing from Type A to Type B, this will mean the risk–benefit analysis for the trial subjects has been changed and therefore the change must[12] be submitted as a substantial amendment to the MHRA.

2.5 Clinical trial authorisation applications requiring expert advice

For certain clinical trials (outlined in section 2.5.1), the MHRA CTU seeks advice from the Clinical Trials Expert Advisory Group (CTEAG) and the Commission on Human Medicines (CHM) before approval for the clinical trial can be given. Sponsors are requested to make contact with the MHRA CTU before submitting the CTA application for such clinical trials and to make available a data package that will allow advice to be obtained. The normal CTA application timeline will then follow receipt of a valid application. The sponsor should ensure that the REC is informed of the substance of the advice from the CTEAG or CHM, either in the REC application or by providing further information during the ethical review process, depending on the timing of the applications.

Sponsors of all FIH trials should take account of the 'Guideline on strategies to identify and mitigate risks for first-in-human clinical trials with investigational medicinal products' (CHMP/SWP/28367/07) available on the EMA website.

For those planning a FIH clinical trial, both sponsors and investigators should identify the factors of risk and apply risk mitigation strategies accordingly as laid down in the guideline (see section 12.5 for further details).

2.5.1   When will expert advice be sought?

The decision to refer applications for expert advice will be based on the assessment of risk factors and the proposed mitigation strategy. Areas for consideration when determining risk factors include the mode of action, nature of the target and the relevance of animal species and models. Some examples of clinical trials where expert advice may be sought include FIH clinical trials with novel compounds:

- where the mode of action involves a target that is connected to multiple signalling pathways (target with pleiotropic effects), for example, leading to various physiological effects or targets that are ubiquitously expressed
- acting (directly or indirectly) via a cascade system where there may be an amplification effect which might not be sufficiently controlled by a physiological feedback mechanism
- acting (directly or indirectly) via the immune system with a target or mechanism of action which is novel or currently not well characterised
- where there is novelty in the structure of the active substance; for example, a new type of engineered structural format such as those with enhanced receptor interaction as compared with the parent compound
- where the level of expression and biological function of the target receptor may differ between healthy volunteers and subjects with the relevant disease
- where there is insufficient available knowledge of the structure, tissue distribution, cell specificity, disease specificity, regulation, level of expression and biological function of the human target, including downstream effects
- acting via a possible or likely species-specific mechanism or where animal data are unlikely to be predictive of activity in humans.

In addition, the MHRA CTU may refer other applications if particular issues are identified during the assessment process.

2.5.2   Required areas for discussion

The sponsor for a clinical trial requiring expert advice should consider the following and provide the relevant information on each point as appropriate:

- a discussion of the function of the target in humans
- a discussion of the ability of the subject to maintain a normal physiological response to challenge in the presence of the IMP

- a discussion for the transition from non-clinical to human testing, particularly with regard to highly species-specific molecules
- a discussion of the potential for on-target and off-target effects and how this will be handled in the clinic
- a discussion of the doses used in the relevant animal species (particularly with regard to the testing in the animal model of the starting dose to be administered to humans)
- a rationale for the starting dose in humans (including, for example, receptor occupancy)
- a rationale for the trial population (particularly for the use of healthy volunteers)
- a rationale for the administration schedule for the initial and subsequent cohorts (this should include the time interval between doses administered to individual subjects)
- a rationale for the dose escalation, particularly with regard to potential adverse effects
- a rationale for the proposed trial site, including the facilities available.

2.6 Voluntary Harmonisation Procedure

In April 2009, the Clinical Trials Facilitation Group (CTFG) launched the Voluntary Harmonisation Procedure (VHP). This procedure allows sponsors of EU multinational clinical trials to obtain a harmonised assessment of their CTA application (and subsequent amendments) by all the competent authorities involved. The sponsor receives a single, harmonised set of questions which have been consolidated following scientific discussion between the lead Member State and the other concerned Member States. Further details are available on the Heads of Medicines Agencies (HMA) website (www.hma.eu).

2.6.1 Voluntary Harmonisation Procedure process

The VHP process consists of three steps or phases. Phase 1 consists of the request for a VHP and validation of the CTA application. Core documentation (protocol, IB, IMPD, manufacturer's authorisation and labelling) is submitted electronically to the VHP coordinator and potential participating Member States are identified. The competent authorities of the participating Member States accept or decline to validate the submission within three days. One competent authority then agrees to act as the Reference Member State for the application.

Phase 2 is the assessment step where the CTA application and supporting data are assessed by the competent authorities of the participating Member States. The Reference Member State provides a draft assessment report, together with GNA points, to the VHP coordinator, who circulates the assessment report to the other participating Member States for comment. Additional GNA points may be raised and these are consolidated by the Reference Member State and are then forwarded to the sponsor for response. The GNA response is assessed by the Reference Member State, which makes a recommendation for approval or decides that GNA points have not been fully resolved. Participating Member States comment on the Reference Member State's recommendation and, once the GNA points have been resolved, the VHP is approved.

Phase 3 consists of the national step, where the CTA application is formally submitted to each participating Member State. Phase 3 is usually a formality as all the issues and requests for further information should have been dealt with during Phase 2.

2.6.2 Advantages for the sponsor

There are several potential advantages for sponsors submitting CTA applications using the VHP. Firstly, only one set of core documentation is required and there are no Member State specific requirements. Secondly, if GNA points are raised, they are consolidated by the Reference Member State, which can result in a reduction of around half the GNA points raised by Member States. Most importantly, a single decision is arrived at by all the participating Member States. The sponsor can decide not to submit a national application if a Member State raises a specific condition that is unacceptable to the sponsor.

Other advantages include:

- VHP applications are given priority by competent authorities
- the electronic submission only has to be sent to one address
- there are fixed timelines for the Member States to assess the application and send out a consolidated response to the sponsor
- the scientific discussion of points between the Member States should result in increasingly harmonised application reviews in the Member States.

2.7   Chapter legislative references

Throughout this chapter, specific terminology – 'must', 'required' or 'requirement' – has been used to interpret activities that are legislative requirements. These terms have been number-coded in the text where used, and the corresponding reference in the legislation can be found below.

1.   Schedule 3, Part 2 of SI 2004/1031
2.   Regulation 17 (2) of SI 2004/1031
3.   Regulation 36 of SI 2004/1031
4.   Regulations 32 to 35 of SI 2004/1031
5.   Regulation 18 (2) of SI 2004/1031
6.   Regulation 19 (5) of SI 2004/1031
7.   Regulation 18 (6) of SI 2004/1031
8.   Regulation 18 (5) of SI 2004/1031
9.   Regulation 19 (7) of SI 2004/1031
10. Regulation 18 (4) of SI 2004/1031
11. Regulation 31A (4) of SI 2004/1031
12. Regulation 24 of SI 2004/1031
13. Regulation 30 of SI 2004/1031
14. Regulation 27 of SI 2004/1031

Ethical review

3

Editor's note

The Clinical Trials Directive 2001/20/EC requires a favourable opinion to be obtained from a research ethics committee (REC) before a clinical trial, or any advertising or recruitment relating to the trial, can start. A favourable opinion is required from a single REC, irrespective of the number of sites at which the trial will be conducted. As part of its ethical review of an application, the REC considers (among other aspects) the relevance of the clinical trial and its design, whether the evaluation of the anticipated benefits and risks is satisfactory, and the adequacy and completeness of the written information to be given and the procedures to be followed, for the purpose of obtaining informed consent to the subjects' participation in the trial. As part of its favourable opinion for a trial, the REC also confirms its approval of the suitability of trial sites and investigators.

This chapter describes the process within the UK for applying for ethical review, the requirements for a valid application, and which updates and reports are required by the RECs during the live phase of the clinical trial. The ethical requirements for informed consent are detailed, including the principles relating to the inclusion of minors and adults lacking capacity for informed consent. The Health Research Authority (HRA) website (www.hra.nhs.uk) should be consulted for up-to-date guidance on procedures and requirements, including guidance issued by the National Research Ethics Service (NRES) and the National Research Ethics Advisors' Panel.

3.1   Appointment of research ethics committees

RECs reviewing clinical trial applications must[1] be recognised for this purpose by the United Kingdom Ethics Committee Authority (UKECA) and must[2] comply with the legislation relating to the membership and operation of such committees. In addition, RECs also have standard operating procedures (SOPs) to follow; these SOPs are published on the HRA website.

3.1.1   United Kingdom Ethics Committee Authority

The UKECA is a body consisting of:

- England – Secretary of State for Health
- Wales – National Assembly for Wales
- Scotland – Scottish Ministers
- Northern Ireland – Department for Health, Social Services and Public Safety.

The members of the UKECA may act alone in relation to the region of the UK for which they are responsible, or jointly. Arrangements can also be made for the functions of the UKECA to be exercised by other public authorities on its behalf; for example, the functions of the UKECA in relation to England have been delegated by the Department of Health to the HRA.

The UKECA may recognise a REC if it is satisfied that the arrangements for its membership and operation would enable the committee to perform its functions adequately and comply with the legislative requirements[2]. Application for recognition is made by the REC's appointing authority (see section 3.1.2).

When recognising a committee, the UKECA must[3] specify:

- whether the committee may act for the entire UK or only for a particular area
- the description or type of clinical trial in relation to which it may act
- any other conditions or limitations that apply to the committee.

Since 2004, recognition of RECs by the UKECA has been in one or more of the following categories:

- **Type 1** Committees recognised to review Phase I trials taking place at any site in the UK, where the sponsor has no knowledge that the product has effects likely to be beneficial to the subjects of the trial, and the subjects are healthy volunteers or subjects not suffering from the disease or condition to which the trial relates.

- **Type 2** Committees recognised to review clinical trials in subjects taking place only at sites within the domain of the REC – that is, an area defined by the geographical remit of the REC's appointing authority. (*Note: New applications are no longer allocated for review by Type 2 committees. However, they have continuing recognition to review substantial amendments and undertake other business relating to active trials for which they previously gave a favourable opinion.*)

- **Type 3** Committees recognised to review clinical trials in subjects taking place at any site in the UK.

Recognition of a REC may be revoked if the committee fails to perform its functions adequately, or does not comply with the provisions of Schedule 2 to SI 2004/1031.

The UKECA is also responsible for monitoring the performance of RECs, and for providing advice and assistance to them. Provision of advice and assistance was delegated by the UKECA to the NRES, as part of the HRA, as of 1 December 2011.

The Gene Therapy Advisory Committee (GTAC), part of NRES within HRA, is the national REC for gene therapy clinical trials, trials using advanced therapy investigational medicinal products (ATIMPs; see Annex 3 for further details of these trials) and trials of stem therapy involving cells derived from cell lines. GTAC has Type 1 and Type 3 category recognition from the UKECA. Clinical trials involving medicinal products for gene therapy must[4] be submitted to GTAC, although low-risk gene therapy trials may be transferred to other RECs.

3.1.2   Appointing authorities for research ethics committees

The REC's appointing authority is the body that establishes the REC, appoints its members and officers, provides its staff, premises and facilities, monitors its performance through the provision of annual reports, and generally takes responsibility for its governance. The responsibilities of an appointing authority are set out in detail in the UK Health Departments' 'Governance arrangements for research ethics committees' (GAfREC). A harmonised UK-wide edition of GAfREC came into effect on 1 September 2011.

The current appointing authorities for recognised RECs in the UK are:

- England – HRA, except for:
  - » GTAC – Department of Health
  - » Ministry of Defence Research Ethics Committee (MoDREC) – Ministry of Defence
- Wales – All Wales Business Centre
- Scotland – NHS Health Boards
- Northern Ireland – Health and Social Care Business Services Organisation.

Note that, following the winding up of the Appointing Authority for Phase I Ethics Committees (AAPEC) on 31 January 2012, operational responsibility for RECs previously appointed by AAPEC was transferred to NRES and the HRA became the appointing authority.

3.2 Application to research ethics committees

An application to a recognised REC must[5] be made by the chief investigator for the trial. (Chapter 11 provides the definition of a chief investigator and the details of their role and responsibilities in a trial.) All applications to RECs in the UK are made using the online Integrated Research Application System (IRAS) at https://www.myresearchproject.org.uk. Detailed guidance is available within IRAS on completion of the REC application form and the online process for booking and submission of the application to an appropriate REC.

3.2.1 Requirements for a valid application

The particulars and documents to be submitted as part of a valid application are set out in Part 1 of Schedule 3 to SI 2004/1031. The standard application form and document checklist within IRAS incorporate all the necessary requirements. IRAS provides detailed guidance next to each question in the application form on the ethical issues and other information of potential interest to the REC. A summary of key points is set out in Table 3.1. The application must[6] be signed by the chief investigator. Electronic authorisation of the chief investigator declaration in IRAS is considered to comply with this requirement.

Table 3.1 Practical guidance on the research ethics committee application process

Research ethics committee (REC) application
Using IRAS – general points
Take advantage of the guidance within IRAS. It is based on common issues and questions raised in previous applications.
Ensure the project filter is completed correctly so that IRAS generates an appropriate version of the application form, including all relevant sections. In particular, applicants must declare where a trial includes the administration of any ionising radiation, use of tissue samples, or inclusion of minors or adults lacking capacity to consent for themselves.
If further advice is required, contact the HRA Queries Line.
Help the REC to understand the trial
Describe the scientific background, purpose and methodology of the trial in language comprehensible to both expert and lay members of the REC. Any acronyms or technical terms should be defined.
For complex studies, such as those with multiple arms and repeat visits, it can be helpful to include a diagram summarising the trial procedures to help REC members understand what is involved for subjects.
Ensure that details given in the application form are consistent with the protocol – for example, in the schedule of visits and examinations.
Dealing with more complex ethical issues
Many clinical trials are similar in the way they address typical ethical issues (for example, methods of recruitment, informed consent, data protection, payments and incentives). However, some trials may propose unusual procedures to address particular issues arising from the circumstances of the trial. These are not necessarily unethical simply because they do not fit with established practice. Raise these issues with the REC and explain the reasons for the proposal and any alternatives you may have considered. Mention any precedents you are aware of. It is part of the role of the REC to facilitate ethical research by advising on how difficult issues can be addressed.
Subject information sheets and consent forms
HRA guidance on information sheets gives detailed guidance on style, format and content, including recommended templates and wordings. The REC will expect you to take this into account. Not all sections are relevant to every trial and the template may need to be tailored to provide clear, appropriate information. However, if you propose to depart significantly from the recommended approach, justify this in the application.
It can be helpful to test the information sheet and other materials to be used by subjects with a group of patients, representatives or members of the general public.
You should prepare separate information sheets and consent forms where subjects have the option of taking part in sub-studies or donating samples and data for future research use in addition to the main trial.

Table continues

Table 3.1 *continued*

Adults lacking capacity
Proposals to include adults lacking capacity should be carefully justified in Part B Section 6 of IRAS.
Describe the procedures for identifying and seeking consent from legal representatives. Where it is not possible to identify a personal legal representative, strategies should be in place for contacting nominated legal representatives appointed by the host organisation.
Where consent could be given either by subjects (if capable, or following recovery) or by legal representatives, separate information sheets and consent forms should be prepared for use as appropriate. The HRA guidance on information sheets includes templates for legal representative materials.
If proposing to recruit subjects prior to consent due to the need for urgent treatment as part of the trial, justify this and say how decisions on enrolment will be made and by whom. Give details of how consent will be sought following enrolment.
These procedures should also be clearly set out in the protocol for reference by trial sites and monitors.

Minors
In addition to the information sheet and consent form for parents, consider whether age-appropriate information should be provided to the child. The HRA guidance on information sheets includes guidance on materials for children with examples. If applicable, say how the child would be involved in discussion about their participation.

Radiation
Where a protocol involves administration of X-rays, CT scans or any other ionising radiation (including where the radiation is the same as a subject would receive outside the trial), this must be specifically approved by the REC under the Ionising Radiation (Medical Exposure) Regulations 2000 (IRMER).
Ensure this is declared in the IRAS filter and the radiation section generated.
It is advisable to identify a lead medical physics expert and lead clinical radiation expert at an early stage to advise on the protocol and contribute to the assessments required in IRAS.
For trials involving exposure to radioactive materials (for example, PET, bone scans), nuclear medicine professionals at each trial site must hold appropriate certification issued on behalf of health ministers by the Administration of Radioactive Substances Advisory Committee (ARSAC; www.arsac.org.uk). ARSAC reviews the suitability of the exposures to the objectives of the trial and advises the sponsor and the REC on any issues arising. The ARSAC application can be submitted from IRAS in parallel with the REC application.

Insurance and indemnity for non-NHS sponsors and investigators
For sponsors, co-sponsors and investigators outside the NHS, the application should include details of the insurance or indemnity cover to meet any liabilities arising from the trial.
State clearly the quantum of cover that will be in place, and any maximum amount payable to a single subject.
The REC should be notified of any exclusions in the policy that could affect the availability of cover, other than standard conditions, such as the requirement to obtain regulatory approvals and to notify the insurer of any claims.

Insurance and indemnity for non-NHS sponsors and investigators *continued*

Applications should normally include the certificate of insurance (whether block cover or a trial-specific policy). If the policy has not yet commenced, assure the REC that the certificate will be provided before the trial starts.

Sponsors outside the EEA

For any sponsor or co-sponsor established outside the European Economic Area (EEA), a legal representative based in the EEA must be named on the application. Further guidance is available within IRAS.

Supporting documentation

Supporting documentation should carry version numbers and dates where applicable, including the protocol, subject information sheet, consent form, letters to subjects and other clinicians, diary card and other subject-related documentation.

Submit any advertising material to be used in recruiting subjects to the trial, including webpages, blogs etc. (It is not necessary to include the correspondence to be used in recruiting sites.)

A cover letter is only required when re-submitting an application (to explain how it addresses issues raised in a previous review) or to provide other information or clarification in support of the application.

Submitting the application

IRAS gives step-by-step guidance on the online submission process.

Ensure all required declarations (for example, chief investigator, sponsor representative, radiation experts) are signed using electronic authorisation in IRAS before proceeding with submission.

REC meeting

Attendance of the chief investigator and sponsor's representative at the REC meeting is welcomed as it facilitates the REC review and enables questions to be resolved more quickly. Therefore, attendance is recommended if possible.

During the review process

Notify the REC of any significant changes arising from review by other bodies (for example, by the MHRA, or from new safety information).

Issues raised by the REC can be addressed in correspondence. It is not normally necessary to re-submit the application form unless a whole section is missing due to an error in completing the filter.

However, the applicant is free to update the dataset in IRAS at any time so that up-to-date information is included in any future applications (for example, to R&D offices).

Further guidance

A range of further guidance is available on the HRA website, including guidance developed by the National Research Ethics Advisers' Panel.

CT, computerised tomography; HRA, Health Research Authority; IRAS, Integrated Research Application System; NRES, National Research Ethics Service; PET, positron emission tomography; REC, research ethics committee

It is important to ensure that all relevant documents are submitted to the REC for review and that there is consistency between any documents submitted and the application form. If this is not done there may be issues with the application. For example, if the eligibility criteria in the protocol differed significantly from that detailed in the REC application form, it would not be clear to the REC how eligibility would be determined. Another issue might be where written information was provided to or completed by the subject but had not received favourable ethical opinion (for example, where pain diaries, subject information cards or visual analogue scales (VAS) have not been submitted to the REC).

3.2.2   Time period for ethical review

The REC is normally required[7] to give an opinion on an application within 60 calendar days of receipt of a valid application. Where it considers that further information is required in order to give an opinion, the REC may give a provisional opinion and make one request in writing for further information from the applicant. A clock stop period will be applied while waiting for receipt of this information.

In the case of a clinical trial involving a medicinal product for gene therapy or somatic cell therapy or a medicinal product containing a genetically modified organism or tissue-engineered product, the normal time period for review is extended to 90 days. This may be extended by a further 90 days (that is, to 180 days in total) where the REC needs to consult a specialist group or committee about the application.

3.2.3   Review of an application by the research ethics committee

3.2.3.1   Scope of ethical review

The REC must[8] consider and give an opinion on any issue relating to a clinical trial raised by the applicant that, in the opinion of the REC, is relevant to matters the REC is required to consider as part of its ethical review. The REC is required[9] to consider a number of specific matters:

- the relevance of the clinical trial and its design, including statistical elements
- whether the evaluation of the anticipated benefits and risks is satisfactory and the conclusions are justified
- the protocol
- the suitability of the investigator and supporting staff

- the investigator's brochure or summary of product characteristics (as applicable)
- the quality of the facilities for the trial
- the adequacy and completeness of the written information to be given, and the procedures to be followed, for the purpose of obtaining informed consent to the subjects' participation in the trial
- if the subjects are to include minors (aged under 16) or adults incapable of giving informed consent due to physical or mental incapacity, whether the research is justified having regard to the conditions or principles specified in Part 4 or Part 5 of Schedule 1 to SI 2004/1031
- provision for indemnity or compensation in the event of injury or death attributable to the clinical trial
- any insurance or indemnity to cover the liability of the investigator or sponsor
- the amounts and, where appropriate, the arrangements for rewarding or compensating investigators and subjects
- the terms of any agreement between the sponsor and the owner or occupier of the trial site which are relevant to the arrangements referred to in the point above
- the arrangements for the recruitment of subjects.

The REC is not limited to consideration of these issues. Typically, ethical review of a clinical trial will also include consideration of the following:

- advertising materials
- fairness of the selection criteria
- screening procedures
- arrangements for checking the health status of healthy volunteers
- arrangements for checking the simultaneous or recent involvement of potential subjects in other trials
- justification for interventional and non-interventional procedures to be undertaken with subjects over and above those required for normal clinical care, including sample taking, imaging and questionnaires or interviews
- justification for withholding any treatment that would be part of the normal care received by subjects outside the trial
- any 'stopping rules' and criteria for withdrawal of individual subjects from the trial

- safety monitoring arrangements, including the justification for appointing an independent data monitoring committee
- arrangements for access to confidential data about subjects and for protecting their privacy
- retention and proposed future uses of biological samples
- arrangements for notifying other healthcare professionals of the subject's participation
- continuing care of subjects at the end of the trial
- subject/public involvement in the design of the trial
- any potential conflicts of interest for investigators
- publication and dissemination of the trial results
- sponsorship arrangements (including the appointment of legal representatives for sponsors based outside the European Economic Area (EEA))
- non-interventional sub-studies submitted as part of, or alongside, the main trial application (for example, genetics).

3.2.3.2   Requirement for review at a full meeting

Applications for ethical review of a clinical trial must[2] be reviewed at a 'full meeting' of the REC. A 'full meeting' is a meeting of the committee attended by at least seven members of the committee, including the following:

- one lay member who is not and never has been a healthcare professional or a chairman, member, director, officer or employee of a health service body
- one expert member.

Deputy members attending the meeting in place of the member for which they have been appointed to deputise count towards the quorum requirement. A maximum of two co-opted members may also attend.

Where a quorum is not present, the committee may not give either a provisional or a final opinion on any new application for review of a clinical trial. The committee may discuss applications on the agenda and give preliminary advice to applicants, but the applications will need to be reconsidered at a further full meeting before an opinion is given. The applicant is usually formally invited to the meeting to present the trial and answer any pertinent questions. The applicant is not required to attend, but it is recommended that they do so.

3.2.3.3 Decisions available to the research ethics committee

A full meeting of a REC may reach either a final opinion, favourable or unfavourable, or a provisional opinion on an application.

(i) Favourable opinion

When giving a favourable opinion, the committee may specify any conditions to be met prior to the start of the trial (or the start at each site). These should be clearly set out in the favourable opinion letter. The conditions must[10] be fully met before the trial starts, otherwise it will be considered that the trial does not have a favourable opinion in place.

Examples of conditions a REC might include in its opinion are:

- requirement to obtain management permission from host organisations before starting the trial at any site (a standard condition included with all favourable opinions)

- requirement to obtain clinical trial authorisation (CTA) from the MHRA (a standard condition included with all favourable opinions)

- specified additions or amendments to be made to the subject information sheet or other trial documentation

- requirement for the chief investigator to undertake training in informed consent or Good Clinical Practice (GCP)

- ensuring that investigators and other research staff have been trained to undertake interventions or procedures outside their routine competence

- reaching agreement with the responsible care organisation(s) on responsibilities for funding the plan for continuing care of subjects at the end of the trial

- ensuring data encryption is in place on the personal computers or laptops to be used in the research

- obtaining or renewing a final certificate of insurance or indemnity to provide the cover specified in the REC application.

It is recommended that the committee is notified for information once the conditions have been met (except for management permission from individual host organisations at individual sites) and is provided with copies of final documentation for reference purposes, where appropriate. It is the responsibility of the sponsor to ensure that the conditions have been complied with.

The REC may also give advice or make suggestions alongside its opinion that are not binding on the applicant. These should be clearly distinguished from any conditions specified as part of the favourable opinion.

(ii) Unfavourable opinion
Where the final opinion is unfavourable, the applicant should be given a full explanation of the committee's reasons.

(iii) Provisional opinion
A full meeting of a REC may decide that a final opinion cannot be issued until further information or clarification has been received from the applicant and/or advice has been sought from a referee. In this case, it should indicate a provisional opinion based on its initial review.

Where the committee gives a provisional opinion, it should be clearly agreed whose responsibility it is to consider the further information or advice and to issue the committee's final opinion. Responsibility may be delegated to the chairman or vice-chairman acting alone, or to a sub-committee of specified members including at least the chairman or vice-chairman.

Requests for further information or clarification may include recommendations for revision of any of the supporting documentation (for example, the subject information sheet and consent form).

3.2.3.4 Letters giving the research ethics committee's opinion
The REC must[11] set out its opinion, including any conditions, in writing to the chief investigator. The following information should be included in the letter or in enclosures in all cases:

- a summary of the ethical issues considered by the committee
- a list of all documents reviewed at the meeting, giving version numbers and dates
- a list of the members who were present for the discussion of the application or who submitted written comments on the application prior to the meeting; the list should indicate lay members and give the profession in the case of expert members
- any declarations of interest by members which are material to the application
- the names of any observers present at the meeting

- (in the letter) the committee's view on any relevant issues on which the applicant has specifically asked for its opinion.

RECs also issue an NRES guidance document 'After ethical review: guidance for sponsor and investigators' with all favourable opinion letters. This is not part of the opinion but provides advice on further reporting to the REC during the trial. The guidance is updated from time to time and is available on the HRA website.

3.2.3.5 Duration of a favourable opinion

Where a favourable opinion is given by the REC this remains in place for the duration of the trial as described in the application, protocol and any amendments made by the sponsor. There is no requirement to notify the REC of an extension to the planned end date for the trial stated in the application to the REC, except where the extension is a result of a substantial amendment (for example, an increase in target recruitment, addition of new procedures or sub-studies, or extension of follow-up).

3.2.3.6 Further review following an unfavourable opinion

Where a REC has given an unfavourable opinion on an application for ethical review, the applicant has the following options for seeking further review:

- the applicant may submit another application, which will be reviewed as a new application
- the applicant may appeal against the decision of the first REC (this must[12] be to the UKECA) and seek a second opinion from another REC on the same application ('the second committee').

Where a new application is submitted, the assumption is that this will be modified to take account of the reasons for the unfavourable opinion. The modifications should be clearly indicated in the application and summarised in a cover letter. The new application may be re-submitted to the same REC or to a different committee. If it is sent to a different committee, it is a requirement in IRAS that the applicant declares whether the trial has been reviewed previously; this enables the REC to review the relevant documents and correspondence relating to the previous application.

The functions of the UKECA relating to appeals are delegated to the HRA. Notices of appeal should be sent in writing to the senior manager responsible for managing appeals within NRES, who will consider whether there are reasonable grounds for appeal and, if so, make arrangements for review by a second committee within 60 days of receipt of the notice of appeal. The second committee will be provided with copies of all relevant correspondence on the review by the first committee. Additional written representations may be made, and the second committee will also invite the chief investigator and sponsor's representative to attend the review meeting in the normal way.

If the second committee gives a favourable opinion, it becomes the responsible REC and should be the recipient of all required notifications and reports during the trial. If the second committee also gives an unfavourable opinion, there is no provision for further appeal, but this does not exclude the possibility of a new application being submitted which has been modified to take account of the reasons for the opinion.

3.2.3.7 Review of general advertising and screening procedures at clinical trial units

Clinical trial units, particularly Phase I units, may undertake general, non-trial-specific advertising and screening procedures to recruit potential trial subjects, prior to inviting them to participate in a specific trial. This activity constitutes preparations for undertaking a trial and is not part of the conduct of a trial as defined in Regulation 2 of SI 2004/1031, provided that it does not include any recruitment or screening procedures relating to a particular trial. It is therefore not a legal requirement for the procedures and materials to be reviewed by a REC and a favourable opinion obtained. However, such trial units may seek ethical advice on the procedures from a REC on a voluntary basis and are encouraged to do so by the HRA as a matter of good practice. Requests for such advice are clearly separated from applications for an opinion on a particular trial. It is recommended that records of the correspondence with the REC are retained and that it is clear from the correspondence which versions of the advertising material and screening protocol have been reviewed and approved by the REC.

3.2.4   Site-specific assessments

The REC is required[9] to consider the following site-specific issues, including:

- the suitability of the investigator and supporting staff
- the quality of the facilities
- any insurance or indemnity to cover the liability of local investigators
- the terms of any agreement between the sponsor and the trial site which are relevant to arrangements for compensating investigators and subjects.

As part of its favourable opinion for a trial, the REC must[9] therefore confirm its approval of the suitability of trial sites and investigators. All planned UK trial sites must[13] be listed in the REC application. Where sites are added during the trial, these must[14] be notified to the REC as a substantial amendment (section 3.4 provides further details on amendments).

The arrangements for undertaking site-specific assessment (SSA) in the UK depend on whether the site is within the NHS, that is, whether subjects are recruited into the trial in or through the NHS and a duty of care is owed by the NHS organisation(s) in respect of their treatment and care under the protocol.

A trial site is defined as a hospital, health centre, surgery or other establishment or facility at or from which a clinical trial, or any part of such a trial, is conducted (Regulation 2 of SI 2004/1031). For the purpose of SSA, NRES considers a site to be the single organisation responsible for recruiting subjects and conducting protocol procedures at a particular locality. Each site must[15] have a single (or 'principal') investigator who is responsible for the local conduct of the trial and to whom other sub-investigators and research team members are accountable (see Chapter 11 for the definition of a principal investigator and details of their role and responsibilities in a trial). Therefore, an NHS Trust would be considered a single site, though the trial may involve procedures being conducted at more than one location or department within the NHS Trust. In the primary-care setting, the GP practice would be the trial site if subjects are being recruited and treated by the practice. Where procedures are conducted 'off-site', that is, at a subject's home or mobile clinic, the site would be responsible for the conduct of those procedures.

The application for SSA must[13] clearly list all locations where procedures will be undertaken and for which the principal investigator is responsible as part of the trial site.

3.2.4.1   Site-specific assessment of NHS sites

The review of site-specific issues at NHS sites is no longer undertaken by the main REC or by any local RECs. Instead, it is now the responsibility of the appropriate NHS research and development (R&D) office, and it is integrated into the normal research governance review required for all research conducted in or through the NHS. The favourable opinion from the main REC includes approval for all NHS sites named in the application on condition that management permission for the trial is given by the R&D office. This means that the favourable opinion for each site is only in place once R&D permission has been obtained.

It is the sponsor's responsibility to ensure that this is in place as part of its duty to satisfy the conditions of the opinion. Under guidance from NRES, it is not necessary for the REC to be informed of permissions at each site, but the sponsor must[16] keep the relevant records.

Application for SSA at NHS sites is made by including the site-specific information (SSI) form for the site as part of the NHS R&D application prepared in IRAS.

3.2.4.2 Site-specific assessment of non-NHS sites

This is the responsibility of the REC system. The REC undertaking the SSA is known as the 'SSA REC' and may be either the main REC or an appropriate local REC. Designated SSA RECs may be appointed by NRES for specialist research units outside the NHS such as units conducting Phase I trials. The SSA REC does not need to be a UKECA-recognised REC as its role is to advise the main REC, which remains responsible for the opinion.

Application for SSA at non-NHS sites is made by submitting the SSI form and any supporting documentation to the SSA REC using IRAS. The application can be made as soon as the main REC application has been declared valid. If there is any doubt about whether SSA is required, the REC operational manager should be consulted.

Under the NRES SOPs, the SSA REC has 14 days (for a Phase I trial) or 25 days (for other trials) from receipt of a valid SSA application to notify the main REC of the outcome of the assessment. The main REC will then confirm to the chief investigator whether or not the site is approved as part of its favourable opinion.

3.2.4.3 Site-specific assessment of subsidiary sites

The main sites undertaking recruitment and administering the trial interventions will always require SSA; however, it may be necessary for the main site to arrange for routine procedures required by the protocol to be carried out by other organisations under contractual arrangements with the recruiting organisation (for example, MRI imaging or laboratory analysis using standard protocols may be undertaken on premises owned by universities, research charities or private companies; or arrangements may be made for blood samples required as part of follow-up monitoring to be collected at a GP surgery close to a subject's home).

The main site and partner organisation(s) may be considered as a single NHS site if all of the following conditions apply:

- all the subjects are NHS patients recruited at the main site

- the relevant NHS R&D office (which may be a joint research office acting for both an NHS Trust and a university partner) assumes full responsibility under the Research Governance Framework for all procedures involving subjects recruited at the site, including those undertaken by non-NHS organisations

- indemnity for all procedures is in place under the Clinical Negligence Scheme for Trusts ('NHS indemnity').

Where these criteria are met, ethical approval for the partner organisation is not required; however, the arrangements must[13] still be described in the application for SSA and reviewed by the R&D office responsible for the recruiting site. Where any of the above criteria are not met, the partner organisation must[13] be considered a separate research site or 'subsidiary site', and be listed in the REC application, or notified subsequently as a substantial amendment.

Where the subsidiary site is a non-NHS site, the chief investigator or sponsor may request exemption of the site from the normal requirement for SSA by writing to the main REC giving the name and address of the subsidiary site, details of the routine procedures to be conducted and the name of the person who will act as local principal investigator (that is, take responsibility for the conduct of these procedures). The REC will confirm any such exemption in writing.

It is therefore important for sponsors and chief investigators to be aware of any partner organisations or subsidiary sites involved in the trial and ensure that these are appropriately notified to the REC, either as part of an SSA or request for exemption. Issues in this area have been identified on inspection or reported as serious breaches. For example, one trial had used over 20 subsidiary sites for assessments such as scans and ECGs; however, there had been no consideration as to whether these sites required R&D approval or SSAs.

3.2.4.4   Site-specific assessment of patient identification centres

Subject or patient identification centres (PICs) are not considered to be trial sites. PICs are organisations from which clinicians or clinical units refer potential subjects to the investigational team in another organisation for assessment and possible recruitment to a trial. Responsibility for recruitment, informed consent and further procedures as set out in the protocol lies with the trial site rather than the PIC. There is no requirement for SSA and approval of PICs. Local management permission for the involvement of the organisation should be sought from the R&D office under the separate governance arrangements for PICs.

3.3   Informed consent

3.3.1   Definition of informed consent

Informed consent must[17] be given by each subject or from a person with parental responsibility or a legal representative. In most circumstances, informed consent must[18] be in place prior to the enrolment of the subject concerned. However, in exceptional circumstances, enrolment may take place prior to informed consent where urgent treatment needs to be provided.

'Informed consent' means that the decision to take part in the trial is given freely after the subject (or person with parental responsibility or a legal representative) has been informed of the nature, significance, implications and risks of the trial. This information will be set out in written information sheet(s), which must[13] be approved by the REC as part of its favourable opinion. The regulations specifically require[17] potential subjects to be informed of the right to withdraw from the trial at any time without being subject to any resulting detriment, and require[17] subjects to be given a contact point where further information about the trial can be obtained.

Detailed guidance on the recommended format and content of information sheets and consent forms has been developed by NRES and is available on the HRA website. The production of these documents is described in Chapter 4.

3.3.2   Recording of informed consent

Informed consent must[19] be evidenced in writing. In general, this will be done by inviting the person giving consent to sign and date the consent form. The consent form must[13] have been approved by the REC as part of its favourable opinion. Where the person giving consent is unable to sign or mark a document to indicate consent, they may give their consent orally in the presence of at least one witness, who must[19] sign the consent form as evidence that the information was accurately explained to and understood by the subject and that consent was freely given.

The requirement[18] for written consent to be in place prior to enrolment means that it is not permitted for consent to be given by telephone, unless this is evidenced in writing – for example, by faxing a signed consent form to the site or sending an email with an electronic signature.

3.3.3   Who can seek informed consent?

The person giving consent must[20] have had an interview with the investigator or another member of the investigational team at the site, at which they have had the opportunity to understand the objectives, risks and inconveniences of the trial and the conditions under which it is to be conducted. The requirement[20] for an interview does not exclude procedures for briefing potential subjects as a group in certain circumstances (for example, volunteers at a Phase I trial site). However, each individual must[20] also be given the opportunity to be interviewed privately to ensure that they do not want to raise any further questions and this is the context in which they will be invited to confirm their consent in writing.

The UK regulations allow for the interview with a potential subject (or other person giving consent) to be undertaken by any member of the investigational team at the site. The application form submitted to the main REC must[13] set out the general policy for the trial in terms of what types of personnel will be involved (for example, the principal investigator, medical sub-investigators and/or research nurses) and the procedures that will be followed. All personnel involved in the consent process must[21] have had appropriate training for this role.

3.3.4   Loss of capacity following initial decision

If a capable adult gives informed consent to take part in a trial, but subsequently becomes unable to give informed consent by virtue of physical or mental incapacity, the consent previously given when capable remains legally valid.

If a capable adult refuses informed consent, and subsequently becomes unable to give informed consent, the refusal is legally binding. The individual cannot be entered into the trial by seeking consent from a legal representative.

3.3.5   Withdrawal of consent

A subject has the right to withdraw from the trial at any time without being subject to resulting detriment. Following withdrawal, no further protocol procedures should be undertaken unless the subject agrees to being followed up for their own safety. Otherwise, any further treatment should continue outside the protocol.

It is generally understood that any data and samples already collected at the point of withdrawal may be retained and used in the trial analysis. The subject may request that no further data are added to the database, that any retained samples be destroyed and (on rare occasions) that previous data collected are not used. This should be documented.

3.3.6   Inclusion of minors and incapacitated adults in trials

Directive 2001/20/EC sets out fundamental principles relating to the inclusion of minors and adults lacking capacity to give informed consent in clinical trials. Persons who are incapable of giving legal consent to clinical trials should be given special protection. Such persons may not be included in clinical trials if the same results can be obtained using persons capable of giving consent. Normally these persons should be included in clinical trials only when there are grounds for expecting that administering the medicinal product would be of direct benefit to the subject, thereby outweighing the risks.

However, there is a need for clinical trials involving children to improve the treatment available to them. Children represent a vulnerable population with developmental, physiological and psychological differences from adults, which make age- and development-related research important for their benefit. Medicinal products, including vaccines, for children need to be tested scientifically before widespread use. This can only be achieved by ensuring that medicinal products which are likely to be of significant value for children are fully studied. The clinical trials for this purpose should be carried out under conditions affording the best possible protection for the subjects. Criteria for the protection of children in clinical trials therefore need to be laid down.

In the case of adults incapable of giving their consent, such as persons with dementia or psychiatric patients, Directive 2001/20/EC states that inclusion in clinical trials should be on an even more restrictive basis. Investigational medicinal products may be administered to such individuals only where there are grounds for assuming that the direct benefit to the subject outweighs the risks. The written consent of the subject's legal representative is required.[17]

Directive 2001/20/EC leaves it to the national law of Member States to define a 'minor' and a 'legal representative', and to lay down the detailed criteria for including minors and adults lacking capacity in clinical trials.

3.3.6.1 Conditions and principles applying to minors and incapacitated adults

All the conditions and principles listed in Part 4 of Schedule 1 to SI 2004/1031 must normally be satisfied if a minor is to be included in a clinical trial. Similarly, all the conditions and principles listed in Part 5 of Schedule 1 to SI 2004/1031 must normally be satisfied if an incapacitated adult is to be included in a clinical trial. In both trials including minors and trials involving adults lacking capacity, where the emergency provisions apply, Part 3 (1) to (5) of Schedule 1 to SI 2004/1031 relating to the informed consent process does not apply until the emergency has passed.

The conditions address the justification for carrying out clinical trials involving minors. The trial must[22] relate directly to a clinical condition from which the minor suffers, or be of such a nature that it can only be carried out on minors, and some direct benefit must[22] be expected to the group of subjects involved in the trial. This does not necessarily exclude placebo-controlled trials provided there is evidence of potential benefit to subjects in the interventional arm and no recognised effective therapy is being withheld. However, the REC will look closely at the risk–benefit profile of the trial and the justification for a placebo arm. Additionally, the trial must[22] be necessary to validate data obtained in other clinical trials with persons able to give consent or by other research methods.

As with minors, the conditions address the justification for including adults lacking capacity in a clinical trial. The trial must[23] relate directly to a life-threatening or debilitating clinical condition from which the adult suffers, and there must[23] be grounds for expecting that administering the investigational medicinal product (IMP) will produce a benefit to the subject outweighing the risk, or produce no risk at all. The trial must[23] also be necessary to validate data obtained in other clinical trials involving persons able to give consent, or by other research methods. These conditions rule out including adults lacking capacity in non-therapeutic trials where they do not have the disease or condition the IMP is intended to treat (that is, Phase I healthy volunteer trials).

The conditions require[22,23] that minors and adults lacking capacity receive information according to their capacity of understanding about the trial, its risks and benefits; and, in the case of minors, from staff with experience with minors. Where minors or incapacitated adults are capable of assessing the information and forming an opinion, any explicit wish to refuse participation in the trial or be withdrawn at any time must[22, 23] be considered by the investigator. This also means that, in addition to the legal consent required, it will be appropriate in some cases to explore whether the subject 'assents' or does not object to participating in the trial.

No incentives or financial inducements must[22, 23] be given to a minor or to a subject lacking capacity (or to a person with parental responsibility or legal representative), except for compensation in the event of injury or loss. Reimbursement of travelling and other expenses is normally appropriate, and RECs may also consider allowing small non-monetary gifts to minors as a thank you for participation (provided these are not considered an inducement). Monetary payments are generally considered unacceptable.

Further guidance on inclusion of minors in clinical trials is available in 'Medical research involving children' on the Medical Research Council (MRC) website and from the Royal College of Paediatrics and Child Health website (www.rcpch.ac.uk). NRES guidance on subject information sheets includes age-appropriate materials for use in involving 6–10 and 11–15 year olds in decisions about their participation. It also summarises the published literature and guidance on children's research.

Guidance on clinical trials and other research involving adults lacking capacity is available in an online toolkit on the HRA website. NRES guidance on subject information sheets includes materials for use in trials involving adults lacking capacity.

3.3.6.2   Definition of a legal representative in the UK

The definition of a legal representative depends on whether the subject is a minor or an adult with incapacity. The definition also varies where the subject is an adult with incapacity in Scotland. The detailed provisions for who may give consent are set out in Tables 3.2 and 3.3.

Common to the definition of the legal representative in any scenario is that the individual concerned must[24] not be *a person connected with the conduct of the trial'.*

3.3.6.3   Consent of a minor

A minor is defined as a person under the age of 16 years (Regulation 2 of SI 2004/1031). Table 3.2 prescribes a hierarchy for determining who should be approached to give informed consent on behalf of a minor prior to their inclusion in the trial. The provisions for informed consent by a legal representative only

3

Table 3.2 Hierarchy of informed consent for a minor

Person who may give consent	Definition	Commentary
Parent	A parent or person with parental responsibility in law	Should always be approached if available. Under the Children Act 1989, parental responsibility may be acquired by an unmarried father, step-parent, second female parent or appointed guardian.
Personal legal representative	A person not connected with the conduct of the trial who is: • suitable to act as the legal representative by virtue of their relationship with the minor, and • available and willing to do so	May be approached if no person with parental responsibility can be contacted prior to the proposed inclusion of the minor, by reason of the emergency nature of the treatment provided as part of the trial. The investigator must be satisfied that the person has sufficient knowledge of the minor and an interest in their welfare.
Professional legal representative	A person not connected with the conduct of the trial who is: • the doctor primarily responsible for the medical treatment of the minor, or • a person nominated by the relevant health care provider (for example, an acute NHS Trust or Health Board)	May be approached if no person suitable to act as a personal legal representative is available. Informed consent must be given before the minor is entered into the trial. Care organisations should have arrangements for appointing professional legal representatives where required.

apply if, by reason of the emergency nature of the treatment provided as part of the trial, no person with parental responsibility can be contacted prior to the proposed inclusion of the minor (see section 3.3.6.5 on emergency situations where it is also not possible to contact a legal representative). The regulations relating to minors apply to England, Wales, Scotland and Northern Ireland without distinction.

3

> **Relevant law in England and Wales against which decision-making capacity should be assessed**
>
> In England and Wales, the Mental Capacity Act 2005 makes provisions relating to the care, treatment and decisions made on behalf of people who lack capacity. Although the provisions for approving research under sections 30–33 of the Mental Capacity Act 2005 do not apply to clinical trials, the remainder of the Act does apply insofar as it is relevant to the conduct of a clinical trial. Investigators should be aware in particular of the core principles set out in section 1 and the definition of incapacity in sections 2–3 of the Mental Capacity Act 2005, which are based on English common law – that is, case law developed by the courts.
>
> Under section 1, a person must be assumed to have capacity unless it is established that he lacks capacity, and is not to be treated as unable to make a decision unless all practicable steps to help him do so have been taken without success. Therefore the recruitment procedures and materials should be designed to enable potential trial subjects to give informed consent for themselves wherever possible.
>
> Under section 2, a person is considered to lack capacity where he is unable to make a decision for himself in relation to a particular matter at the material time (that is, when a particular decision needs to be made), due to an impairment of or disturbance in the functioning of the mind or brain. The impairment or disturbance could be temporary (for example, due to trauma or an episode of mental illness) or permanent (for example, serious brain injury or dementia).
>
> Under section 3, a person is unable to make a decision for himself if he is unable to understand the information relevant to the decision, retain the information, use or weigh up the information in making the decision, or communicate his decision (by any means).
>
> The statutory Code of Practice on the Mental Capacity Act 2005 describes the provisions of the Act in more depth and gives practical guidance on assessing capacity and helping people make decisions. The Act is available on the following website: www.justice.gov.uk

3.3.6.4 Consent of incapacitated adults

The term used in the regulations to refer to an adult lacking capacity is 'an adult unable by virtue of physical or mental incapacity to give informed consent' (Part 1 (4a) of Schedule 1 to SI 2004/1031). An adult refers to a person aged 16 or over. Beyond this, the regulations do not define capacity or incapacity to give consent. Investigators and other research team members involved in enrolment of trial subjects are responsible for assessing decision-making capacity in accordance with the law in the relevant part of the UK.

Table 3.3 sets out the hierarchy for determining what type of legal representative should be approached to give informed consent on behalf of an adult who lacks capacity to give informed consent by virtue of physical or mental incapacity prior to inclusion of the subject in the trial. The provisions in England, Wales and Northern Ireland differ from those in Scotland.

Relevant law in Scotland and Northern Ireland against which decision-making capacity should be assessed

Scotland

In Scotland, the legislation equivalent to the Mental Capacity Act 2005 in England and Wales is the Adults with Incapacity (Scotland) Act 2000. Under section 1 (6) of the Act, a person is 'incapable' if he is incapable of:

    (a)   acting

    (b)   making decisions

    (c)   communicating decisions

    (d)   understanding decisions, or

    (e)   retaining the memory of decisions

due to mental disorder or inability to communicate because of physical disability; but people should not be treated as unable to communicate if they can be assisted to do so by any means.

Further guidance is available from the Scottish Government in 'Adults with Incapacity (Scotland) Act 2000: communication and assessing capacity: guidance for social work and healthcare staff', available at www.scotland.gov.uk/.

Northern Ireland

In Northern Ireland, there is no equivalent legislation, and matters relating to capacity and incapacity would be determined by the common law.

3.3.6.5 Emergency situations in trials involving minors and incapacitated adults

Where, as part of the trial, the treatment needs to be administered urgently to a minor or to an adult lacking capacity, time may not allow for written consent to be obtained first from a person with parental responsibility (in the case of minors) or a legal representative. Minors or adults lacking capacity are allowed to be entered into a trial prior to informed consent being obtained, provided that:

- having regard to the nature of the trial and the particular circumstances of the case, it is necessary to take action for the purpose of the trial as a matter of urgency, but

- it is not reasonably practicable to obtain informed consent prior to entering the subject, and

- the action to be taken is carried out in accordance with a procedure approved by the REC.

Table 3.3 Hierarchy of informed consent for an incapacitated adult

Person who may give consent	England, Wales and Northern Ireland	Scotland
Personal legal representative	A person not connected with the conduct of the trial who is: • suitable to act as the legal representative by virtue of their relationship with the adult, and • available and willing to do so. Note that the regulations for these countries do not specify next of kin and there is no hierarchy specifying the order in which relatives or friends are to be approached. Responsibility lies with the investigating team to identify a suitable person after consulting the patient's usual care staff and health records. A personal legal representative could include someone with a Lasting Power of Attorney under the Mental Capacity Act 2005 in respect of welfare decisions.	1A. Any guardian or welfare attorney who has power to consent to the adult's participation in research. 1B. If there is no such person, the adult's nearest relative as defined in Section 87 (1) of the Adults with Incapacity (Scotland) Act 2000.
Professional legal representative (care organisations should have arrangements for appointing professional legal representatives where required)	A person not connected with the conduct of the trial who is: • the doctor primarily responsible for the adult's medical treatment, or • a person nominated by the relevant healthcare provider (for example, an acute NHS Trust or Health Board). A professional legal representative may be approached if no suitable personal legal representative is available.	A person not connected with the conduct of the trial who is: • the doctor primarily responsible for the adult's medical treatment, or • a person nominated by the relevant healthcare provider. A professional legal representative may be approached if it is not reasonably practicable to contact a personal legal representative (either 1A or 1B above) before the decision to enter the adult into the trial is made.

Where a minor is recruited in an emergency situation without prior informed consent, steps must[22] be taken to seek informed consent from a person with parental responsibility or a legal representative as soon as practicable after the initial emergency has passed. Where consent is withheld, the subject must[22] be withdrawn from the trial; samples and data collected up to this point may be retained with the consent of the person with parental responsibility or legal representative.

Where an incapacitated adult is recruited in an emergency situation without prior informed consent, steps must[23] be taken to seek informed consent either from the subject (if capacity has been recovered) or from a legal representative as soon as practicable after the initial emergency has passed. Where consent is withheld, the subject must[23] be withdrawn from the trial; samples and data collected up to this point may be retained with the consent of the subject or legal representative.

Issues with emergency consenting procedures have been seen on inspection. For example:

- In a trial, an NHS Trust had not appointed a professional legal representative, required as part of the consent process, at the start of the trial. As a result, consent forms were subsequently signed retrospectively by the R&D manager a year after the subjects had entered the trial. In addition, there was no formal document available to demonstrate that the NHS Trust had appointed this individual as the professional legal representative, and that the person was appropriate to perform the role.
- In another trial a number of subjects had their consent forms signed by the treating medically qualified doctor who randomised them onto the trial. This process was not as described or intended by the trial protocol. Subjects were also not subsequently asked for personal consent to continue in the trial following the emergency and their return to capacity.

3.3.6.6 Responsibilities of research ethics committees in trials involving minors and incapacitated adults

In trials involving minors and incapacitated adults, the application to the REC must[13] include:

- justification for including minors or adults lacking capacity
- the trial policy for identifying and approaching persons with parental responsibility or legal representatives, including scenarios where a professional legal representative may need to be appointed

- if applicable, the justification for proceeding with enrolment prior to consent where emergency treatment needs to be given, how and by whom enrolment decisions would be made, and follow-up consent procedures
- written information to be given to persons with parental responsibility or legal representatives for the purpose of seeking informed consent
- any written information to be given to the subjects prior to recruitment, where they have some capacity for understanding (there may be multiple versions depending on the age range included)
- written information to be given to adults who regain capacity following recruitment without prior informed consent in an emergency situation
- a copy of the form to be used to record consent (and assent, if applicable).

If the REC does not have a member with suitable expertise, it must[25] obtain expert advice before giving its opinion on a clinical trial involving minors or incapacitated adults. Procedures for obtaining advice from expert referees are included in the NRES SOPs for RECs, which are available on the HRA website.

3.4   Amendments

3.4.1   Substantial or non-substantial, authorisation or ethical opinion?

There are two types of changes to clinical trials and their associated documentation: substantial and non-substantial amendments. Except when taking urgent safety measures (see section 3.5.1), the sponsor of a clinical trial is required[14] to obtain authorisation from the competent authority and/or a favourable opinion from the REC before implementing any amendment that is considered to be substantial. Amendments that do not meet the criteria for a substantial amendment do not require notification to either body, but such changes must[14] be recorded by the sponsor (ideally including the sponsor's rationale as to why the amendment is non-substantial) and made available upon request. Non-substantial amendments may be notified for information only at the sponsor's discretion, but do not require a favourable opinion before being implemented.

The definition of a substantial amendment, together with examples, is provided in the European Commission 'Detailed guidance on the request to the competent authorities for authorisation of a clinical trial on a medicinal product for human use, the notification of substantial amendments and the declaration of the end of the trial' (hereinafter 'detailed guidance CT-1'). A substantial amendment is a change that is likely to have a significant impact on the safety or physical or mental integrity of the clinical trial subjects, or the scientific value of the clinical trial. It is up to the sponsor of the clinical trial to assess whether an amendment is to be regarded as substantial or not. It is also the responsibility of the sponsor to decide whether a substantial amendment requires authorisation, or an ethical opinion, or both (such decisions may be reviewed during a GCP inspection). The general guidance in Table 2.1 (Chapter 2) has been agreed between NRES and the MHRA, taking account of the detailed guidance CT-1.

Where a substantial amendment only requires authorisation by the competent authority, it is not necessary to notify the REC for information. Similarly, where a substantial amendment only requires a favourable opinion by the REC, it is not necessary to notify the competent authority for information.

Further guidance is also available within the NRES SOPs for RECs and on the HRA website.

3.4.2 Notifying substantial amendments to the research ethics committee

The sponsor or chief investigator should submit the amendment to the REC using the notice of substantial amendment form within IRAS, which is updated from time to time in line with the format prescribed by the European Commission. Any necessary supporting documentation must[26] be provided (for example, a revised protocol, subject information sheet or consent form). Changes of wording should be clearly highlighted, either as tracked changes or in a separate list of changes.

3.4.3 Ethical review of substantial amendments

Where a substantial amendment is notified for ethical review, the REC must[14] give an opinion within 35 days of receiving a valid notice of amendment.

Substantial amendments are not required to be reviewed at a full meeting of the REC. Under the NRES SOPs, amendments may be reviewed by a sub-committee, either at a face-to-face meeting, telephone meeting or in correspondence. The sub-committee must[2] include at least an officer of the committee and one other member. One member may be co-opted to a sub-committee.

The REC may request further information from the sponsor or chief investigator on the amendment, but unlike for new applications there is no provision for the 35-day clock to stop while a reply is awaited.

The decision reached should be either a favourable or unfavourable opinion of the amendment. The regulations do not allow the REC to give a favourable opinion for part of the amendment only; however, when giving an unfavourable opinion the committee may indicate which parts of the amendment would have been acceptable and give guidance on the submission of a modified amendment taking account of its concerns.

Where sponsors plan to make a large number of amendments covering various aspects of the trial, consideration should be given to dividing them into two or more separate notifications. This may enable the REC to give a favourable opinion more quickly to relatively straightforward changes; for example, the addition of new sites or changes of principal investigator.

3.4.4 Modified amendments

If the opinion is unfavourable, the sponsor may then modify the proposed amendment. A written notice of the modification should be sent to the REC at least 14 days before it is due to be implemented, using the same form as for the initial notification and indicating the modifications that have been made. The amendment may be divided into more than one modified amendment to allow for separate opinions to be given on each part of the package. The REC must[27] give an unfavourable opinion on a modified amendment within 14 days, otherwise it may be implemented.

Modified amendments may be reviewed by a sub-committee in the same way as other substantial amendments. However, when giving an unfavourable opinion a sub-committee may delegate responsibility to the chairman to give a favourable opinion of the modified amendment if it is subsequently amended in such a way that meets its concerns.

3.4.5 Appeal against unfavourable opinion of substantial amendments

There is no provision in the legislation for appeal against an unfavourable opinion for a substantial amendment. However, provisions for appeal are included in the NRES SOPs.

3.5   Safety reporting to the research ethics committee

3.5.1   Urgent safety measures

Where the sponsor or an investigator takes urgent safety measures in order to protect the subjects of a trial against any immediate hazard to their health or safety, the REC (and the competent authority, see section 2.3.7) must[28] be notified immediately and in any event within 3 days that such measures have been taken and the reasons be given why they have been taken. The initial notification to the REC should be by telephone. Notice in writing must[28] be sent within 3 days. The notice must[28] set out the reasons for the urgent safety measures and the plan for further action.

The REC is not required to approve urgent safety measures. However, the committee will review such notifications and consider whether the measures taken are appropriate in relation to the apparent risk to subjects, and what further action the sponsor and investigator(s) propose to take – for example, the submission of substantial amendments to the protocol. Where any concern arises about the safety or welfare of subjects or the conduct of the research, the REC may address these with the sponsor and chief investigator.

3.5.2   Expedited reporting of individual SUSARs in the UK

The sponsor must[29] notify the REC in an expedited fashion of any suspected unexpected serious adverse reactions (SUSARs) occurring in the concerned trial in the UK. There is no requirement to report SUSARs occurring in the trial outside the UK, or in other UK trials of the same IMP.

Expedited SUSAR reports should be sent to RECs electronically in accordance with NRES procedures.

There is no requirement to include SUSAR reports with the documentation submitted to a REC as part of a new trial application. The protocol and application form should provide the REC with an up-to-date summary of the safety profile of the IMP. However, where the sponsor subsequently receives safety data during the ethical review process or prior to the start of the trial in the UK which materially changes the safety profile of the IMP as described in the application and could affect the risk–benefit assessment and information to be provided to potential subjects, this must[30] be notified to the committee.

3.5.3   Annual safety reporting

It is a legislative requirement[31] in the UK that, for each IMP being tested in the trial, the sponsor should provide the competent authority and REC with an annual report on the safety of subjects in all clinical trials of the product for which the sponsor is responsible, whether in the UK or elsewhere. All annual safety reports (ASRs) should be in the format of development safety update reports (DSURs) (see section 5.15 for further details of the content and format of DSURs). The DSUR should be sent to the REC as soon as practicable after the end of the reporting period, and within 60 days at the latest.

The REC is required to receive the full DSUR including the line listing of suspected serious adverse reactions. However, as per NRES guidance, the REC is only expected to review the executive summary of the DSUR.

3.6   Other required reports to the research ethics committee

3.6.1   Annual progress reports

There is no requirement under the regulations to provide progress reports, other than DSURs (see section 3.5.3). It is, however, considered to be good practice for the sponsor to provide an annual progress report to the REC, and this is requested in the NRES guidance issued alongside the favourable opinion letter. A standard template for the annual progress report is published on the HRA website.

3.6.2   Temporary halt of the trial

When the sponsor temporarily halts a trial, for any reason, whether it is a halt of the whole trial or at individual trial site(s), the REC (and competent authority; see section 2.3.8) should be notified within 15 days by submission of the notification of substantial amendment form. The form should clearly explain the reasons for the halt and the scope (for example, stopping recruitment and/or interrupting the treatment of subjects already included). The substantial amendment will be reviewed by the REC in the normal way.

If the sponsor has submitted a substantial amendment to halt the trial and subsequently wishes to restart the trial, it must[14] submit a further notification of substantial amendment form requesting a favourable opinion. Evidence should be provided that it is safe to restart the trial. If the sponsor decides not to recommence the trial after a temporary halt, the conclusion of the trial must[32] be declared (see section 3.6.3).

3.6.3 Declaration of the conclusion or early termination of the trial

The sponsor must[32] notify the REC (and the competent authority; see section 2.3.10) in writing that a trial has ended within 90 days of the conclusion of the trial. If the trial is terminated early, the sponsor must[32] notify the REC (and competent authority; see section 2.3.9) within 15 days of the date of termination. An explanation of the reasons for early termination should be given; examples may include difficulty with recruitment or funding, or safety issues. A notice of substantial amendment could be submitted alongside a declaration of early termination where it is necessary to seek ethical review of related actions such as informing subjects and arranging continuing care and follow-up outside the trial.

It has been seen on inspection that trials have terminated early due to lack of recruitment, or even lack of funding, but have not been notified as early terminations. This is largely due to a common misconception that early termination refers only to safety-related terminations. This is not the case and early termination of a trial for any reason should be notified.

Once the end of the trial has been declared, it is no longer possible to submit notices of substantial amendment.

It is recommended that, if a trial is abandoned prior to commencement, the chief investigator or sponsor notifies the main REC and the MHRA by letter, outlining the reasons for abandoning the trial.

3.6.4 Serious breaches

There is no legal requirement to notify serious breaches of the protocol or GCP (as defined in Regulation 29A of SI 2004/1031) to the REC. However, it is recommended that sponsors notify the REC by copy of the report sent to the MHRA, that is, within 7 days of becoming aware of the breach (reporting to the

MHRA is described in section 1.3.5). This is not a condition of the favourable opinion, but is requested in the NRES guidance issued with favourable opinion letters.

It is helpful to the REC to be aware of serious breaches as they may raise issues on which ethical advice is required – for example, where there have been deficiencies in the informed consent process and consideration needs to be given to providing further information and/or seeking fresh consent from subjects, potentially requiring notification of a substantial amendment to the REC. There have also been examples seen on inspection where corrective and preventative actions implemented in response to a serious breach had involved the provision of information to subjects or their relatives; however, the REC had not been informed of this action, nor approved the written information that was provided.

As well as advising the sponsor where requested, the REC may also contact the MHRA under the memorandum of understanding in place between NRES and the MHRA. NRES and the MHRA GCP Inspectorate routinely share information about serious breach reports so that consistent and coordinated advice can be provided to sponsors on any follow-up action required.

3.6.5   Final reports

The clinical trial summary report should be sent to the REC within one year of the conclusion of the research (that is, one year from the notification of the end of trial). In the case of early termination, provision of this report is at the discretion of the sponsor. At a minimum, the REC should receive information on whether the trial achieved its objectives, the main findings, and arrangements for publication or dissemination of the research including any feedback to subjects. If the trial will not be published, this should be explained and justified.

3.7   Retention of documentation by the research ethics committee

The REC is required[2] to retain all the documentation relating to a clinical trial on which it gives an opinion for at least 3 years from the conclusion or early termination of the trial. Where the trial does not proceed (for example, it is given an unfavourable opinion, or does not start following a favourable opinion), the

REC is required to retain the documentation for at least 3 years from the date of the opinion. There is no requirement to retain documentation relating to applications that are withdrawn prior to giving an opinion.

Documentation is considered to be retained where it is held in electronic form and can be accessed when necessary. It is not necessary to retain original paper copies. RECs in the UK normally retain documentation electronically within the NRES Research Ethics Database.

3.8 GCP inspections and ethical review

The MHRA does not inspect either HRA or RECs as part of the GCP inspection remit. Compliance with regulatory requirements related to ethical approvals by the research site is inspected, however. This could include checks on:

- ethics approvals (both initial and amendments)
- informed consent process (for example, checks to ensure that the approved versions of the subject information sheet and consent forms are being used, and used in accordance with the process described in the ethics application)
- annual and expedited safety reporting to RECs
- the trial conduct to ensure, in practice, it matches the information provided to the RECs in the ethics application form
- end-of-trial reporting.

3.9 Chapter legislative references

Throughout this chapter, specific terminology – 'must', 'required' or 'requirement' – has been used to interpret activities that are legislative requirements. These terms have been number-coded in the text where used, and the corresponding reference in the legislation can be found below.

1. Regulation 5 of SI 2004/1031
2. Schedule 2 of SI 2004/1031
3. Regulation 7 of SI 2004/1031
4. Regulation 14 (5) of SI 2004/1031
5. Regulation 14 (1) of SI 2004/1031

6.   Regulation 14 (6) of SI 2004/1031

7.   Regulation 15 (10) of SI 2004/1031

8.   Regulation 15 (8) of SI 2004/1031

9.   Regulation 15 (5) of SI 2004/1031

10. Regulation 15 (3B) of SI 2004/1031

11. Regulation 15 (3A) of SI 2004/1031

12. Regulation 16 of SI 2004/1031

13. Schedule 3, Part 1 of SI 2004/1031

14. Regulation 24 of SI 2004/1031

15. Regulation 2 of SI 2004/1031

16. Regulation 31A (4) of SI 2004/1031

17. Schedule 1 of SI 2004/1031

18. Article 3 of Directive 2001/20/EC

19. Schedule 1, Part 1 (3) of SI 2004/1031

20. Schedule 1, Part 3 of SI 2004/1031

21. Schedule 1, Part 2 (2) of SI 2004/1031

22. Schedule 1, Part 4 of SI 2004/1031

23. Schedule 1, Part 5 of SI 2004/1031

24. Schedule 1, Part 1 (2) of SI 2004/1031

25. Regulation 15 (6) and (7) of SI 2004/1031

26. Schedule 3, Part 3 of SI 2004/1031

27. Regulation 25 of SI 2004/1031

28. Regulation 30 of SI 2004/1031

29. Regulation 33 of SI 2004/1031

30. Schedule 1, Part 2 (10) and Schedule 3, Part 1 (1r) of SI 2004/1031

31. Regulation 35 of SI 2004/1031

32. Regulation 27 of SI 2004/1031

Key trial documentation

4

Editor's note

Regulatory documentation can be described as those documents that are required to be produced and submitted to the competent authority. However, in the context of clinical trials, this definition also includes those essential supporting documents required to be submitted to the research ethics committees (RECs) for the main REC opinion, as well as those documents submitted to either the nominated REC or research and development (R&D) office for site-specific assessments. In addition to regulatory documentation, a number of ancillary documents may also be prepared during the course of a clinical trial; these may be key to ensuring that the study is conducted accurately, consistently and according to the protocol, legislation and Good Clinical Practice (GCP).

The term 'key trial documents' is taken to include all the document types indicated above. If these key trial documents are not managed appropriately, this could affect the safety of the subjects, the credibility of the data and the trial results. Therefore, organisations should consider applying the principles described in this chapter to the preparation and control of each of these types of documents. This will help ensure the management of the clinical trial is consistent (particularly when conducting large, global, multi-centre clinical trials) and help ensure that the trial data collected are accurate.

4.1   Expectations and legislative requirements

An organisation should have clear formalised procedures detailing how key trial documents are prepared, reviewed, approved and implemented. This ensures quality for every aspect of the trial and these procedures must[1] be complied with.

There is also specific guidance available in relation to the content of a number of key trial documents. For example:

- protocol and investigator's brochure (IB): ICH Topic E6 (R1) – 'Guideline for Good Clinical Practice' (hereinafter 'ICH GCP')
- investigational medicinal product dossier (IMPD): CHMP – 'Guideline on the requirements to the chemical and pharmaceutical quality documentation concerning investigational medicinal products in clinical trials' (CHMP/QWP/185401/2004)
- subject information sheet and consent form: ICH GCP, Health Research Authority (HRA) website
- clinical study report (CSR): ICH Topic E3 – 'Structure and content of clinical study reports' (hereinafter 'ICH E3')
- development safety update report (DSUR): ICH Topic E2F – 'Development safety update report'.

Therefore, this guide will not discuss in detail the content of the key trial documents, but will provide some additional information in relation to their production and control.

Table 4.1 provides a list of some examples of key trial documents essential to the consistency and accuracy of the management of the clinical trial and credibility of the data collected. This is not an exhaustive list and it may differ for each trial and also from country to country, depending on each country's own legislative requirements. This guide will focus on those required in the UK.

It is also important to remember that other organisations employed by the sponsor (for example, vendors, consultants and investigator sites) may also produce documentation to facilitate the conduct of their designated tasks and activities. The sponsor should always be aware of these documents and decide what impact they have on trial conduct and accuracy. Refer to section 4.6 for considerations in relation to these types of documents.

4.2   Generation of key trial documentation

A written procedure should be in place for the preparation, review, approval, version control and updating of key trial documents. This may be a generic procedure that covers all or a range of documents. Alternatively, there may be individual procedures in place for each particular type of document, or for some single-centre trials it may be appropriate to include procedures within the protocol

Table 4.1 Examples of key trial documentation

Key trial documentation[a]		
Competent authority documentation[b]	**Research ethics committee documentation[c]**	**Ancillary documentation[d]**
Protocol and subsequent amendments	Protocol and subsequent amendments	Risk-adaptive risk assessment
Clinical trial authorisation application form and amendments	Ethics application form and amendments	Risk assessment mitigation plan
Investigator's brochure	Investigator's brochure	Case report form
Development safety update report	Development safety update report	Safety management plan
Clinical trial summary report/clinical study report	Clinical trial summary report/clinical study report	Publications
End-of-trial notification form	End-of-trial notification form	Instruction manuals (for example, laboratory, pharmacy)
Urgent safety measures	Urgent safety measures	Statistical analysis plan
Serious breaches	Subject information sheets	Data management plan
Investigational medicinal product dossier	Consent and assent forms	Monitoring plan
Sample labelling	Advertisements/recruitment material (for example, newspaper, magazine, radio)	Contracts
	Any information given to subjects or their carers (for example, diaries, questionnaires, instructions)	
	Evidence of insurance or indemnity	

[a] This is not a comprehensive list and is only intended to provide a list of examples.

[b] Documentation required by the competent authority.

[c] Documents required by the research ethics committee (REC).

[d] Non-regulatory documentation, but key in terms of the outcome of the clinical trial. These documents, if produced, may be essential in terms of management of the clinical trial.

(Chapter 14). This will depend on the organisation's quality system and business need. It is recommended that any procedures in place explain how these documents are prepared and approved, who is responsible for these tasks, how they are version-controlled, and how they are issued, updated and implemented.

The use of template documents is recommended to ensure key sections or wording are included, where applicable, and to ensure consistency between documents. For example, there are certain elements which must[2] be included in documents (for example, protocols). Templates can ensure that these areas are always covered, thereby streamlining the documents' production and approval and ensuring their quality and consistency.

The retention requirements of all documents, including draft and superseded versions, are described in section 10.7.1.

An overview of the process for producing and amending key trial documents is illustrated in Figure 4.1.

4.2.1   Preparation of key trial documents

When planning a new clinical trial, it is advised that there is an assessment of which key trial documents are required.

The author must[1] use any procedure(s) available to instruct them in the preparation of the relevant document(s). If a template is available, the author must[1] ensure that it is the current version. Any deviation from the procedure and/or template must[1, 3] be clearly justified and documented. The author is recommended to refer to any existing key trial documents for that trial to ensure consistency (see section 4.5).

Once prepared, the document(s) is usually circulated to appropriate members of the trial team for review and comment.

4.2.2   Review of key trial documents

Selection of appropriate reviewers and approvers will vary depending on the type of clinical trial being conducted. For all trials, regardless of type, there is likely to be a set of core trial team roles involved in document review and approval (for example, trial manager, regulatory affairs, statistics, data management, medical/safety, chief investigator, clinical supplies/pharmacy, R&D office; the roles depend on the set-up of the organisation). However, there may also be additional

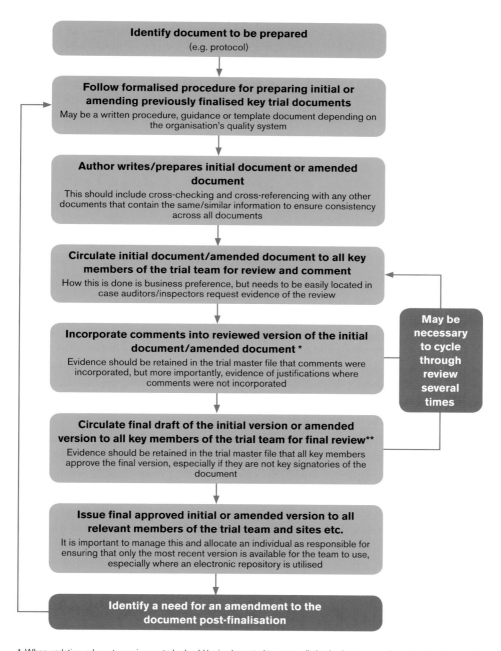

4

Identify document to be prepared
(e.g. protocol)

Follow formalised procedure for preparing initial or amending previously finalised key trial documents
May be a written procedure, guidance or template document depending on the organisation's quality system

Author writes/prepares initial document or amended document
This should include cross-checking and cross-referencing with any other documents that contain the same/similar information to ensure consistency across all documents

Circulate initial document/amended document to all key members of the trial team for review and comment
How this is done is business preference, but needs to be easily located in case auditors/inspectors request evidence of the review

Incorporate comments into reviewed version of the initial document/amended document *
Evidence should be retained in the trial master file that comments were incorporated, but more importantly, evidence of justifications where comments were not incorporated

May be necessary to cycle through review several times

Circulate final draft of the initial version or amended version to all key members of the trial team for final review**
Evidence should be retained in the trial master file that all key members approve the final version, especially if they are not key signatories of the document

Issue final approved initial or amended version to all relevant members of the trial team and sites etc.
It is important to manage this and allocate an individual as responsible for ensuring that only the most recent version is available for the team to use, especially where an electronic repository is utilised

Identify a need for an amendment to the document post-finalisation

* When updating, adequate version controls should be implemented to ensure distinction between each version of a document. Also, consideration should be given to restricting editing access depending on document and circulation.

** Prior to finalising the document, there should be a documented quality control process to ensure correctness and consistency.

Figure 4.1 Flowchart of process for generating and amending key trial documentation

persons involved in review and/or approval of documents for particular types of clinical trials where specialist input is needed, such as for pharmacokinetic trials. Selection of appropriate persons for review and approval of documents will also vary depending on the document type. A particular document may not need to be reviewed and/or approved by all trial team members, and thus consideration should be given to the input each role will have depending on the activities being described within the document.

It is recommended that the review and incorporation of comments is documented and retained as evidence that all relevant team members had the opportunity to review the document and that all comments were assessed appropriately. This can be by email, tracked changes in the electronic format of the document, a hand-amended hard copy, meeting minutes or formal review forms. This step can be repeated until there is a consensus on the final document.

A quality control (QC) step should be built into the review and approval process of key trial documents and this step must[3] be formally documented. See section 4.5 for details on QC processes.

A peer review may also be useful for some documents such as the protocol and CSR or publications. Risks associated with clinical trials can include trial design errors (that is, inadequate sample sizing, flawed randomisation, potential unblinding or even inadequate follow-up or collection of end-point data) and analytical errors (that is, incorrect interpretation of the results, errors regarding the interpretation of analyses, such as mistaking a lack of statistical significance as an ineffective treatment rather than insufficient subject numbers). A peer review process for the protocol and CSR or publications may identify any such potential risks prior to finalising these documents. Peer review is conducted by qualified and experienced persons; sometimes it is done by the trials steering committee or data monitoring committee or, alternatively, by independent experts. Again, it is recommended that there is clear documentation of any peer reviews along with evidence that their recommendations have been assessed and incorporated. This must[3] be retained in the trial master file (TMF).

4.2.3   Approval and issue of key trial documents

It is good practice for an organisation to approve each document type by means of a formal sign-off and, if so, to define who are the required signatories. Consideration could also be given to documenting evidence of review and approval of other team members who are not official signatories. Signatory requirements will depend on the type of document. For example, the protocol is a regulatory document that should be signed off, at a minimum, by the sponsor as evidence that the sponsor has 'authorised' the protocol (paragraph 52 of the detailed guidance CT-1) and by the investigator(s) (or chief investigator for a multi-centre trial) as confirmation that they agree to comply with the protocol. The case report form (CRF), on the other hand, does not necessarily need to be a signed document; however, it is recommended that there is documented evidence of approval of the final version by relevant personnel to ensure that it is fit to collect the data required, so that it meets the objectives of the clinical trial.

How an organisation documents review comments and approvals will vary greatly. Some examples are provided below:

- retention of annotated documents (such as documents incorporating tracked changes)
- use of a document (for example, a table) to track which comments were accepted or rejected and why
- use of a generic approval form that clearly identifies the document being approved (including its version)
- approval forms for specific documents
- email/use of voting buttons on emails with retention of the final email (it is worth considering where emails used to approve documents are retained in the TMF; for example, it may be more efficient to file these with the document, rather than in a large section under correspondence).

4.3   Updating and amending key trial documents

Updating and amending key trial documents generally follows the same process as for the initial preparation of the document (refer to Figure 4.1), although it is recommended that there is a documented rationale for each change made to the document. It may also be appropriate to prepare a summary of changes for the document (either incorporated into the document or as a stand-alone document) so that those reviewing or using the document can easily identify what changes have been made.

A clearly documented instruction by a responsible individual can be helpful as it can inform stakeholders that all relevant approvals have been received and the updated version of the document can be implemented. It is recommended that a mechanism is put in place to track amended documents including when these have been circulated and implemented to ensure clear reconstruction of the trial.

It has been observed on inspection that amended documents were not formally implemented; therefore assumptions have to be made as to when they were followed. This can result in the incorrect use of documents, such as continuing to use superseded subject information sheets and consent forms.

Tracking can also facilitate the timely update of key trial documents in line with legislative requirements. For example, it is a requirement[4] to review the IB on an annual basis (see section 4.7.3 for further details on this type of document). Methods of tracking can range from the use of a calendar reminder or an MS Excel® spreadsheet to a trial management system.

4.4   Version control

Key trial documents (in particular those that are in electronic format) will form part of the TMF and therefore must[5] be protected from unauthorised access and unauthorised or accidental editing. This may be achieved by restricting access to certain trial team members or roles, or by changing the document to a non-editable format.

Key trial documents should also have some means of unique document identifier so that different versions of a particular document can be distinguished from each other. The document identifier may indicate the document's lifecycle status (for example, draft, final, version number) and the date of the document. It is suggested that the identifying version control is on every page of the document and the document is paginated.

All versions of a document used during the lifetime of the trial must[3] be kept to allow reconstruction of the trial. It is recommended that files clearly indicate document versions that have been superseded, so that these documents are not inadvertently used.

A situation where there are no or inadequate version controls for documents may give rise to problems when it comes to reconstructing the clinical trial, if the following cannot be established:

- which version(s) was submitted to the competent authority and REC, or sent to the contract research organisation (CRO) or investigator sites
- that the correct version of a document was implemented before a version-specific activity was undertaken
- when a document was updated and implemented in relation to changes in the clinical trial

- that the correct version of the document was being used at any given time during the clinical trial.

Common findings related to version control include:

- documents exist with a complete lack of version control
- multiple documents with the same version number exist, but with different version dates
- documents have different text, but there has been no change to the version number
- the version number or date changes throughout the pages of the document.

A lack of version control can lead to significant issues for the conduct of the trial. For example, it has been seen on inspection that ineligible subjects have been recruited for a trial because the eligibility checklist used by investigator site staff was not version-controlled and therefore was not updated when a protocol amendment changed the eligibility criteria.

4.5   Cross-checking and quality control

Some key trial documents contain the same information and therefore there should be a system in place for cross-checking the documents during their preparation, including a formal QC step, to ensure that the information and message is consistent and accurate. An organisation's quality system should clearly identify who is responsible for ensuring the consistency check across all the documents. Ideally an audit trail should show who performed this check and when (see section 14.3 for further information on QC processes). See Table 4.2 for examples of areas and information that cross over between key trial documents.

It is not the responsibility of the competent authority or REC to identify discrepancies in the consistency of the documentation submitted to them. It is the responsibility of the sponsor (or delegated representative) to ensure consistency prior to making the submission. Therefore, implementing a formal QC step prior to making a submission or implementing documents can ensure that there is consistency built in from the start, and that as documents are amended the information is updated consistently across all other relevant documents.

It has been identified on inspection that information contained within different documents is sometimes inconsistent. For example:

- On review, a trial was found to have different inclusion and exclusion criteria detailed in the protocol, REC application form and clinical trial authorisation (CTA) application form. Therefore, it could not be established which of the criteria were correct and therefore which should be followed.
- The safety information was not consistent across the protocol, IB and subject information sheet for a trial. This could have resulted in expectedness being incorrectly assessed and important safety signals being missed.

4.6   Sponsor oversight of third-party key trial documents

During the course of a clinical trial there may be a number of other organisations involved that are employed by the sponsor to conduct certain functions (such as vendors, consultants or investigator sites). There may be occasions when these other parties prepare documents in order to facilitate the conduct of these functions – for example, production of documents as determined by their own

Table 4.2 Examples of documents requiring cross-checking

Information Key trial document	Eligibility criteria	Safety data for IMP	IMP	Trial restrictions (for example, prohibited medications or foods)	Trial procedures	Delegated functions	Safety reporting requirements
Protocol	✓	✓	✓	✓	✓	✓	✓
IB		✓	✓				✓
IMPD			✓				
Subject information sheet/consent		✓	✓	✓	✓		
CTA	✓	✓	✓		✓	✓	✓
IRAS	✓	✓		✓	✓		
Risk assessment/plan	✓	✓	✓	✓	✓	✓	✓
CRF	✓			✓	✓		✓
Contract[a]		✓			✓	✓	
MP/DMP/SAP					✓	✓	
SAE report							✓

[a] Contracts may relate to sponsor, investigator site and vendors (for example, laboratories, niche providers, manufacturing sites, medics, freelancers). Contracts are discussed in Chapter 1.
CRF, case report form; CTA, clinical trial authorisation; DMP, data management plan; IB, investigator's brochure; IMP, investigational medicinal product; IMPD, investigational medicinal product dossier; IRAS, Integrated Research Application System; MP, monitoring plan; SAE, serious adverse event; SAP, statistical analysis plan

formal procedures. These documents are also key trial documents. Common examples at an investigator site are source worksheets, accountability logs or pharmacy dispensing guidelines. If an organisation is preparing such documents, the sponsor should have adequate oversight either by review and approval of the documents themselves or the methods employed by the organisation to prepare these documents, as otherwise the trial activities conducted at that organisation could be jeopardised. Therefore, identification of these documents by the sponsor's representatives managing the organisation (for example, the monitor or trial manager) is essential. There have been numerous examples where the sponsor was unaware of documents produced by third parties, and as a result had failed to identify non-compliances, which could have been avoided with adequate sponsor oversight of these documents. For example:

- At an investigator site, it was identified by the inspector that some of the paediatric subjects had been under-dosed according to the protocol. It became apparent that the investigator had prepared an 'investigator protocol' which changed the dosing regimen to mg/kg with a maximum dose at a particular weight, as per standard hospital practice, rather than the protocol-defined regimen of mg/kg with no upper dose limit. The sponsor had not been aware of this document and had not identified the dosing non-compliances during monitoring, which could have impacted on the results and potentially the conclusion of the trial.

- An investigator site pharmacy used its local standard accountability forms rather than the forms provided by the sponsor. The sponsor had agreed to this without reviewing the local forms against its own template and requirements. As a result, key information for full subject-level traceability of the investigational medicinal product (IMP) (that is, which subjects received particular doses/batches, and on which dates) could not be reconstructed at that site from the documentation.

4.7 Key trial document considerations

4.7.1 Risk assessment

It is a requirement of units that are accredited as part of the Voluntary MHRA Phase I Accreditation Scheme to produce a risk assessment for all proposed trials (see Chapter 12). For those clinical trials that apply the risk-adapted approach (see section 2.4), a risk assessment should be conducted. However, it is recommended that a full bespoke risk assessment is completed for all trials.

A risk assessment can:

- identify the potential risks to trial subjects and to the reliability of trial results, and the actions necessary to mitigate them
- assist in determining which key trial documents may be needed
- identify input required from the members of the trial team or external experts
- identify requirements for safety monitoring
- identify trial management requirements, which can assist in the planning and resource aspects of the trial (for example, identification of trial monitoring requirements so that these can be budgeted for in any funding application)
- categorise the risk associated with the IMP and its use; for lower-risk category trials this may simplify the requirements for both obtaining regulatory approvals and conducting the trial
- identify the potential for adverse event monitoring, record keeping, IMP storage and documentation requirements to be adapted.

The risk assessment should be clearly documented. Ideally, it should be a separate document in its own right and it is therefore considered a key trial document; however, it could be included as part of the protocol. It is recommended that the risk assessment is produced prior to finalisation of the protocol as the risk assessment and mitigation may influence the trial design and trial procedures.

The risk assessment would typically be undertaken by a multi-disciplinary team able to consider all the various aspects of the trial. This team may include:

- a medically qualified doctor with understanding of the therapeutic area and the therapeutic use of the proposed IMP (for example, medical monitor or chief investigator)
- a pharmacist/toxicologist/pharmacologist who has a detailed understanding of the IMP (particularly important for potential Type B and C category trials)
- a statistician with relevant experience of medical statistics
- a person with an appropriate level of understanding of applicable regulatory, legal and GCP requirements (for example, regulatory affairs, quality assurance or research governance personnel)
- other personnel as necessary (for example, research nurses, data management personnel, trial managers or medical writers).

The real risk of the trial is obtained by an evaluation of the potential risks associated with all the interventions in the trial protocol and not just from the IMP authorisation status. Appendix 2 of the 'risk-adapted approach guidance' indicates areas for consideration in conducting this risk assessment. This risk assessment would identify the specific risks and vulnerabilities in the trial and identify actions to mitigate them. For example, a trial may be assessed as category Type A based on the risk of the IMP and its use; however, there may be other risks associated with the trial procedures or the use of a vulnerable population that would mean that there were other important risks to consider and the trial may not necessarily be overall a lower-risk trial. Conversely, the risk assessment process can also identify areas where traditional GCP practice could be adapted, as no particular risk is identified. For example, for an IMP used as per normal clinical practice, there may be no requirement to monitor temperature during storage.

Aspects an organisation may consider when conducting the risk assessment include:

- IMP requirements of the trial (for example, sourcing, manufacturing, packaging strategies, labelling requirements, dosing strengths, blinding requirements)
- any country-specific risks (for example, differences in clinical practice, local regulations)
- investigator site staff experience and training requirements in the protocol, GCP and in use of the IMP at both a generic site level and an individual site level (for example, if specific risks were identified at the site assessment visit).

Implementing a process to define the risk for the various areas assessed is recommended. There are already published methodologies that may be suitable for application to clinical trials, but as yet there are no specific validated methods for clinical trials. The process may be quantitative or qualitative, but it is suggested that it includes an assessment of the impact of the hazard and the probability/likelihood of occurrence. (Caution is advised when using any scoring system for categorising overall levels of risk as high, medium or low, to ensure that a specific high-risk vulnerability is not missed which may require a specific risk mitigation.) Additionally, it is recommended that the risk assessment includes a summary of the discussion of the area assessed as this may be the rationale for implementing adapted traditional GCP practices. Examples of 'real-life' risk assessments are available on the GCP Forum page of the MHRA website.

Once the risk assessment or risk mitigation plan is finalised and approved, the documents must[3] be retained in the TMF. However, it is advisable to circulate the documents (where appropriate) to relevant trial personnel, so that they are aware of their content. It is also recommended that one person has responsibility for overseeing that the mitigations or actions planned from the risk assessment have been implemented and undertaken; this would typically be the responsibility of the project manager or chief investigator.

The sponsor should undertake a continual review of the risk assessment, which is particularly important when new information becomes available. For example, the risk assessment should be re-examined following a protocol amendment, after serious breaches or when new data are obtained (new summary of product characteristics (SPC), related non-clinical/clinical trial results are released, a data monitoring committee meeting or interim analysis takes place). Ideally, any review of the risk assessment would be documented to ensure that there is evidence that it was assessed (even when no changes were required).

4.7.2   Clinical trial protocol and amendments

There should be a defined process for the development of the protocol and how the document is ultimately approved by the sponsor. Ideally, there will also be a template that the project team can use to facilitate the production of protocols consistently containing all the required[2] elements. The process should define who is responsible for overseeing the production of the protocol and for coordinating input from other members of the project team; this may be the project manager or chief investigator.

The production of the protocol will involve a number of parties; this should include at a minimum a medically qualified doctor (and ideally the chief investigator or a principal investigator), a biostatistician and a clinical pharmacologist. It is recommended that it should also include the clinical supplies function or pharmacy, the safety, data management and clinical operations function, and other ancillary parties depending on the nature of the trial (for example, toxicologist, medical physicist or clinical radiation expert).

Any amendment to the clinical protocol should follow a similar preparation, review and sign-off process, although, depending on the reason and content of the amendment, it may not require input from all the original functions.

4.7.3 Investigator's brochure

The IB documents all relevant information about the IMP, including chemical structure, non-clinical trials and clinical trials. The IB should also detail which adverse reactions are expected and their frequency of occurrence, giving valuable safety information and guidance to the investigator, as this will be used for assessing expectedness and will determine the expedited reporting requirements of any suspected unexpected serious adverse reactions (SUSARs).

As with the protocol, there should be a defined process for the development of the IB, including who is responsible for overseeing the production and coordinating input from other members of the project team (this may be the trial manager or the regulatory affairs function) and how the document is ultimately approved by the sponsor. The sponsor may also have a template that can be used to facilitate its production.

The production of the IB will usually involve input from a number of functions, including non-clinical/translational scientists, safety function, medical advisors, clinical operations and the regulatory function.

The IB must[4] be reviewed on an annual basis. This review must[3] be documented, even if it was decided that no updates to the document were necessary. This is especially important, as the IB may be relevant across multiple clinical trials using the same product. Documentation of the review can be achieved in a number of ways, for example:

- issuing a file note
- using a form to document both the review and the decision to continue using the existing version of the IB or the decision to change the document
- re-issuing an up-versioned IB on an annual basis.

In the non-commercial sector, a full IB is not always required as authorised products are more commonly used in these clinical trials. Where an IB is not required, the appropriate section of the SPC may be used as the reference safety information for assessments of expectedness. However, where an IB is produced (for example, where an authorised product is being used outside its licensed indication or subject population), it may be appropriate to prepare an abbreviated IB to cover any data regarding its use in the new indication or subject population and to append the SPC. If this is the case, the same responsibilities as above would apply; however, it is likely that there might only be input from the chief investigator.

4.7.4   Investigational medicinal product dossier

An IMPD is a highly technical document, usually produced by the regulatory function in conjunction with the clinical supplies team. It contains full details of the chemical and pharmaceutical quality of the IMP (for example, the formulation, manufacturing processes and stability data). See section 2.2.5 for further details on the content of this document.

4.7.5   Subject information sheet and informed consent documentation

Alongside the development of the protocol, the subject information sheet and informed consent form should be produced.

As with the protocol and IB, there should be a defined process for the development of these documents, which should include who is responsible for overseeing their production (for example, this may be the trial manager, chief investigator or R&D office) and how the document is approved by the sponsor. The sponsor may have a template that can be used to facilitate the production of these documents or use a checklist to ensure that all the relevant content is present.

Production of these documents usually involves input from a number of functions, including the clinical operations function, a medically qualified doctor and the safety function. It is also useful for commercial sponsors to involve one of the investigators (either the chief or a principal investigator) in the review. An individual should be responsible for ensuring the information in the subject information sheet and informed consent form is consistent with that in the protocol and IB/SPC.

The information to be included in the subject information sheet and consent form will be determined by the subject population being recruited into the trial (for example, if they are minors or incapacitated adults there are special requirements for the informed consent process; see section 3.3.6 for further details) as well as the type of IMP under investigation and trial activities being conducted. For example:

- in gene therapy IMP trials, additional genotyping samples may be required which the subject will need to be notified about and provide consent for

- mandatory or optional blood sampling (that is, optional pharmacokinetic or genotyping)
- adverse reactions for any procedures being undertaken (for example, MRI, blood sampling and endoscopy)
- who is taking consent (that is, if this is not a medically qualified doctor, is this apparent, and how will access to a medically qualified doctor be described/documented if required)?
- who is giving consent (for example, someone with parental responsibility for a minor or a legal representative for an incapacitated adult)?

4

4.7.6   Clinical study report

The final outcome of the clinical trial is the production of the clinical study report (CSR) or a publication. This document should accurately reflect the objectives of the trial, the summary of what happened and the outcome or results. This should ideally follow the format and concept detailed in ICH GCP.

There should be a defined process for the development of the CSR, including who is responsible for overseeing its production and how the document is reviewed, QC checked and then approved by the sponsor. The sponsor may have a template that can be used to facilitate the production of the CSR.

The QC step is important in the production of the CSR. Data listings are generally produced directly from the database; however, the CSR may also contain data within in-text tables. It is therefore recommended that the process for the development of the CSR also considers the production and accuracy of any in-text tables to ensure these are correct (that is, provided as part of the statistical output or, if manually produced, showing evidence of QC of the in-text tables).

As the CSR or publication reflects the conduct of the trial and provides the summary of the results, it is important that it contains a listing of all the significant non-compliances that occurred during the trial and how these contributed to the analysis. As described in section 1.3.5, it is important that there is a definition of which non-compliances are considered significant and non-significant and that there is a mechanism for the collection and assessment of non-compliances. In addition there should be a process for ensuring that significant non-compliances are provided to the statistician (to assess the impact on the population for inclusion in the analysis) and also provided to those writing the CSR for inclusion in the report.

It has been a common finding on inspection that it has not been apparent whether all the protocol and GCP non-compliances have been documented in the CSR. For example:

- Subjects had not met the eligibility criteria but had been waived into the study. The CSR, however, stated that all subjects had been eligible.
- Only a selected number of non-compliances (that is, those identified from the CRF) were included in the CSR as there was no process to collect, circulate and assess deviations from other sources (for example, those identified at site by the trial team or by monitoring activities, or identified during analysis of samples by clinical laboratories).
- The CSR and protocol deviation logs were inconsistent.
- There was no definition of significant non-compliances, and there was no documented review of the non-compliances to verify that all those considered significant were actually listed in the CSR.

A statement of compliance with GCP is usually included in the CSR. If this is included, there should be an assessment of whether this statement requires qualification based on the conduct of the trial and any departures from the protocol and GCP non-compliance that occurred.

4.7.7   Other documents

Other key trial documents not covered in this chapter, but described elsewhere in this guide include:

- monitoring plan – section 7.3.4
- development update safety reports (DSURs) – section 5.15
- drug accountability forms – section 6.13
- statistical analysis plan – section 9.7.

4.8   Chapter legislative references

Throughout this chapter, specific terminology – 'must', 'required' or 'requirement' – has been used to interpret activities that are legislative requirements. These terms have been number-coded in the text where used, and the corresponding reference in the legislation can be found below.

1.   Schedule 1, Part 2 (4) of SI 2004/1031

2.   Schedule 1, Part 2 (7) of SI 2004/1031

3.   Regulation 31A (4) of SI 2004/1031

4.   Regulation 3A of SI 2004/1031

5.   Regulation 31A (6) and (9) of SI 2004/1031

4

Pharmacovigilance for clinical trials

5

5.1 Relevant terminology

To determine the safety reporting requirements that apply to a trial, it must first be established whether the trial is interventional or non-interventional (Chapter 2). Only interventional trials fall within the remit of the Clinical Trials Regulations, and therefore this chapter is limited to the safety reporting requirements for such trials.

While the chapter includes guidance for trials that are investigating the use of authorised products (that is, products that have a licence or authorisation), it does not include pharmacovigilance requirements for non-interventional studies conducted on authorised products used in the post-authorisation setting (such as non-interventional post-authorisation safety studies), which fall outside the remit of the Directive 2001/20/EC and the SI 2004/1031. Pharmacovigilance requirements for such post-authorisation safety studies are covered by the pharmacovigilance regulations (Regulation 726/2004 as amended by 1235/2010, Directive 2001/83/EC as amended by 2010/84/EU), relevant implementing measures and EU Good Pharmacovigilance Practice Guidance.

The definitions given in Table 5.1 may further assist in the clarification of safety reporting requirements.

5.2 Introduction to safety reporting

Clinical trials may be designed to look at the safety and tolerability of a single drug, or may look at the efficacy of the product in comparison with similar treatments or placebos. In terms of ensuring that the safety of trial subjects is protected, all drugs involved in clinical trials are relevant. Throughout this chapter, in addition to the Clinical Trials Regulations, the revised European Commission 'Detailed guidance on the collection, verification and presentation of adverse event/reaction reports arising from clinical trials on medicinal products for human use' (hereinafter 'detailed guidance CT-3') has been referenced. In addition to EudraLex Volume 10 (where detailed guidance CT-3 can be found), the MHRA website and EudraVigilance website (http://eudravigilance.ema.europa.eu) should also be consulted for up-to-date guidance.

As per the definition of an investigational medicinal product (IMP), all drugs used in clinical trials as comparators, even those with a marketing authorisation, are considered IMPs. Comparators are therefore subject to the same reporting requirements as the test drug, and it is the responsibility of the sponsor, not the marketing authorisation holder (MAH), to report adverse events in relation to comparators. There are also situations where non-investigational medicinal products (nIMPs) are subject to reporting requirements (see section 5.10).

The reporting requirements[1] for interventional clinical trials are described below, including guidance on how adverse events should be recorded. Within Part 5 of SI 2004/1031, the majority of the pharmacovigilance responsibilities are documented as being the responsibility of the sponsor. It is possible for the sponsor to delegate

Table 5.1 Definitions of terms used in clinical trial safety reporting

Term	Definition
Adverse event	Any untoward medical occurrence in a subject to whom a medicinal product has been administered, including occurrences which are not necessarily caused by or related to that product.
Adverse reaction	Any untoward and unintended response in a subject to an investigational medicinal product which is related to any dose administered to that subject.
Suspected unexpected serious adverse reaction	A serious adverse reaction, the nature and severity of which is not consistent with the information about the medicinal product in question set out: • in the case of a product with a marketing authorisation, in the summary of product characteristics for that product • in the case of any other investigational medicinal product, in the investigator's brochure relating to the trial in question.
Serious adverse event, serious adverse reaction or unexpected serious adverse reaction	Any adverse event, adverse reaction or unexpected adverse reaction respectively that: • results in death • is life-threatening • requires hospitalisation or prolongation of existing hospitalisation • results in persistent or significant disability or incapacity • consists of a congenital anomaly or birth defect. 'Important medical events' may also be considered serious if they jeopardise the subject or require an intervention to prevent one of the above consequences. The term 'life-threatening' in the definition of 'serious' refers to an event in which the patient was at risk of death at the time of the event; it does not refer to an event which hypothetically might have caused death if it were more severe.
Reference safety information	The information used for assessing whether an adverse reaction is expected. This is contained in either the investigator's brochure or the summary of product characteristics.

some or all of these functions; however, this should be clearly defined in writing. For example, a commercial pharmaceutical company may contract pharmacovigilance reporting functions to a contract research organisation (CRO), in which case the responsibilities for reporting should be clearly defined in agreements. In the non-commercial sector, safety reporting functions are often delegated to the chief investigator of the trial. It is important in this scenario that the investigator is fully and formally informed of those delegated functions, and that the procedures in place within the sponsor organisation are clear as to who is responsible for what. This should include a clear definition of who is responsible for reporting to the competent authorities, research ethics committees (RECs) and investigators, and the required timelines for this reporting (Chapter 1 describes mechanisms to maintain oversight of pharmacovigilance activities).

For all aspects of safety reporting for clinical trials, there should be clear procedures in place within the sponsor organisation to ensure that the regulatory requirements described in Part 5 of SI 2004/1031 and the associated EU guidance are complied with (see paragraph 17 of the detailed guidance CT-3). This should be considered in relation to all of the requirements described in this chapter. The clinical trial protocol should include a clear safety section, with definitions, procedures and responsibilities for recording and reporting adverse events and serious adverse events (SAEs). Sponsors may want to consider developing standard templates to ensure that all these elements are included in each protocol.

An overview of the flow of adverse event assessment and reporting is provided in Figure 5.1. This chapter will discuss each step in detail.

5.3   Adverse events – recording and notification

The investigator is required[2] to report to the sponsor any adverse events (including abnormal laboratory results) that are identified in the protocol as critical to evaluations of the safety of the trial. The sponsor is required[3] to keep detailed records of all adverse events relating to a clinical trial that are reported to it by the investigators for that trial. There is also a requirement[4] for the sponsor to produce an annual report which includes a listing of all serious adverse reactions (SARs) and a summary report of the subjects' safety. In many trials, in particular for those with unlicensed medicines, it is expected that the investigator keeps a record of all adverse events that occur for a trial subject and that all of these are reported to the sponsor, either immediately as an SAE, or as defined in the protocol. The investigator should assess adverse events for seriousness and also for causality in relation to the IMP(s) and/or comparator therapy in accordance with the protocol. This enables the collection of all the safety data during the trial, which will assist sponsors and competent authorities in gaining an understanding of the safety profile of the IMP.

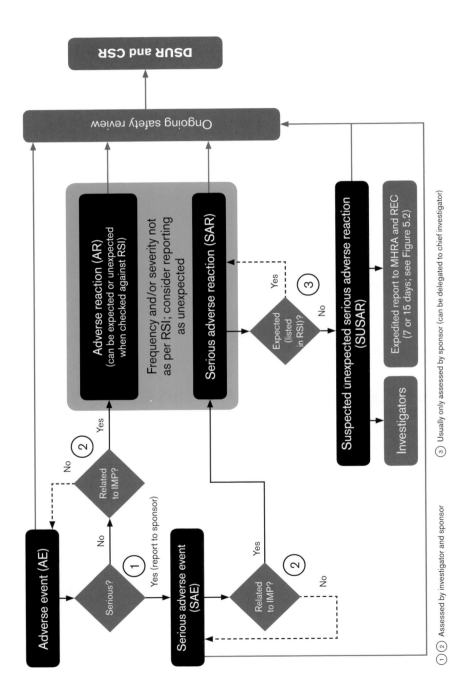

Figure 5.1 Overview of collection and reporting of adverse events

① ② Assessed by investigator and sponsor   ③ Usually only assessed by sponsor (can be delegated to chief investigator)

CSR, clinical summary report; DSUR, development safety update report; IMP, investigational medicinal product; REC, research ethics committee; RSI, reference safety information

While there is no legal requirement for investigators to record all non-serious adverse events from a trial, when sponsors are determining what adverse events require recording and reporting, the principles of Good Clinical Practice (GCP) referred to in SI 2004/1031, in particular those relating to the safety of the subject and the integrity of the data, must[5] be considered. This could be documented, for example, in the trial risk assessment.

However, in the context of the clinical care of the patient, it is routine practice to record adverse events in the patient's medical notes. It is also recommended that this includes the documentation of the assessment of causality, severity and seriousness. In the case where the patient is a subject in a clinical trial, these adverse events are also recorded in the case report forms (CRFs), if used (unless the protocol stipulates otherwise). An ongoing log of adverse events is often kept in the CRFs at the investigator site, which can be used by the sponsor to pick up new trends – for example an increased frequency of a non-serious expected event that may be linked to the IMP (see section 5.8).

In some trials there may be non-serious adverse events that the sponsor has identified as being adverse events of interest, or important to the evaluation of the safety of the trial. These may be related to a specific safety concern that non-clinical work has identified and may require close monitoring (for example, changes in ECGs, changes in liver function tests). These must[2] be defined in the protocol, and must[6] then be reported to the sponsor in accordance with the reporting requirements and timeframes described in the protocol. These events may not meet the requirements for expedited reporting to competent authorities but may be of special interest to the sponsor, or may even be part of the stopping criteria for a Phase I study. Such events are likely to be study- or IMP-specific and dependent on the known data on the IMP under investigation.

For trials in licensed medicines falling into the Type A and Type B categories as defined in the MRC/DH/MHRA paper 'Risk-adapted approaches to the management of clinical trials of investigational medicinal products' (hereinafter 'risk-adapted approach guidance'), there is some potential for the trial protocol to clarify any recording and reporting requirements for adverse events that may have been adapted based on a risk assessment. For example, some trials in IMPs that have a marketing authorisation may be considered low risk and extensive safety data on the product may already be available. As it is therefore highly unlikely that the trial will reveal any new safety information on the product, there may be little benefit in the investigator recording all adverse events beyond normal clinical practice. Trials more likely to be suitable for taking a risk-adapted approach are those trials in medicines that have been authorised for a long time and that have been used extensively. In particular, this may apply to 'P' products (a category of medicine which does not require a prescription but which has to be sold under the supervision of a pharmacist; 'P' appears on the label) and 'OTC' (over the counter) products. The trial may be identical to using the medicine in normal clinical practice; the only difference may be randomisation. Any modification to the expectation of recording and reporting all adverse events must[7] be explicitly justified in the safety monitoring plan or protocol. The safety monitoring plan should be provided to the MHRA in the application (or notification) for the clinical trial authorisation (CTA). This would enable the MHRA Clinical Trials Unit (CTU) to assess the planned safety monitoring on a case-by-case basis. When taking a risk-adapted approach, potential modifications could include specifying SAEs that do not require[7] immediate reporting, and reduced recording and reporting of certain adverse events – for example, non-serious adverse reactions listed in the summary of product characteristics (SPC).

NHS Trusts also operate incident reporting systems. Reporting systems are vital in helping NHS organisations analyse the type, frequency and severity of incidents and the organisations can then use that information to make changes to improve patient care. Incident reporting systems may also capture adverse events; it is therefore recommended that the system is considered as part of the safety reporting process.

5.4   Serious adverse events

5.4.1   Serious adverse events – recording and reporting

The investigator must[8] immediately report to the sponsor any SAE that occurs for a subject at a trial site at which they are responsible for the conduct of a clinical trial. It is therefore expected that trial protocols stipulate immediate reporting of SAEs to the sponsor in order to fulfil this requirement. In practice, this means reporting within 24 hours of the investigator's knowledge of the event (paragraph 29 of the detailed guidance CT-3 specifies that in no circumstances should this period be longer than 24 hours).

This report can be made either verbally or in writing; however, following the immediate report, the investigator must[9] make a detailed written report on the event. Typically, immediate reporting is done by fax or email, but the protocol should describe the reporting mechanism, and it is recommended that this also includes any back-up procedures for SAE reporting within either the sponsor organisation or the designated vendor. The out-of-hours contact process for advice on safety and unblinding, as appropriate to the trial, would also be described here (see section 5.11). Whatever mechanism is used for reporting, there should be sufficient cover of, for example, the fax machine or email inbox, to ensure that events are picked up and processed in a timely manner by the sponsor or CRO (this includes during holiday periods). There should also be a process in place for triage of these events when received to ensure that those that meet expedited reporting requirements are identified and processed without delay.

The timelines for suspected unexpected serious adverse reaction (SUSAR) reporting purposes (see section 5.5) start at 'day 0', which is the day that the sponsor actually receives the information containing the minimum reporting criteria (rather than the day that the sponsor picks up and processes this information, which could lead to late reporting if there is a delay in this). If reporting has been contracted out, 'day 0' would be the date of receipt by the contracted organisation. It is recommended that this is specified in the sponsor's or vendor's written procedure(s) to facilitate timely reporting.

Where trial end-points are adjudicated and reviewed by a committee, there should be a procedure in place to ensure that this is done in a timely manner. If an event was judged by the committee to be an SAE and not a trial end-point (as defined in the protocol) this may be reported late in the absence of timely review, which would become a more serious issue if it led to late SUSAR reporting. This is a relatively common issue seen with such committees.

SAEs do not in general need to be actively sought out once the trial has ended, unless this has been specified as required in the protocol (paragraph 32 of the detailed guidance CT-3). However, SAEs experienced by a subject after the treatment of that subject has ended should be reported to the sponsor if the investigator becomes aware of them.

There are specific long-term follow-up requirements for trials of advanced therapy medicinal products; these arrangements should be covered in the protocol (or associated document) submitted during the trial authorisation process (see section 5.13).

Within the protocol, it is possible to define certain SAEs that do not require immediate reporting to the sponsor, despite their meeting the definition of an SAE. For example, there may be justification to adapt the safety reporting according to the risk assessment for the trial. This may be because the IMP is a well-established medicine for which a great deal of safety information already exists. The nature and extent of safety monitoring should be based on the risk assessment and a safety monitoring plan should be developed (see Appendix 2 of the risk-adapted approach guidance). This safety monitoring plan should be included with the CTA application, either within the protocol or in the cover letter, and approved by the MHRA as part of the authorisation process.

In addition, other events such as pre-planned hospitalisation, trial end-points or disease-defining events may also be stipulated in the protocol as not requiring immediate reporting. For example:

- hospitalisation for routine pre-planned events (such as hip replacement, labour and birth, routine transfusions), an operation that was planned as part of eligibility for the trial (for example, knee replacement, fibroid treatments) and chemotherapy
- prolongation of hospitalisation without an associated adverse event (for example, prolonged hospitalisation while appropriate social care is set up for elderly patients)
- adverse reactions considered expected as part of the trial treatment (as per the SPC), such as the standard expected side effects of chemotherapy in an oncology trial or anticipated adverse events related to trial procedures (for example, low blood pressure during dialysis, tiredness or sore skin following radiotherapy) – unless the frequency or severity of such events is unusual
- anticipated events from disease progression – for example, AIDS-defining events in an HIV trial or disease progression in oncology trials
- end-points such as re-infarction or death in a myocardial infarction study.

Such events should still be recorded by the trial team in the subjects' notes and CRF (if required).

Abnormal laboratory parameters may also require reporting within the same timeframes as SAEs. These must[10] be specified in the protocol and made clear to the concerned laboratory to ensure that these 'alert values' are reported immediately to the investigator for onward reporting to the sponsor.

There are also a number of safety issues that do not require expedited reporting, such as new events that are related to the conduct of the trial (for example, an SAE associated with the trial procedure, lack of efficacy or a major safety finding in relation to non-clinical studies). These are still important safety events and may affect the trial. Although they do not meet the definition of a SUSAR, other actions may be appropriate (for example, an urgent safety measure, a substantial amendment or early termination).

The sponsor organisation's SAE reporting requirements should be described in a written procedure (in addition to a description within the trial protocol). This could include providing a template for the SAE reporting form. This ensures consistency of the data captured in SAE forms across all sponsored trials. Any study-specific SAE forms adapted from the template should be reviewed by the sponsor against the standard sponsor form, to ensure that it captures all of the required data elements (see section 5.6.3). This is also recommended in non-commercial organisations when, for example, SAE forms are developed at a departmental level, such as the research and development (R&D) office or within oncology trial centres. Examples have been seen on inspection where SAE forms were not designed to capture the seriousness and the causality of adverse events, thus making it impossible to identify SUSARs which required expedited reporting.

It is common within the non-commercial sector and in smaller organisations for pharmacovigilance functions to be delegated by the sponsor to the investigator and trial team, often due to a lack of medical expertise or limited resource at the sponsor's R&D office. Research nurses in trial teams often perform many pharmacovigilance activities, such as completing the SAE form and obtaining follow-up information about the outcome of the SAE or SUSAR. Often the research nurse will complete the initial SAE details for the form to be sent to the sponsor; however, a medical review and assessment of the SAE (particularly with regard to causality and seriousness) is also required[11], and this assessment must[12] be clearly documented. This is usually achieved by the investigator (or another delegated medically qualified doctor from the trial team) signing the SAE form to confirm their review. It is important that all key trial activities are fully captured in the trial paperwork.

5.4.2   Serious adverse event follow-up

If the trial team has initially been unable to obtain all the necessary information from the subject and/or the treating medically qualified doctor, the basic minimum information on the SAE should still be transmitted to the sponsor (for the minimum information needed for a report, see section 5.6.3). Attempts should be made by the trial team to obtain further follow-up information on the SAE to ensure that a complete record of the events has been captured, and this information should be transferred to the sponsor.

Sponsors should ensure that there is appropriate follow-up for SAEs that are reported to them. On a practical level, tracking and follow-up of SAE reports could be done, for example, using a spreadsheet or simply through making electronic calendar entries and associated alerts. It is not necessary to put in place a complicated technical system for such follow-ups, but whatever system is used should ensure that SAE reports missing any key information are followed up in a timely manner to complete the dataset and track the welfare of the subject.

It is recommended that a record of all follow-up attempts is maintained as, in the event of the information not being received, this would demonstrate due diligence on the part of the trial team and the sponsor.

5.4.3 Pregnancy

Pregnancy does not meet the definition of an SAE. A congenital anomaly or birth defect is, however, considered an SAE. When a pregnancy occurs in a trial, either in a female subject or the female partner of a male subject, this should be followed up until at least the end of the pregnancy, whether that is a live birth, abortion etc. It is recommended that pregnancy cases are followed up initially as soon as the sponsor is notified, and then tracked in order to be able to request further follow-up near term, to allow collection of information on the pregnancy outcome. Without follow-up of the pregnancy, it would not be possible for the trial team to know if a congenital anomaly or birth defect occurred, and therefore if there was an SAE that must[8] be included in the safety evaluation of the IMP. Follow-up is of course dependent on obtaining informed consent for this from the subject (or their partner in the case of male trial subjects). It may not be necessary for all trials to collect information on pregnant partners of male subjects; however, if there is a known or suspected effect on spermatogenesis or if there is potential for the IMP to be transferred to the foetus in the seminal fluid, follow-up would be necessary. This should therefore be dealt with in the protocol (and risk assessment) and also included in the trial consent form. Methods for managing follow-up of SAEs also apply to follow-up of pregnancies and are described in section 5.4.2.

5.5 Suspected unexpected serious adverse reactions

5.5.1 SUSAR recording and reporting

The purpose of reporting adverse events in an expedited manner to the competent authority is to provide an early warning of any potential issues with IMPs or with the conduct of the trial in the time between the annual reviews of the risk–benefit profile of the IMP in the development safety update reports (DSURs).

Therefore it is a legislative requirement[13] that the sponsor must ensure that all relevant information about a SUSAR that occurs during the course of a clinical trial in the UK, and that is fatal or life-threatening, is recorded and reported as soon as possible to:

- the competent authority in the UK
- the competent authorities of any European Economic Area (EEA) state other than the UK in which the trial is being conducted
- the relevant REC in the UK.

5

This report must[13] be no later than 7 calendar days after the sponsor first becomes aware of the reaction.

A further follow-up report regarding any additional information relevant to the SUSAR is required[13] within 8 calendar days of submitting the initial report. It should be noted that only deaths associated with a SUSAR need to be reported in an expedited manner; there is no requirement to report, in an expedited manner, all deaths on a clinical trial.

All other SUSARs, that is, those that are not fatal or life-threatening, must[13] be reported no later than 15 calendar days after the sponsor is first aware of the reaction. This reporting is required to both the competent authority and the REC. Where significant new information on an already reported case is received by the sponsor, the clock starts again at 'day 0', that is, the date when new information is received. This new information is then reported as the follow-up report within the 15-day timeframe (or 7 days for fatal and life-threatening events). These requirements should be covered within the sponsor's procedures for safety reporting, including the timelines of reporting, and how and by whom the reporting is to be done.

It should be noted that paragraph 41 of the detailed guidance CT-3 specifies that the purpose of the reporting obligation of SUSARs to the RECs is to make them aware of SUSARs that have occurred in the territory of the Member State concerned. This effectively means that, in the UK, there is no longer a requirement in global trials for the sponsor to submit regular line listings of all SUSARs that originate outside the Member State concerned (six-monthly line listings were commonly submitted in the past).

The sponsor is also required[13] to ensure that the investigators responsible for the conduct of a trial are informed of any SUSARs that occur in relation to an IMP used in the trials they are involved with. This is the case whether that SUSAR occurs in the trial that the investigator is involved in, or another trial using the same IMP for which the sponsor is responsible. No timelines are specified in the regulations for reporting to investigators; however, this should be done in a timely manner to ensure that investigators are kept fully informed of all safety information. Should new safety information arise that may impact on the ongoing safety of trial subjects, then concerned investigators should be informed immediately.

It is recommended that information relating to SUSARs is provided in a concise and practical way to investigators, such as by collating SUSARs into a line listing in periods warranted by the nature of the research or clinical development project and the volume of SUSARs generated. It is expected that this will vary between different IMPs and clinical development programmes and this decision should be documented (for example, in the trial risk assessment). Therefore, if an organisation has a procedure that states, for example, that for all trials investigators will be informed on a six-monthly basis, this would not necessarily be acceptable as this does not take into account the differing nature of the trials and IMPs. Investigator listings should be accompanied by a concise summary of the evolving safety profile of the IMP (see the detailed guidance CT-3).

It is recommended that sponsors also consider how it can be demonstrated that these reports have been reviewed by the investigator, as they may be sent electronically or made accessible through an internet portal. Typically, investigators sign and date paper reports to confirm their review, so this system would need to be replicated electronically. If reports are made available via an internet portal, the sponsor should ensure that concerned investigators have access to the portal and have been trained on how to access the information, before the trial commences. For example, in one trial using such a portal, the inspectors found that the email notifications to alert the investigator of new information in the portal were all being held by the hospital's spam filter and the investigator was unaware of their existence. It has also been found that the safety reports at an investigator site were incomplete or had been recently added to the investigator site file by the trial monitor prior to the inspection, indicating that there had been a failure of the process for ongoing communication to and review of safety issues by the investigator.

5.5.2   SUSAR reporting – sponsor or investigator?

Some organisations are structured so that the sponsor (for example, an R&D office) takes responsibility for reporting SUSARs to competent authorities. In some situations, the chief investigator or trial team reports SUSARs on behalf of the sponsor. It is important that when sponsor responsibilities are delegated to the chief investigator, clear and detailed arrangements and/or procedures are put in place prior to the start of the trial outlining the transfer of tasks (see section 1.1.4).

In the scenario where the capture of SAEs is carried out by the investigator but the reporting of the SUSARs is performed by the non-commercial sponsor, it is still of great importance that the medically qualified investigator (or other delegated medically qualified doctor) performs the relevant seriousness and causality assessments.

In commercial organisations, reporting to the competent authorities and to the RECs may be performed by different departments; for example, the pharmacovigilance or regulatory department may interact with the competent authorities while the clinical operations department may interact with the RECs and investigators. Reporting to the REC necessitates maintenance of the names and contact details of the RECs involved in the trials of the IMP, and a robust process should be in place to track this. Inadequacies in this process have led to SUSARs being submitted on time to competent authorities, but submitted late to the RECs by the same sponsor.

5.6 Assessments and information required for reporting purposes

Reporting requirements for clinical trial adverse event reports are dependent on certain assessments, including seriousness, causality and expectedness. Seriousness and causality must[11] always be assessed by a medically qualified doctor; this is usually the investigator. Expectedness is then usually assessed by the sponsor, but may be delegated to the principal investigator or chief investigator by the sponsor.

5.6.1 Seriousness and causality assessments

Seriousness must be assessed against the standard definition in Regulation 2 of SI 2004/1031 (Table 5.1). Some medical events may jeopardise the subject or may require an intervention to prevent one of the defined criteria of seriousness. Such events (commonly referred to as 'important medical events') should also be considered as 'serious' in accordance with the definition. Examples of such events would be intensive treatment for allergic bronchospasm in an emergency room or at home; blood dyscrasias or convulsions that do not result in hospitalisation; or development of drug dependency or drug abuse.

Sponsors may use different scales to record the causality of an event. For example, a simple two-point scale may be used where the options for the suspected causal relationship are 'yes' or 'no'. Alternatively, more complex scales can be used that include terms such as 'definitely related', 'probably related', 'possibly related', 'unlikely to be related' or 'not related'. It is recommended that guidance is included in the protocol for investigators on the causality scale used. Where more than two options are available, a definition for each option can be provided together with which options equate to an adverse reaction and which equate to an adverse event (that is, which terms map to 'yes' and which to 'no' for reporting purposes).

It is important for the sponsor to ensure that, if safety reporting procedures contain a template SAE reporting form, any protocol-specific causality assessment scales are not in conflict with that used on the template SAE form. Processes should be in place to ensure consistency between documents such as the protocol, SAE forms and the CRF.

If the investigator states that the event is not related, it is recommended (where appropriate and practical) that the SAE form prompts the investigator to provide details of an alternative explanation for the event (for example, an underlying disease). If the investigator assigns the causality as 'not assessable', it is expected that the sponsor adopts a conservative approach whereby the event is deemed a suspected adverse reaction until follow-up information is received from the investigator. This also applies if the investigator does not supply a causality assessment on initial reporting, that is, the event is considered as causally related. It is important that if key information is missing from a report made to the sponsor, follow-up of this information is actively pursued, and the associated reports are updated with this follow-up information once received.

5.6.1.1 Who should make the causality assessment?

Causality assessment decisions must[11] be made by a medically qualified doctor, as these decisions require medical and scientific judgement to be used as well as knowledge of the subject concerned. If the investigator is not a medically qualified doctor, this task must[11] be formally delegated to a medically qualified doctor who is a member of the research team. The trial delegation log should reflect this. Documentation to verify that the assessment has been made by a medically qualified doctor must[12] be retained; for example, the reports could be signed and dated by the person making the assessment. If initial reports are not completed by an investigator (for example, if they are completed by the study research nurse), the follow-up reports should then contain documented evidence that the assessment decisions were made by a medically qualified doctor. It is recommended that this is supported by countersigning the SAE form and by the entries made by the medically qualified doctor in the subject's medical notes.

All adverse events judged by either the investigator or the sponsor as having a reasonable suspected causal relationship to an IMP qualify as adverse reactions. The sponsor may also make an assessment of causality. The investigator's decision should be independent of the sponsor – that is, the assessment should not be influenced by the sponsor. In the case where the sponsor assessment differs from that of the investigators' assessment, the most conservative approach should be taken when it comes to regulatory reporting. Under no circumstances should the sponsor downgrade the investigator's opinion or put the investigator under pressure to change their assessment. If the sponsor disagrees with the investigator's causality assessment, both the opinion of the investigator and the sponsor should be provided on the report (see paragraph 59 of the detailed guidance CT-3). This disagreement should be fully documented.

5.6.2   Expectedness assessments

The reference safety information (RSI) used for a clinical trial, against which expectedness assessments are made, should be clearly identified in the protocol and specified in the cover letter with the CTA application. Protocols often lack clarity on this, stating only that the 'SPC or IB' is to be used (wording potentially remaining from the protocol template text). The RSI is part of a document (investigator's brochure (IB) or SPC) that specifically references what adverse events are considered to be expected for that IMP. If the trial is international, it should be consistent in all the territories where the trial is taking place (that is, the same RSI must be used across the trial regardless of where trial sites are based). For IMPs that do not have a marketing authorisation, the reference document for safety and assessment of expectedness should be an IB. At the start of the trial, checks should be made to ensure that the risks and side effects listed in the subject information sheet given to trial subjects are consistent with those listed in the IB and/or SPC.

Generally, the sponsor will perform the assessment of expectedness; however, if this task is delegated to investigators or the chief investigator, then there should be processes in place to ensure that the individuals have access to the most appropriate, up-to-date RSI, and that the RSI is correctly understood and assessments are performed consistently. Failure to ensure this can lead to issues in safety reporting. For example, in a large multi-centre study, expectedness was delegated to individual investigators; however, as the investigators did not receive consistent training in the interpretation of expectedness, some investigators did not understand that expectedness related to what was expected for side effects of the IMP, not to what was anticipated for the particular disease area. As a result, a large number of SUSARs were under-reported as events were deemed to be expected when in fact these events were not listed in the RSI and should therefore have been assessed as unexpected.

Expectedness decisions must[14] be based purely on the content of the RSI in either the IB or SPC; other factors, such as the subject population and subject history, should not be taken into account. Expectedness is not related to what is an anticipated event within a particular disease. For example, in a trial of fluticasone in subjects with asthma, an adverse event of exacerbation of asthma may be reported. Exacerbation of asthma is not listed as an undesirable effect in the SPC, but it is certainly an anticipated event in an individual with asthma. However, if exacerbation of asthma is not in the RSI, then the event, if considered related to the IMP (and not in relation to the underlying disease), is classed as unexpected.

Many trials are conducted with more than one IMP; therefore, expectedness assessments apply to all suspect IMPs in the trial. If an SAE is suspected of being causally related to one or a number of IMPs, then expectedness will also need to be assessed for each of the IMPs in relation to the requirements for expedited reporting.

Reports which add significant information on specificity or severity of a known, already documented adverse event constitute unexpected events. For example, an event more specific or more severe than that described in the RSI would be considered unexpected. Specific examples would be acute renal failure as an expected adverse reaction with a subsequent new report of interstitial nephritis, and hepatitis with a first report of fulminant hepatitis.

Where the SPC is the RSI and the sponsor of the clinical trial is not the MAH, there should be a mechanism in place for the sponsor to check for any updates to the SPC (for example, via alerts on regulatory websites) at intervals defined in the risk assessment and it is recommended that this includes clear responsibility assigned for this activity. It is important to have a process in place to ensure that the most relevant version of the SPC is being used for the trial to make expectedness decisions. In situations where the MAH may be providing product to a sponsor for use in a trial, the agreement with the MAH may include a caveat that the sponsor must be informed when safety-related changes are made to the SPC by the MAH. The version of the SPC being used in the trial should be dated and any superseded versions should be retained with the trial documents.

For those IMPs that have a marketing authorisation, but are not being used in accordance with that marketing authorisation (for example, in a different indication), the sponsor will need to decide whether it is appropriate to use an SPC or an IB as a reference document or whether this information can be included in the protocol. It is possible, under certain circumstances, for SPCs to be used when the IMP is being used in a different indication; however, this must[15] be approved at the trial authorisation stage. Where there are significant differences between the SPC and the IB with regard to the description of those events that are considered to be expected reactions (for an IMP with a marketing authorisation in the EU), the sponsor should have a documented rationale for these differences based on available data.

A sponsor should have a robust rationale for classifying events as expected within the RSI, taking into account factors such as the type of event and possible causal relationship. In addition, the frequency with which the event is seen in the general population or population under study, together with the frequency with which the event is reported in subjects receiving the IMP compared with subjects receiving a placebo, are all considerations when assessing whether to class a reaction as expected.

If sponsors are not clear about which section of the IB is to be used as the RSI, under-reporting of SUSARs could occur. An example was seen on inspection, where an organisation had failed to report a myocardial infarction considered to be related to the IMP as a SUSAR because it used the adverse events listing in the IB; this listing contained myocardial infarction which was considered unrelated to the IMP. The listing containing adverse reactions should have been used to assess expectedness.

There should be appropriate procedures in place to ensure that SPCs and IBs are reviewed for safety information to ensure consistency. Safety monitoring activities that trigger safety changes to an SPC should lead to the consideration of whether equivalent changes in content or wording are required to the IB and the subject information sheet.

5

Examples of expectedness assessments

A subject in a trial of an anti-hypertensive treatment is hospitalised with a stroke

As the event is serious due to the hospitalisation, the research nurse completes an SAE form. The investigator reviews the SAE and decides that the event is possibly related to the IMP and is expected. The expectedness assessment that the investigator makes, however, is not based on a check against the content of the RSI for the product (in this case, the SPC); instead, it is based on the investigator's knowledge of the subject's medical history as the subject's treating medically qualified doctor. On a subsequent monitoring visit, the monitor reviews the SAE against the SPC and identifies that stroke is not listed in this document. The serious adverse reaction (SAR) is therefore unexpected, and consequently a SUSAR.

This example highlights the importance of always referring to the RSI approved for the trial when assessments of expectedness are made by the investigator, to ensure that any reaction that is unexpected and serious is correctly identified as a SUSAR and reported within the required timeframes. Late reporting of SAEs and SUSARs could lead to delays in appropriate action being taken to protect trial subjects and non-trial patients (where applicable) from newly identified safety concerns.

A subject in a trial experiences a severe rash that is assessed as being related

The treating medically qualified doctor suspects it may be Steven–Johnsons Syndrome (a potentially life-threatening skin condition). As the IMP is licensed in the UK and is being used within the licensed indication, the UK SPC is being used to assess expectedness. The SPC lists 'rash' as a known reaction to the IMP; however, since the event the subject experiences is not consistent with the severity of the terms listed in the SPC, that is, it is far more severe, this event is considered unexpected and therefore a SUSAR, rather than an expected SAR, and requires expedited reporting.

A subject in a trial experiences a seizure following the administration of the IMP

The SPC is used to assess expectedness for the IMP and it lists seizure as a known adverse reaction. However, the subject is hospitalised and dies as a result of the seizure. In this circumstance, the outcome of the adverse event is not in line with the information included in the SPC because a seizure resulting in death is not described in the SPC. Therefore, this adverse reaction should be assessed as unexpected as it is not consistent with the SPC and consequently is a SUSAR.

Some sponsors choose to inform investigators in the IB of all adverse events that have been reported with the product, for general information purposes. A clear distinction needs to be made between events that are included for general information and reactions that are considered by the sponsor to be expected for the product. This could take the form of a tabulation of expected events provided within the IB.

When the sponsor is also the MAH for an authorised product used as an IMP and a new type of adverse reaction is included as expected in the IB, procedures should be in place for the subsequent review of SPCs including consideration of whether it is appropriate to submit a variation to update the SPC. Sponsors of trials with authorised products used outside the licensed indication, and who are not the MAH, will need to monitor any changes to the SPC of the MAH and revise the IB accordingly.

5.6.2.1 When and how should the expectedness reference document be updated?

It is a legislative requirement[16] that the IB is reviewed annually. Any updates to the RSI, in either the IB or the SPC, should be communicated in a timely manner to concerned investigators. Changes to the RSI within the IB are considered as substantial amendments. Such a change would usually occur annually following the DSUR review (see paragraph 55 of the detailed guidance CT-3).

This section applies primarily to IMPs for which there is no marketing authorisation in the EU, and therefore the IB is the document used for making expectedness decisions. As the RSI is the section of the document used to determine whether an event is expected or not, the process by which this is updated is critical to ensuring that expectedness decisions are made appropriately. That is, whether or not an event is added to the RSI as an expected event will affect whether events are reported to the competent authorities and RECs as SUSARs in the future.

The process for updating the RSI can potentially lead to under-reporting of unexpected events. For example, if one occurrence of a particular reaction leads to the sponsor updating the RSI, any subsequent reports of the same reaction would not be reported in an expedited way to the competent authorities or RECs; only the first occurrence would be considered a SUSAR. This could result in reduced expedited SUSAR reporting from clinical trials to competent authorities and therefore could lead to delays in the identification of new safety issues. On the other hand, if the single occurrence is not sufficient to warrant that event being classed as expected in the reference document, then the subsequent cases would also be reported as SUSARs until enough information is held for the RSI to be updated. Similarly, if there is no effective process in place for updating the RSI as necessary, there could be over-reporting of SUSARs if expected events are not included in the document in a timely manner.

Both over-reporting and under-reporting of SUSARs can affect the understanding of the safety profile of the IMP developed by competent authorities in response to expedited reports received. If the IMP goes on to obtain a marketing authorisation, it is good practice for the expected events listed in the IB during the clinical trial stage to contribute to the development of the undesirable effects section in the SPC. It is therefore recommended that this is considered when including events as expected within the IB.

When sponsors send updated IBs to investigators, it must[12] be evident in the trial documentation when these have been received to enable confirmation of the date that the updated IB is being used at the trial site. Old versions of the RSI can be archived to ensure that they are not inadvertently used by the investigator or chief investigator for making expectedness assessments.

An update to the RSI is a substantial amendment, and it is expected that updates will be reviewed in line with the DSUR, when there is a comprehensive review of safety for that IMP. Updates may be made before that time if the new safety information warrants this. However, it should be noted that a substantial amendment of the RSI will therefore change expedited reporting requirements for individual SARs during this period; for reporting in the DSUR, the RSI that was in place at the start of the reporting period will still apply. Therefore, amending the RSI outside the DSUR production process may result in differences between the expectedness assessment of single expedited SARs and their expectedness assessment in the DSUR.

5.6.3   What information needs to go into SAE/SUSAR reports?

The following minimum data elements should be included in SAE reports (for internal processing by the sponsor) and SUSAR reports (for expedited reporting purposes) to enable full reconstruction of the event (see paragraph 97 of the detailed guidance CT-3):

- a valid EudraCT number (where applicable)
- a sponsor study number
- one identifiable coded subject
- one identifiable reporter
- one SAE/SUSAR

- at least one suspect IMP (including active substance, name, code)
- a causality assessment.

It is worth noting that the minimum information needed for reporting purposes includes the causality assessment; however, this assessment may be classed as 'unknown' on the initial report of the event.

In addition, in order for the competent authority to properly process the report electronically, the following administrative information should be provided:

- the sender's (case) safety report unique identifier
- the receipt date of the initial information from the primary source (for example, this may be the date that the investigator is notified that the subject has been admitted to another hospital)
- the receipt date of the most recent information
- the (worldwide) unique case identification number
- the sender identifier.

It is also recommended that the following information is provided as part of the SAE/SUSAR report:

- a full description of the event (or if all the information is not available at the time of the initial report, this could be included in the follow-up), including the event start date, whether or not it is resolved and, if resolved, the date of resolution
- any relevant medical history or relevant concurrent conditions that are not already listed as part of the event
- an assessment of seriousness and expectedness
- dates that the suspect drug was administered to the subject, and whether any changes to administration have been made as a result of the event (such as ceasing the medication, or changing the dose)
- details of any concomitant medications
- in the case of death, the date and cause of death
- the date that the investigator/team became aware of the event, referred to as the receipt date above. This is significant, as if, for example, the subject is admitted to a different hospital from the trial site, there may be a delay in the investigator or study team becoming aware of the event. If the date of awareness is recorded, this enables verification that the event was reported on

time to the sponsor. Without this, the event may appear to have been reported very late in some circumstances
* whether the report is an initial or a follow-up report.

5.6.3.1   Confidentiality issues

SAE reports are one of the most common causes of breaches of subject confidentiality, particularly when the reports are sent from an investigator site to the sponsor organisation. Where appropriate, there should be processes in place to ensure that no subject-identifiable information is included in these reports (unless the subject has specifically consented to this), such that only pseudo-anonymised data (that is, data where the subject code along with another piece of information, held elsewhere, would be required to identify the subject) or anonymised data are sent. In addition, there should be a process in place to remove identifiable data in the event that they are accidentally sent in with safety reports (for example, in laboratory reports, post-mortem reports and imaging results). Investigator sites and trial monitors should be trained in these processes to reduce the potential for error. If subject-identifiable information is received by the sponsor, retraining of those staff concerned should form part of the corrective actions implemented. If the trial is sponsored by the NHS Trust in which it is hosted, identifiable information is less of an issue as the information remains within the NHS Trust. However, it is still good practice to only include pseudo-anonymised or anonymised data.

5.6.4   Electronic SUSAR reporting process

The long-term plan for the European Medicines Agency's (EMA) EudraVigilance Clinical Trial Module (EVCTM) is that sponsors need only report a SUSAR to one place, and the report will then subsequently be made available to all Member States. However, EVCTM currently does not have this functionality. This means that, at the moment, sponsors need to report SUSARs to each concerned Member State separately and also ensure that the report gets into EVCTM. This can either be done by the sponsor directly, or it can be done via the competent authority in the Member State from which the SUSAR originated – for example, via the MHRA for UK SUSARs. It is envisaged that by approximately 2015 (if not before), EudraVigilance will have the required functionalities and will become the single point of reporting in the EU.

SUSAR reports can be submitted electronically to the competent authorities and also to EVCTM via the EudraVigilance Gateway or via EVWEB; both reporting tools have the functionality to direct the report to a competent authority and EVCTM (see Figure 5.2). In addition, in order to assist non-commercial organisations who may lack the technology and resources to be able to report using these options, in September 2010 the MHRA introduced the electronic (e) SUSAR reporting process via the eSUSAR online reporting tool. The eSUSAR system enables all clinical trial sponsors to report all UK-relevant SUSARs to the MHRA. UK-relevant SUSARs are those that occur in any country in a trial where there is a UK site or those that occur in a different trial but with the same IMP. On behalf of sponsors, the MHRA will forward to EVCTM those reports that originate in the UK, or those that are from outside the UK and outside the EEA. The MHRA does not forward those SUSARs that originate in the EEA but are outside the UK. The eSUSAR tool can be used to report these non-UK EEA events to the MHRA, but the sponsor still needs to fulfil its requirement to ensure that the SUSAR is reported to EVCTM (which will need to be achieved via EVWEB or the EudraVigilance Gateway or by agreement with the competent authority in the EEA state in which the SUSAR originated).

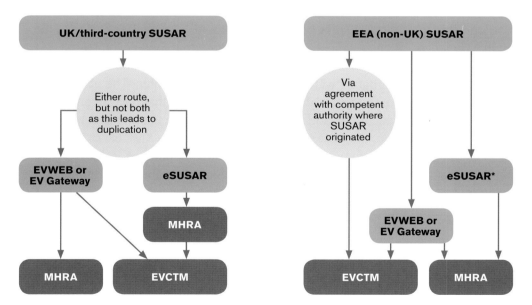

* If eSUSAR is used in this scenario, then sponsors must ensure that these SUSARs are also reported to the EVCTM via the alternative routes outlined in the diagram.

EEA, European Economic Area; EV, EudraVigilance; EVCTM, EudraVigilance Clinical Trial Module; EVWEB, EudraVigilance web interface; MHRA, Medicines and Healthcare products Regulatory Agency; SUSAR, suspected unexpected serious adverse reaction

Figure 5.2 Electronic reporting of SUSARs

5

SUSAR reports that originate in the UK and are submitted to the MHRA via the eSUSAR tool should not be submitted to the EVCTM by the trial sponsor; this will result in duplication.

There is a standard format that should be used for electronic reporting (see ICH Topic E2B 'Clinical safety data management data elements for transmission of individual case safety reports'). In addition MedDRA should be used to code these events. MedDRA stands for the 'Medical Dictionary for Regulatory Activities' and is a standardised medical terminology methodology used to classify adverse event information associated with the use of pharmaceutical products. Further information can be found at www.meddramsso.com.

Electronic reporting is required from both commercial and non-commercial trial sponsors. This can be achieved through the following systems.

5.6.4.1 MHRA eSUSAR tool

The eSUSAR website can be used to report all UK and third-country SUSAR reports to the MHRA (which are subsequently forwarded on to the EVCTM). It is also possible to report SUSARs originating in other EEA Member States to the MHRA; however, sponsors must themselves ensure that these events are reported to EVCTM. Reporting to other EEA Member State competent authorities must be done in accordance with their individual requirements. The eSUSAR website can also be used to maintain a record of reports that have been submitted for each institution, and a PDF print-out can be used to report SUSARs to the REC. In addition, the eSUSAR website produces an XML file of the report in 'E2B' format that can be uploaded into compatible databases. A record (either paper or electronic) can therefore be kept to demonstrate that requirements are being met.

Prior to using the eSUSAR website, sponsors must register their details with the MHRA, nominating an administrator. The administrator is then given a username and password. It is recommended that more than one person is registered at the sponsor, as in the event of a SUSAR occurring only those with a password are able to report. This will prevent any delays in reporting SUSARs and ensure that the sponsor has good oversight of SUSAR submissions. Some non-commercial sponsors delegate SUSAR reporting to the investigators; in this case investigators must be registered on the system to enable them to report.

5.6.4.2 EudraVigilance Gateway

Sponsors that wish to submit SUSAR reports to the MHRA in 'E2B' format via the EudraVigilance Gateway are required to successfully test electronic transmission with the MHRA prior to reporting (further information on 'E2B' reporting can be found on the MHRA website).

5.6.4.3 EVWEB

Alternatively sponsors can use the EMA EVWEB tool to submit SUSAR reports electronically (further details on this can be found on the EMA website). Sponsors that wish to submit SUSAR reports via EVWEB are required to successfully test electronic transmission with the MHRA prior to reporting (further information on 'E2B' reporting can be found on the MHRA website). As with eSUSAR reporting, it is recommended that organisations have more than one registered user for EVWEB.

5.7   Considerations for blinded trials

SUSARs should be unblinded prior to reporting to the competent authority and REC. This is in order to provide meaningful information that can enable a full evaluation of the data in the context of the safety profile of the IMP. Blinded information is not useful to the competent authority and tells it nothing about the IMP; therefore, SUSAR reports where a suspect drug is not unblinded will not be accepted. To reduce the potential for bias to occur following a SUSAR in the continuing trial, the sponsor organisation should put in place procedures to cover how unblinding can be dealt with for expedited reporting purposes without compromising the blinded members of the trial team. It would, however, be appropriate for data monitoring committees (DMCs) or persons performing ongoing safety evaluations during the trial to receive unblinded data.

In commercial organisations, unblinding is usually done by the pharmacovigilance department for reporting purposes. In the non-commercial sector, a comparable arrangement is often set up by delegating unblinding to the pharmacy department or to the R&D office, thereby ensuring that the blind of the investigators and research team is not broken. A clear written procedure should be in place covering unblinding for adverse event reporting purposes. This could include details of who needs to authorise the unblinding before it goes ahead, who must remain blinded and that the blind is only broken for the specific subject concerned. This process would usually be different from unblinding in an emergency for treatment purposes, for which a separate unblinding procedure will be needed (see section 11.4.9).

5

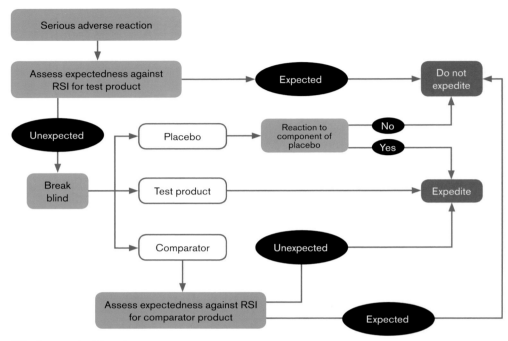

RSI, reference safety information

Figure 5.3 Unblinding in relation to SUSAR reporting

To enable processing of the SAR in a blinded trial, expectedness may be assessed initially using the assumption that the test drug has been given to the subject (see Figure 5.3). If it is assessed as unexpected as per the RSI of the test drug, the SUSAR should be unblinded for reporting. If after unblinding it is evident that the subject received the comparator, but the event still meets the criteria for a SUSAR (that is, unexpected as per the comparator reference document, which should be defined in the protocol), then it must[13] be expedited according to the requirements set out in section 5.5. If following unblinding the subject is found to have received a placebo, this event would not require expedited reporting, unless in the opinion of the investigator or sponsor the event was related to the placebo (for example, an allergic reaction to an excipient).

In some studies there are both open and blinded IMPs, that is, the test IMP is blinded, but the comparators are not. If this is the case and an SAE occurs that is considered to be related to the comparator, and is unexpected, this must[13] be expedited.

For trials in high-morbidity or high-mortality diseases, where efficacy end-points could also be SUSARs, the integrity of the clinical trial may be compromised if

---

An example of an unblinding scenario

The trial has three suspect IMPs – drug A/placebo (blinded) and drugs C and D (not blinded). A SAR of haemorrhage occurs which is unexpected (and therefore a SUSAR) in relation to C and D, but it is an expected event according to the RSI for A. All drugs are listed in the suspect IMP field of the SUSAR report since the investigator or organisation considered the event was related.

Is there a need to unblind for drug A/placebo (even though it is an expected event for A)?

Yes, firstly because it is not possible to list a drug as suspect without unblinding, as all suspect drugs require unblinding prior to reporting to the competent authority and REC. Also once the drug has been unblinded, causality may be reassessed – that is, if unblinding reveals that a placebo was given, the drug may no longer be regarded as suspect.

Therefore, in this scenario if there was only one IMP for which the event was expected, there would be no need to report and no need to unblind. However, because other IMPs were suspect, this was reported as a SUSAR and because the blinded drug was listed as suspect, it has to be unblinded (even though it was an expected event for that IMP). If the blinded drug was not listed as suspect, then it would not have to be unblinded.

5

the blind is systematically broken. Under these and similar circumstances, the sponsor must[7] specify in the protocol and reach agreement at the clinical trial authorisation stage, as to which serious events would be treated as disease-related and would therefore not be subject to systematic unblinding and expedited reporting. For trials such as these, sponsors are strongly recommended to set up an independent DMC to review the safety data in an ongoing manner (see section 5.9).

5.8   Ongoing safety evaluation

An ongoing safety evaluation (often referred to as signal detection or ongoing safety surveillance) should be conducted throughout the trial on the safety data that have been received. It must[4] be reviewed annually. Undertaking such an activity helps to ensure that the most up-to-date safety information is available about the risks of a studied product. New risks or additional information about known risks may have an impact on the conduct of the clinical trial. If new safety information comes to light relating to the product, the conduct of the trial or clinical practice, this may have a broad impact on the use of the IMP (in particular, where the IMP is an authorised product); this may then impact both on subjects in the trial or other trials using the same IMP and those being treated elsewhere (for example, in routine clinical practice).

5

Consider, for example, a trial where subjects were supplied with a range of different-strength tablets to take during different periods of the trial. Ongoing safety monitoring during this trial highlighted that there were a significant number of overdoses occurring, caused by trial subjects mixing up the tablets that they should have been taking. As a result of this safety monitoring, actions were taken to change the labelling and presentation of the IMP, thereby removing the potential for dose confusion and related overdose. This highlights the significance of safety monitoring for those subjects currently on the trial, and also those who will be treated in the future.

In order to undertake signal detection, good pharmacovigilance should be built into the systems from the start; protocols and risk assessments should consider the key elements of safety reporting and facilitate the collection and review and reporting of all relevant safety information.

Where the product is marketed by the sponsor, the ongoing safety review will fit in with the signal detection procedures already in place (however, it should be ensured that these include the clinical trial data, not just the post-marketing information). There is no specific timeframe specified in the legislation for the ongoing safety review, other than what is in place for the production of DSURs. It is recommended that the frequency of analysis is relative to the type of IMP, to the known safety profile of the drug and to the volume of data being received (that is, if no new data have been received during a time period, there is no value in re-analysing the data; if events come in rarely, they could be analysed as they are received). The processes that a sponsor has in place for the ongoing assessment of safety data are likely to be reviewed during a MHRA GCP inspection. This review will include any associated plans and procedures, evidence of meetings, any outcomes and associated protocol amendments.

Where there are specific safety concerns for the trial or IMP, and a DMC is involved, the protocol and DMC guidelines should be clear about any potential stopping criteria for the trial (for example, whether the trial should be stopped after a certain number of specific types of SUSARs have been seen in the trial population).

SAEs should be reviewed in addition to SARs as, for example, an increase in frequency of an SAE may affect the investigator's or sponsor's opinion of causality. Many studies will have a DMC (see section 5.9) that would be responsible for this review, in conjunction with the sponsor.

Non-serious adverse events should also be considered for ongoing safety evaluation. Such events may be reported in an expedited manner to the competent authority and REC in special circumstances if they alter the risk–benefit assessment of the IMP (see section 5.4.1). Currently non-serious adverse events are not part of the DSUR, unless they impact on the risk–benefit of the IMP. If the IMP is an authorised product with a risk management plan, then this plan should be complied with in terms of any specified reporting requirements for non-serious adverse events of interest or more detailed follow-up of specific events of interest.

For example, if there is an increase in non-serious events at a level which is more frequent than expected, then these events may require further assessment by the sponsor. In the commercial setting, this may involve ensuring that the sponsor reviews those specified non-serious events as part of the signal detection process. This will require consideration of how such events are included in the database, as non-serious adverse events would not usually be received in-house until the CRFs have been monitored (although this will depend on the methods used by the organisation as, if electronic data capture is used, receipt of the information will be quicker). Conversely, in Phase I studies involving a dose escalation protocol, all adverse events would be scrutinised at each dose escalation step.

For investigator sites that are hosting trials, the investigator should review all events, both serious and non-serious. However, as the investigator's review would usually not have the same scope, breadth of information and perspective as the sponsor's review, a sponsor assessment is still required[4].

Where the sponsor of the trial is not the MAH, it is still important to perform regular safety reviews and assessments of SAR and SAE frequency, with the review frequency based on risk. In the non-commercial setting, this safety review and assessment is likely to be delegated to the chief investigator responsible for the trial as the R&D office is unlikely to have access to all of the required data to enable a complete assessment to take place and in addition may not have the required medical expertise. It is important that any review that is carried out by the sponsor or trial team is fully documented, including any potential actions that need to be taken, or simply capturing a conclusion that the events reviewed do not constitute a potential safety issue. It is good practice for non-commercial sponsors to report any significant safety data to the MAH. This is often stipulated by pharmaceutical companies as a requirement in the contracts for supplying IMP to the non-commercial sponsor.

> **Examples to illustrate how the results of ongoing safety evaluation can impact subjects on the trial and those who will be treated in the future**
>
> *New safety issue*
>
> A SUSAR of QT prolongation (a QT interval in excess of 0.44 seconds is associated with possible development of ventricular arrhythmia, syncope and sudden death) is received for a clinical trial of an IMP that is not an authorised product. The event is not included in the IB. This could be a new safety issue which may require further investigation by the clinical trial team and the competent authority, with the potential that communication to other principal investigators running trials with this IMP is needed. Some safety issues could halt a trial temporarily or even permanently.
>
> *Cluster of SUSARs*
>
> A cluster of SUSARs of anaphylactic shock is received in a trial of an authorised product. The SPC lists anaphylactic shock as a rare event, but following a number of SARs of anaphylactic shock, the sponsor reports a subsequent reaction as a SUSAR. This is because the sponsor assesses the event as unexpected as it can no longer be justified as a rare reaction. The competent authority may review the SUSARs with a proposal that the MAH(s) for this product should increase the likelihood of occurrence in the wording of the SPC – for example, from rare to common. Ultimately, SUSARs received for authorised products may result in product labelling being strengthened, or even the inclusion of new warnings for prescribers and subjects.

5.9   Data monitoring committees/data safety monitoring boards

There may be occasions when a data safety monitoring board (DSMB) or a data monitoring committee (DMC) forms part of the oversight and management of a trial. The responsibilities of the DMC are usually to review unblinded data to enable monitoring of the safety of the drug under investigation. It would then be the DMC's role to make recommendations to the sponsor on trial conduct, such as the need to amend the protocol, or to terminate the trial early due to safety concerns. If a trial steering committee (see section 7.2.1) has also been set up, the DMC would normally report recommendations to them; if not, the DMC would report directly to the sponsor. By appointing a DMC, decisions can be made on the unblinded trial data without compromising the integrity of the trial. The members of the DMC should be independent of the sponsor (although investigators and sponsor staff can attend at the invitation of the DMC, should this be required), given that their recommendations may affect the future conduct or continuation of the trial.

A DMC is not needed for all clinical trials; it will depend on the complexity and end-points of the trial and can be considered as part of the risk assessment. When deciding if a DMC is necessary, it is recommended that consideration be given to:

- the safety profile of the IMP (that is, any significant potential risk of harm, or unknown or uncertain risks)
- the size of the trial (that is, numerous centres versus a single centre – for a large number of sites, further consideration should be given to the need for an overview of all the data from all the sites)
- end-points and/or other data requiring regular review (for example, review could identify that the end-point has been reached before the end of recruitment, thereby finishing the trial earlier than anticipated)
- the potential for high morbidity or mortality during the trial (that is, subjects with life-threatening illnesses)
- vulnerable populations.

Where it has been decided that a DMC is necessary, there should be formalised procedures in place for the formation, remit and membership of the committee. The requirements should then be described in a formal trial document such as the protocol or a DMC charter prior to the enrolment of trial subjects. This may include details on the following:

- how communication will be managed between the DMC, sponsor and investigator teams, including how the unblinded data will be transferred to the committee (where applicable)
- how often the committee will meet (both planned meetings and the process for triggered meetings)
- how decisions will be taken (what activities should take place during closed sessions and what will be the voting process)
- how reports from the DMC will be produced to safeguard the blind for the trial (for example, by producing closed minutes for the sponsor but open minutes for the DMC)
- how to ensure recommendations made by the DMC are addressed without delay, and in an appropriate manner; if such recommendations require an urgent safety measure to be implemented, it must[17] be ensured that this is reported to both the competent authority and REC in the required timeframe

5

- who is responsible for maintaining the DMC documentation during the course of the trial and how it is maintained as part of the trial master file (in order to comply with Regulation 31A (4) of SI 2004/1031).

It is important that the procedures followed by the DMC and any outputs are clearly documented for a trial to ensure that the data used to make decisions are robust and the decisions themselves are documented and retained to verify compliance. It is advised that this documentation also verifies who prepared and checked any reports and listings for the DMC and when (including the quality control of any data provided). This is especially important if the DMC is conducting any unblinded reviews during the course of the trial to ensure the trial team and investigator sites remain blinded.

Further guidance on data monitoring committees can also be found on the Health Research Authority (HRA) website and in the EMA 'Guideline on data monitoring committees' (EMEA/CHMP/EWP/5872/03).

5.10 Safety reporting requirements for nIMPs

nIMPs are those products that are used in accordance with the trial protocol, but which fall outside the IMP definition (refer to Table 6.1 for the definitions of an IMP and a nIMP). nIMPs can include challenge agents used to induce a physiological effect, such as certain allergens used in respiratory trials; rescue medication used for preventative action, such as salbutamol in asthma trials; or concomitant medications that are required by the protocol or background therapy. Further guidance on nIMPs can be found in Chapter 6 of this publication and EudraLex Volume 10, Chapter III.

Under the detailed guidance CT-3 the following reporting arrangements for nIMPs apply:

- SUSARs related to nIMPs, where there is a possibility of an interaction between a nIMP and an IMP, must[13] be reported as SUSARs (there is therefore no need to report a SUSAR related to a nIMP if there is no suspected interaction between the nIMP and IMP).
- If a SUSAR occurs, and it might be linked to either a nIMP or an IMP, but cannot be attributed to only one of these, the SUSAR must[13] be reported.
- If an adverse reaction associated with the nIMP is likely to affect the safety of the trial subjects, the sponsor must[17, 18, 19] report this to the competent authorities and RECs as an urgent safety measure, a substantial amendment, or via a notification to terminate the trial early, as applicable.

The decision as to whether the reaction is likely to affect the safety of the trial subjects is a sponsor decision (which may be delegated to investigators in some organisations).

For those clinical trials where the trial sponsor is not the MAH for the nIMP, it is recommended that SARs associated with the nIMP are reported to the MAH, so that this information can be used in the MAH's ongoing safety evaluation process. Note that this is no longer required for comparators under the detailed guidance CT-3. If the nIMP does not have a marketing authorisation and is classified as a 'special', then reference to the MHRA website for guidance on reporting of adverse reactions in relation to specials should be made (note this is outside the remit of the Clinical Trials Regulations).

5.11   Out-of-hours medical cover

Provision of out-of-hours medical cover for investigators can be determined by the sponsor using a risk-based approach, depending on the IMP and population under investigation. ICH Topic E6 (R1) – 'Guideline for Good Clinical Practice' states that medical personnel should be readily available to advise on trial-related medical questions or problems. Out-of-hours medical cover ensures that, where investigators need urgent medical advice related to their subjects' participation in a trial, they are able to access this from a medically qualified doctor who has knowledge of the trial and the product(s), even outside standard working hours, and in particular for global trials.

It is often the case that the sponsor has a comprehensive overview of the IMP and of results arising from the same or different trials with the IMP. Therefore, in an emergency the sponsor is potentially in a better position than other parties involved in the trial to provide information relating to the IMP which may be of interest for the care of a trial subject. However, out-of-hours medical advice may be contracted out by sponsors to an external medical advice service. Where this is the case, there should be clear written agreements in place defining responsibilities of the involved parties and appropriate training must[20] be provided. It is recommended that the out-of-hours service of the sponsor or vendor is tested at regular intervals (frequency to be determined by the sponsor) to ensure that contact can be made in a timely manner and out of hours. These tests must[12] be documented. Where out-of-hours cover is delegated to the chief investigator running the trial, as is often the case in the non-commercial sector, it is helpful for the sponsor to have guidance in place in terms of expectations on the cover to be provided. Those medically qualified doctors that are involved in providing out-of-hours cover should have knowledge of or access to the relevant trial protocol and IB or SPC.

Out-of-hours emergency contact for trial subjects is described in section 11.4.8.

5.12 Investigator-initiated trials

After a marketing authorisation has been granted, the MAH may be involved in trials for which it is not the sponsor, such as trials initiated by investigators employed by NHS Trusts or academic institutions. The level of involvement of the MAH may range in these trials from simply providing the product for trial use to providing regulatory support. For example, the MAH may be responsible for the collection and collation of safety data that arise from the trial.

For such trials, it is the sponsor organisation that retains overall responsibility for the trial conduct, rather than the MAH. It is recommended, however, that if the MAH is either supplying the IMP and/or providing funding to the trial, a written agreement is put in place that requires the investigator to report safety information to the MAH, and also requires that the MAH should keep the sponsor/investigator informed of any significant new safety information relating to the IMP during the course of the trial. This would not apply if the investigator is conducting a trial using, for example, standard NHS pharmacy stock, in which case the MAH would have no knowledge of the trial although, as stated previously, it would be good practice for the sponsor to provide the MAH with safety data.

5.13 Specific safety requirements for trials of advanced therapy products

Expedited reporting arrangements for trials using advanced therapy investigational medicinal products (ATIMPs), as detailed in the European Commission's 'Detailed guidelines on Good Clinical Practice specific to advanced therapy medicinal products 2009', differ from that of other clinical trials (refer to Annex 3). The guidance states that new events related to the conduct of the trial or the development of the ATIMP, and likely to affect the safety of the subjects, should be reported according to the existing timelines for expedited reporting. For ATIMP trials, this includes:

- SAEs which could be associated with the trial procedures and which could require modification of the conduct of the trial
- significant hazard to the subject population.

ATIMP trials also have specific requirements in terms of follow-up arrangements over and above those for most trials, although the guidelines do not specify for how long follow-up of safety information should occur. The need for, the duration, and the nature of follow-up should be determined by the sponsor for each clinical trial based on:

- the nature of the ATIMP
- the current state of knowledge regarding that ATIMP
- a risk analysis, including the risk for close contacts and offspring.

The sponsor should also take into account any European Community expertise and guidance on risk assessment and follow-up of subjects treated with particular types of ATIMPs; this may provide more details on the follow-up period and what kind of follow-up is expected. A rationale should be included for choosing the particular follow-up based on knowledge of the level of risk involved with the ATIMP. Follow-up arrangements should be included in the trial protocol and/or associated document and agreed by the competent authority and REC as part of the trial authorisation process. Appropriate information regarding this long-term follow-up should be included in the subject information sheet, to fully enable informed consent for this aspect of the trial.

The following safety issues may be relevant to long-term follow-up:

- suspected or confirmed infection as a result of the disease, concomitant therapy or as a result of the ATIMP therapy
- unexpected reactions (such as hypersensitivity, immunological, toxic or other reaction as a consequence of a change in the construction or function of the viral vector)
- adverse events related to product failure (including lack of efficacy)
- adverse events related to mandatory concomitant medication (such as immunosuppression)
- adverse events related to medical devices which form part of the product or are used for application of the product.

ATIMP trials and associated follow-up requirements are a developing area; therefore, the MHRA, EMA and European Commission websites should be referred to for up-to-date information.

5.14   Pharmacovigilance data collection

In commercial organisations, pharmacovigilance data are often processed and stored in a purpose-built safety database. In the non-commercial setting, pharmacovigilance data may be held centrally by the sponsor R&D office or held by investigators at a trial level, usually in a spreadsheet format (such as MS Excel), or in paper format, or a mix of the two. Either approach is acceptable, as long as there is an appropriate system in place to ensure that all SAEs, SARs and SUSARs are captured by the data collection system for reporting purposes. The system should be fit for purpose and the data held therein must[21] be accurate (for example, subject to a level of quality control) and complete. There should also be a process in place to prevent the safety data being changed by someone not authorised to do so and, if changes are made, these must[21] be evident (that is, there should be an audit trail).

Organisations may choose to use a database specifically designed to manage safety data as these systems allow access to the data from various locations, are readily searchable for use in signal detection and are able to generate listings for reports. When using these systems, sponsors should ensure that they are reliable and, in the event of problems with the associated technology, that there is a back-up plan (that is, if sponsors have no access to the system due to a fault, they are still able to fulfil their legislative requirements for expedited reporting). Paper and spreadsheet systems are simpler to manage, but do not offer the functionality of bespoke electronic systems and generally cannot effectively manage large volumes of data.

If there are separate clinical and pharmacovigilance databases kept for a trial, reconciliation of safety data must[21] be performed between the two. See Chapter 8 for further information on reconciliation activities.

5.15   Development safety update reports

The ICH Topic E2F – 'Development safety update report' (hereinafter 'ICH E2F') came into effect on 1 September 2011 in the EU and relates to the introduction of a common standard for annual reporting for clinical trials across the ICH regions (USA, Japan and Europe). The DSUR replaces the annual safety report (ASR) as the mechanism for periodic safety reporting in clinical trials. It is a legislative requirement[4] in the UK that an annual safety report is submitted to the MHRA and the REC. Submission of these reports is not to be confused with that of the annual progress report to the REC. A report needs to be submitted even when there are no data to include as a statement about ongoing subject safety must[4] be submitted. The main aim of the DSUR is to provide one report for an IMP to be submitted to all authorities across the world in order to reduce the burden on both competent authorities and sponsors.

ICH E2F contains a detailed outline of the key headings for each section of the DSUR to assist with the writing of the DSUR. In addition, an ICH E2F working group compiled two 'model' DSURs to provide further guidance in relation to content and structure of the DSUR (these 'model' DSURs take account of the differing knowledge about a medicine, depending on whether the sponsor holds the marketing authorisation or not). The guideline in its entirety and the accompanying model DSURs can be accessed on the ICH website.

In addition, the Clinical Trials Facilitation Group has developed a question-and-answer document, which is available on the Heads of Medicines Agencies website (www.hma.eu).

5.15.1   Objectives and aims of the DSUR

The objective of the DSUR is to provide competent authorities and RECs with an annual review and evaluation of safety information for an IMP in order to assure regulators that sponsors are adequately monitoring the safety profile of the products under investigation. The DSUR contains safety information obtained by the sponsor from a variety of sources, not only the clinical trials it is sponsoring but also other studies it may be running, such as observational post-marketing studies, registries or non-clinical studies. The DSUR should be a concise document and should focus on the IMP, only including information on comparators where relevant.

The main aim of the DSUR is to present a comprehensive and meaningful review of safety information that has been received during the period of the DSUR. The sponsor should provide an assessment of whether the new information received for the IMP during the reporting period is in accordance with previous knowledge for that product. The DSUR should also summarise the current understanding of the identified and potential risks to clinical trial subjects or to subjects taking the product in the post-marketing setting.

5.15.2 Periodicity

The DSUR should cover a one-year period and no longer, and should be compiled for each IMP, including all trials ongoing or completed in the DSUR period run by the same sponsor. The development international birth date (DIBD) is the first date of authorisation of an interventional trial using that IMP anywhere in the world and the DSUR should start from the date and month of the DIBD. The data lock point (DLP) for the DSUR is the last day of the one-year reporting period from the DIBD. The sponsor, if it is also the MAH for the IMP, may consider aligning the DSUR DIBD with the periodic safety update report (PSUR) international birth date (IBD). However, if the sponsor is planning on synchronising dates, the period of the first DSUR should not exceed one year (although a DSUR covering a period of less than one year can be submitted). PSURs fall outside the scope of the Clinical Trials Regulations.

DSURs should continue to be submitted to competent authorities and RECs 'throughout the clinical trial' (as defined in Article 17 (2) of Directive 2001/20/EC). It is recognised that there is some scope for interpretation of this term, with differences in ICH E2F, the detailed guidance CT-1 and CT-3. The Clinical Trials Facilitation Group Questions and Answers document proposes that, in order to harmonise the approach, information on a particular trial within the DSUR will be submitted until the last visit of the last subject in the Member State concerned for that trial, as defined in the trial protocol. When the sponsor submits the final data in a DSUR for the trial, this should be indicated in the document.

DSURs are not required for studies of short duration, that is, less than one year (for example, many pharmacology studies). However, it is recommended that, if a sponsor conducts several short trials of the same IMP within a one-year period, consideration is given to the production of a DSUR to demonstrate the comprehensive review of safety information.

5.15.3 One DSUR per active substance under investigation

A DSUR should be compiled for each IMP, including all trials ongoing or completed in the DSUR period run by the same sponsor. Therefore, a single DSUR for the IMP should be written with safety data from all clinical trials conducted with the product, for all indications, all dosage forms and all intended populations under study for that sponsor. However, some competent authorities, such as the MHRA, are taking a slightly broader approach to the submission of DSURs by trial instead of by IMP. Although it is strongly recommended to submit one DSUR per IMP, the MHRA has agreed that, where it is appropriate and justified, non-commercial sponsors may submit one DSUR per trial, rather than per IMP (which would incorporate all trials that may be running with that IMP for that individual sponsor). This could apply, for example, where the non-commercial sponsor has several trials running across different institutions and the data are not held centrally. It is important to check both the MHRA and HRA websites for any updates on UK submission requirements prior to submission. Similarly, if sponsors are submitting DSURs to other competent authorities and RECs in other Member States, then it is worth checking whether there are any local requirements in terms of content and submission.

5.15.4 Trials with multiple IMPs

For trials where multiple IMPs are used, a DSUR should generally be prepared for each IMP, unless there is a rationale for why this would not be appropriate (see section 5.15.6). This will be reviewed by individual competent authorities on a case-by-case basis.

Although DSURs are required for IMPs, it is the active substance under investigation that needs to be addressed in the DSUR (as per the definition in ICH E2F). Therefore, there is no requirement to produce a separate DSUR for a comparator, placebo or nIMP. However, it is expected that all SARs are listed in the DSUR, which will include those in relation to comparators, placebos and nIMPs.

5.15.5 Fixed combination products

The guidance states that in general a single DSUR may be produced for fixed combination products (that is, in situations where a product contains at least two active ingredients in a fixed dose which is administered to a subject in a single dosage form). However, the sponsor should include in the DSUR the rationale for producing one DSUR. The sponsor should consider safety information for both the combination and the single ingredients where relevant, which it has become aware of during the DSUR reporting period. For example, the sponsor may become aware of a significant literature article in relation to one of the active ingredients in a fixed combination which may be of relevance to the ongoing risk–benefit review of the combination product. In these circumstances, the sponsor would be expected to include any articles of relevance in the literature section of the DSUR.

5.15.6   Standard combination therapies

In situations where a trial involves multiple products (some of which will be test IMPs, some comparator IMPs and some possibly nIMPs) used together in a well-established treatment regimen (for example, many chemotherapy regimens) where the combination of drugs is not fixed, then it may be more appropriate for the sponsor to prepare one DSUR incorporating the safety data for all products used in the therapy. However, it is important that the sponsor makes a well-thought-out decision about whether to produce one DSUR for each IMP, or to produce one DSUR for the treatment combination, in order to present the safety data in the most appropriate way. The sponsor must include a rationale for why only one DSUR is being prepared. The line listings in the DSUR should include SARs in relation to all IMPs included in the therapy, including any SARs received for the placebos, nIMPs and comparator(s) used in the trials.

5.15.7   Sponsor responsibilities

The sponsor is responsible for the preparation, content and submission of the DSUR. However, the sponsor can delegate the writing of the DSUR to a third party (for example, a CRO) ensuring that a detailed agreement is in place with the vendor describing the activities it will be undertaking. The sponsor would still, however, retain overall responsibility for the quality and content of the document (Chapter 1).

5.15.7.1 Co-sponsorship arrangements

In situations where trials have joint sponsors or co-sponsors, it is important that the responsibilities of each sponsor in relation to the writing, compilation and submission of the DSUR are clearly outlined in an agreement between the various organisations. When a single DSUR cannot be arranged, joint sponsors can agree to prepare separate DSURs for the same IMP – for example, when different indications or routes of administration are being used by different parties. However, the reasoning behind the writing of separate DSURs should be highlighted in the DSUR.

5.15.7.2 Licence partners

It is recognised that some products studied in clinical trials may be out-licensed from the MAH to a licence partner, or companies may be engaged in co-marketing, co-promotional or co-development arrangements. This is a similar scenario to obtaining post-authorisation safety data required to fulfil MAH post-authorisation pharmacovigilance responsibilities, as any safety data that require inclusion in the DSUR should be obtained from the licence partner in a timely fashion to allow for review prior to DSUR submission. To facilitate safety data exchange, a detailed agreement should be in place between licence partners regarding the exchange of clinical trial SAEs and SARs or other data of relevance to the DSUR.

If responsibilities are not clearly defined in agreements, this can lead to problems in meeting regulatory requirements. For example, late submission of SAEs to a sponsor by a co-development partner could result in SUSARs being reported late to the competent authority and the REC as well as relevant SARs not being included in the DSUR.

5.15.8 DSUR content: overview of ICH E2F

The following sub-sections provide an overview of the requirements of the DSUR and highlight some areas of ICH E2F to which sponsors should pay particular attention.

5.15.8.1 Unavailability of data for inclusion in the DSUR

It is recognised that some sponsors will not have access to some of the data required in the guidance. This may particularly affect non-commercial sponsors. For example, all sponsors may not have access to issues relating to manufacturing, non-clinical data and marketing data (such as product authorisation dates or countries where the product is authorised). In this circumstance, the sponsor is encouraged to simply state in the DSUR that it does not have access to these data.

Other sections may not be applicable to sponsors, and it is acceptable to add 'N/A' to the relevant sections. For example, sponsors may not be running any post-authorisation safety studies or registries, in which case, the sponsor should state that this section is not applicable and therefore will not be completed. A simplified document may be acceptable in this case.

5.15.8.2 Reference safety information

The IB or SPC in place at the start of the DSUR reporting period should serve as the RSI to determine whether the information received during the reporting period remains consistent with previous knowledge of the safety profile of the drug under investigation. The IB should contain a discrete section, which is the RSI, allowing the IB to be changed independently of the RSI. Significant changes to the IB or SPC include new information on contraindications, warnings, interactions or new SARs. The IB or SPC in place at the beginning of the reporting period should be appended to the DSUR, regardless of whether the IB or SPC was altered during the period of the DSUR. The RSI in place at the beginning of the reporting period should be the reference for the expectedness assessments in the DSUR line listings, regardless of whether the RSI was updated during that reporting period. If the IB or SPC has been revised during the DSUR reporting period, the sponsor should also submit the current version and list any significant safety-related changes in the relevant section of the DSUR. The DSUR should include the date and version number of the IB or SPC used as the RSI.

5.15.8.3 Regulatory data

The guidance includes a comprehensive overview of the nature of the regulatory information that should be included in the DSUR. For example, this section should include relevant data on marketing authorisation dates, dosage information for the IMP, and whether any regulatory actions have been taken in the reporting period. This could include refusal to obtain a marketing authorisation or clinical trial authorisation, changes to the trial protocol(s) due to safety reasons, and other information in relation to restrictions in the populations or indications.

5.15.8.4 Status of ongoing and completed clinical trials during the DSUR period

The main focus of the DSUR is the presentation of data from interventional trials of the IMP under investigation, whether or not the product has a marketing authorisation. A table should be completed, where necessary, outlining all ongoing and completed clinical trials with the IMP during the DSUR period for which the sponsor is responsible. ICH E2F contains a template table that can be used for this purpose. This table aims to provide the competent authority with an overview of the trials ongoing and completed using the IMP during the reporting period.

5.15.8.5 Estimated cumulative subject exposure

The DSUR should contain a table outlining the estimated cumulative exposure of the IMP from the completed and ongoing trials that the sponsor is responsible for and also exposure data from marketing experience (if relevant and if known when the sponsor is not the MAH). The reason for the inclusion of cumulative exposure data in the DSUR is to assist the competent authority with the overall assessment of the data received during the DSUR period. The cumulative tabulation of exposure provides a context for reviewing any SARs that have been received during the DSUR period by comparing this number with the number of people that may have received the IMP both in trials and in the post-marketing setting (if this is appropriate). The subject exposure table should include a breakdown of subjects exposed to the IMP (including comparators and placebos where appropriate), by particular parameters such as age and sex. ICH E2F provides a template table that can be populated with the estimated number of subjects exposed to the IMP.

5.15.8.6 DSUR line listings

The DSUR must[4] contain line listings of all SARs that have been received by the sponsor during the period of the DSUR for the IMP, any comparator(s), nIMPs and placebos. The listings must[4] include SARs reported to the sponsor from the DLP of the previous DSUR to the DLP of the current DSUR. The listings should include subjects only once regardless of how many SARs they may have experienced. If the trial subjects experienced more than one reaction, the most serious reaction should be listed first in order to drive MedDRA system organ class (SOC) inclusion. If MedDRA has been utilised by the sponsor for the coding of the adverse event or reaction terms reported, then the preferred term level should be presented in the listings and tabulations. ICH E2F contains a template table that can be used to organise the line listings. Note that it is not mandatory to use MedDRA classification for the DSUR.

5.15.8.7 Summary tabulations

The DSUR should also contain a cumulative summary tabulation of all SAEs that have been received by the sponsor for the IMP since the DIBD. This includes SAEs reported to the sponsor for all trials that the sponsor is responsible for with that IMP. If MedDRA is used, the tabulation should be organised by MedDRA SOC. MedDRA SOCs are publicly available to help sponsors who do not have a MedDRA licence so that the SAE can be manually added to the relevant SOC, for example 'Psychiatric Disorders SOC', or 'Infections and Infestations SOC'.

The guidance stresses that, although causality assessments assist with the evaluation of adverse reactions for expedited reporting purposes (that is, for SUSAR reporting), the aggregation of SAEs in the DSUR tabulation provides an overall summary of all events of a serious nature reported to the sponsor.

If the sponsor does not have access to some or all of the cumulative SAE data, this should be stated by the sponsor. For example, cumulative SAE data may not be available in the situation where the company is now the MAH for the product under investigation, but the MAH acquired the licence from another company and was not provided with historical data. However, the sponsor should explain any missing data in the DSUR. The summary tabulations and line listings should be attached as an appendix.

5.15.8.8 Protocol-exempt SAEs/SARs

The line listings and summary tabulations need not include any SAEs or SARs that have been defined in the protocol as not requiring reporting to the sponsor, such as disease end-points or well-established events for products used within the authorised indications (see section 5.4.1).

5.15.8.9 Safety data received from sources other than interventional trials

The DSUR should contain any data that become available to the sponsor, which have been identified from non-interventional studies, epidemiological studies or registries. In addition, if the sponsor becomes aware of any non-clinical data, such as immunotoxicity studies that may be ongoing or completed during the DSUR reporting period, these should also be included. The sponsor should also summarise any significant new safety issues identified through the scientific literature of which it becomes aware. The guidance does not stipulate that the sponsor should actively search the literature in order to complete the DSUR.

For trials sponsored by NHS Trust or academic organisations, the investigator may become aware of significant publications in the literature or abstracts from other research relating to the IMP through ongoing reading in their area of interest and through attendance at conferences. In this case, it may be relevant to discuss and present this information in the DSUR. The sponsor should have a mechanism for including such articles in the DSUR.

5.15.8.10 Trials with authorised medicinal products

In the situation where an IMP has a marketing authorisation (a licence), the sponsor (if also the MAH) may become aware of any safety issues arising from post-marketing use. For example, use in the post-marketing setting may provide further information on situations such as use in pregnancy or off-label use.

5.15.8.11 Late-breaking information

The sponsor may receive significant safety information after the DLP of the DSUR in the 60-day period before submission. The sponsor should summarise any important safety data received, such as individual SUSARs that have been reported, or important findings from non-clinical studies.

5.15.8.12 Blinded trials

If individual SUSARs have been unblinded for the purposes of expedited reporting, these cases should be included in the DSUR in the unblinded format. Therefore, listings and summary tabulations appended to the DSUR could include blinded and unblinded data. The sponsor is not required to unblind reports for the purposes of DSUR writing; any cases which remain blinded should be highlighted in the line listings.

As the DSUR may contain unblinded data, it is important that the sponsor has a mechanism for continuing to conceal the unblinded data from staff who are working on the trial so that the integrity of the trial is not jeopardised. This is of particular concern in a non-commercial organisation where the chief investigator may have been delegated pharmacovigilance responsibilities, including production of the DSUR. It is recommended that the sponsor includes a cautionary note on the front title page of the DSUR to warn of the potential exposure to unblinded data. The sponsor should also have a robust process in place for ensuring that the DSURs are stored in a controlled manner to avoid inadvertent access by trial staff or statisticians (for example, a password-protected folder or storage on a restricted access area of the server).

5.15.8.13 Overall safety assessment

The DSUR must[4] include an overall safety assessment, which should be concise and provide a summary of the information received in the reporting period, comparing it with previous knowledge of the IMP. The sponsor should include an analysis of any newly identified safety concerns, such as the receipt of new and/ or significant SUSARs, or an increase in the frequency of known reactions or in the severity of known reactions. Section 3.1.8.1 of ICH E2F contains for consideration a comprehensive list of potential safety concerns which may arise through clinical trials, non-clinical studies or post-marketing experience.

The sponsor should provide a final statement in relation to the balance between the risks and benefits of the IMP. In addition, the DSUR should include any important or potential risks identified by the sponsor, such as new or potential contraindications or warnings in use. If the sponsor is also an MAH for the product, then this section can be similar in content to the safety specification section of a product risk management plan. Note that risk management plans are outside the remit of the Clinical Trials Regulations. The sponsor should provide a conclusion in the DSUR that highlights whether the knowledge regarding safety of the IMP has changed since the previous DSUR.

5.15.9 DSUR submission

The DSUR (and the required appendices that are outlined in section 3.20 of ICH E2F) should be submitted to the competent authorities where authorisation has been granted for that clinical trial, within 60 calendar days of the DLP. In the EU, a copy of the DSUR should be submitted to the REC that provided the approval for the trial in each country. It is important to note that there may be different or additional local requirements for RECs in individual countries. All local requirements should therefore be checked prior to submission. The MHRA and HRA websites should be checked for up-to-date UK submission requirements at the time of DSUR submission.

5.15.10 DSURs and PSURs

Where MAHs are also sponsoring clinical trials involving a licensed product, there will be some overlap in the content of the DSUR and the PSUR. The focus of the DSUR is on the IMP, while the PSUR is a periodic report for each active substance required to be submitted to competent authorities where marketing authorisations have been granted. The PSUR is an overview of the post-marketing safety experience in a defined period. However, it is important that there is communication between authors of the DSUR and PSUR (if they are different) to ensure consistency in the risk–benefit review that is carried out in relation to the product. Some data will need to be included in both documents; for example, relevant information on post-marketing experience should be captured in the DSUR, and the PSUR should also contain safety findings from interventional trials. Despite the fact that the same staff may be writing a DSUR and a PSUR, the two documents should be stand-alone.

5.15.11 DSUR authors

The DSUR should be compiled and written by individuals who are familiar with the IMP under review, and who are in the position to provide a comprehensive risk–benefit assessment of the safety data received for the period of that DSUR, and put them in context with any data that may have already been received for that product from other trials in the past. It is likely that a medical review of the DSUR would aid the risk–benefit review of the data, but the sponsor should decide if this is necessary depending on many factors, such as the volume and nature of safety data received in the DSUR period. For example, for some established IMPs there is the potential that no SARs may be received during the reporting period, in which case the DSUR should reflect this and a medical assessment may not be necessary. It is important that if a medical review of the DSUR does occur, this review should be documented to reflect any dialogue between authors and medical reviewers that may have taken place.

5.15.12 Quality control

It is important that the DSUR is a correct and accurate document, which contains all the necessary cases in the line listings and cumulative summary tabulations (refer to Chapter 4 for general information in relation to preparing key trial documents). If a large number of SARs have been received in the reporting period, sponsors should ensure there is a mechanism in place to assure themselves that all necessary cases have been included (such as quality control checks). Larger organisations may have a safety database that has the functionality to produce validated line listings to enable the sponsor to be confident that all relevant cases have been included, both in line listings and in cumulative summary tabulations. Effective quality control will also ensure that the conclusions accurately reflect the data that have been included.

However, smaller organisations may be using spreadsheets or paper SAE forms, in which case more manual quality control checks may be appropriate. Quality control steps undertaken as part of the DSUR compilation process should be described in written procedures, and should be documented.

5.16 Chapter legislative references

Throughout this chapter, specific terminology – 'must', 'required' or 'requirement' – has been used to interpret activities that are legislative requirements. These terms have been number-coded in the text where used, and the corresponding reference in the legislation can be found below.

1. Regulations 32 to 35 of SI 2004/1031
2. Regulation 32 (5) of SI 2004/1031
3. Regulation 32 (9) of SI 2004/1031
4. Regulation 35 of SI 2004/1031
5. Regulation 28 (1) of SI 2004/1031
6. Regulation 29 of SI 2004/1031
7. Regulation 32 (4) of SI 2004/1031
8. Regulation 32 (1) of SI 2004/1031
9. Regulation 32 (3) of SI 2004/1031
10. Article 16 of Directive 2001/20/EC
11. Schedule 1, Part 2 (11) of SI 2004/1031
12. Regulation 31A (4) of SI 2004/1031
13. Regulation 33 of SI 2004/1031
14. Regulation 2 of SI 2004/1031
15. Schedule 3, Part 2 (11) of SI 2004/1031
16. Regulation 3A of SI 2004/1031
17. Regulation 30 of SI 2004/1031
18. Regulation 24 of SI 2004/1031
19. Regulation 27 of SI 2004/1031
20. Schedule 1, Part 2 (2) of SI 2004/1031
21. Schedule 1, Part 2 (9) of SI 2004/1031

CHAPTER 6

Investigational medicinal products

Editor's note

In addition to authorisation from the competent authority to conduct a clinical trial, authorisation is also required for the manufacture and importation of medicinal products that are tested in clinical trials – that is, investigational medicinal products (IMPs). The legislation surrounding IMPs ensures that the product is of sufficient quality and is manufactured and labelled in accordance with the terms of the clinical trial authorisation (CTA), to ensure the safety of the subjects and the quality of the data.

This chapter addresses the manufacture and/or importation of IMPs and its associated requirements. The products known as non-investigational medicinal products (nIMPs) are also discussed. These are products that are adjuncts to the product under investigation (for example, rescue medications or standard background therapy).

The EU legislation associated with the manufacture and importation of IMPs is found in Article 13 of Directive 2001/20/EC. The relevant UK legislation can be found in Parts 6 and 7 of SI 2004/1031. Reference to this legislation and associated guidance should be made where required.

6.1 Requirements for a manufacturing authorisation for investigational medicinal products

IMPs, whatever their source, will need to go through a manufacturing or importation step. The manufacturing step includes any manipulations performed on a product, including assembly (packaging and labelling; including the re-packaging and additional labelling of authorised product) but with certain specific exceptions (see section 6.2). Importation essentially means the bringing of an IMP into the EU from a third country (that is, a country outside the European Economic Area (EEA)). Any organisation engaged upon either manufacturing or importation activities must[1] hold a manufacturing authorisation. In the UK this is a specific manufacturer's authorisation for investigational medicinal products, MIA(IMP), with appropriate authorisations. In other EU countries this may be authorised and identified differently by the competent authority; however, throughout this chapter the term 'MIA(IMP)' will be used to describe the manufacturing authorisation in relation to IMPs.

IMP manufacture and importation must be performed in accordance with the EU 'Rules governing medicinal products in the European Union' – EudraLex Volume 4, EU Guidelines to Good Manufacturing Practice (GMP) (in particular Annex 13 and Annex 16) and the *Rules and Guidance for Pharmaceutical Manufacturers and Distributors* (hereinafter the 'Orange Guide'), which applies to IMPs as much as it does to the manufacture of authorised medicines. In particular, Annex 13 contains requirements specific to IMP manufacture and MIA(IMP) holders will need to be familiar with these, as they will be inspected against these standards by the MHRA GMP Inspectorate upon application for an MIA(IMP) and at regular intervals thereafter. Good Clinical Practice (GCP) inspectors will also review appropriate Annex 13 training for those individuals involved in some IMP-related aspects; for example, trial managers or regulatory affairs staff approving IMP labels.

The sponsor of a trial retains ultimate responsibility for that trial, but responsibility for the quality of the IMPs used is generally delegated to the MIA(IMP) holder. Therefore, there should be a technical agreement between the sponsor and the IMP manufacturer(s) that lays out respective responsibilities for manufacture (including packaging and labelling), storage, shipment, batch certification and testing of the IMPs together with responsibilities for handling of complaints, recalls, quality deviations, returns, regulatory issues etc. This document should be signed by both parties prior to undertaking these tasks and kept up to date following any change affecting IMP supplies.

The definitions listed in Table 6.1 may further assist in the clarification of terminology used throughout this chapter.

Table 6.1 Terms used in investigational medicinal product management

Term	Definition
Investigational medicinal product	A pharmaceutical form of an active substance or placebo being tested or used as a reference in a clinical trial, including products already with an authorisation, but used or assembled (formulated or packaged) in a way different from the authorised form, or when used for an unauthorised indication, or when used to gain further information about the authorised form.
Non-investigational medicinal product (medicinal product falling outside the definition of an investigational medicinal product)	Products which are not the object of investigation (other than the tested product, placebo or active comparator) may be supplied to subjects participating in a trial and used in accordance with the protocol. For instance, some clinical trial protocols require the use of medicinal products, such as support or rescue/escape medication for preventive, diagnostic or therapeutic reasons and/or to ensure that adequate medical care is provided for the subject. They may also be used in accordance with the protocol to induce a physiological response. These medicinal products do not fall within the definition of investigational medicinal products (IMPs) in Directive 2001/20/EC and are called non-investigational medicinal products (nIMPs). They may be supplied by the sponsor who provides details of these nIMPs and their proposed use in the trial protocol and ensures that they are of the necessary quality for human use. nIMPs may be supplied by the investigator site.
QP declaration	The declaration by a Qualified Person that the manufacture of an IMP in a third country has been carried out to standards equivalent to EU GMP manufacture (Article 39 of Annex 13). This is required in the CTA application.
QP certification	The QP has a legal responsibility as laid out in Article 13 of Directive 2001/20/EC to ensure that the IMP has been manufactured in accordance with EU GMP and meets the conditions of the clinical trial authorisation and the product specification file.
Regulatory release	Under Article 9 of Directive 2001/20/EC, the sponsor may not start a clinical trial until the clinical trial authorisation and a favourable REC opinion has been granted for the trial and all conditions of the authorisation and favourable REC opinion have been met, and each trial site has been approved.

CTA, clinical trial authorisation; EU, European Union; GMP, Good Manufacturing Practice; IMP, investigational medicinal product; nIMP, non-investigational medicinal product; QP, Qualified Person; REC, research ethics committee

6

6.2 Exemptions from the need for an MIA(IMP)

There is a specific exemption from the need for an MIA(IMP), which is described in Regulation 37 of SI 2004/1031 (hereinafter 'Regulation 37 exemption'). It applies to hospitals or health centres engaged upon assembly only. Such an institution does not require an MIA(IMP) if the assembled IMP is to be used in a clinical trial within that hospital or health centre, or another hospital or health centre named as an investigator site within that same trial. However, this does not exempt the organisations from good practice and from following GMP guidance for assembly (packaging and labelling) activities, only the need for an MIA(IMP) and therefore Qualified Person (QP) certification.

When assembly is performed using the Regulation 37 exemption, the sponsor needs to be clear about the definition of 'hospital' or 'health centre'. Under the Clinical Trials Regulations this includes clinics, nursing homes and similar institutions that are regulated by the Care Quality Commission; it does not include community pharmacies or Phase I units.

A hospital or health centre may not make use of this exemption to supply assembled IMPs on a contract basis. Issues have arisen when organisations, usually with no dedicated pharmacy department or manufacturing unit, wrongly assume that the Regulation 37 exemption applies to all hospital pharmacies and, as such, contract a pharmacy outside the NHS Trust to perform assembly on their behalf. The assembling organisation must[2] be named as an investigator site for that particular clinical trial, otherwise an MIA(IMP) will be required to perform such activities.

The Regulation 37 exemption does not apply to manufacturing units that are located within the hospital but are legally not part of that hospital; for example, 'specials' licence holders and some Phase I units fall into this category. Conversely, the manufacturing unit for a large NHS Trust may reside in a different location from where the clinical activity is based, but as long as the unit is part of the NHS Trust that is named as an investigator site in the CTA application, the location is irrelevant.

For a trial in which the IMPs are authorised products and a risk assessment has determined that a normal dispensing label is appropriate and an additional clinical trial label is not necessary, this activity would not require an MIA(IMP) nor would the Regulation 37 exemption apply. Therefore the IMP could be supplied by a pharmacy under a normal prescription. This activity is covered by Regulation 46 (2) of SI 2004/1031.

6.3   Declaration, certification and release

QP certification and the responsibilities of the QP are defined in Regulation 43 of SI 2004/1031. Article 43 of Annex 13 requires IMPs to remain under the control of the sponsor until after completion of a two-step procedure:

- certification by a QP that the requirements of Article 13(3) of Directive 2001/20/EC have been met ('technical release'), and

- release by the sponsor for use in a clinical trial following fulfilment of the requirements of Article 9 of Directive 2001/20/EC and Regulation 13 of SI 2004/1031 ('regulatory release').

This two-step procedure is depicted in Figure 6.1.

The sponsor is responsible for ensuring that both steps are completed prior to authorising the commencement of a clinical trial. The QP certification must[3] be provided by a QP named on the MIA(IMP) authorisation specified in the CTA application as responsible for the manufacturing and importation of the IMP. The regulatory release may be delegated by the sponsor to the QP, regulatory affairs or trial manager. However, the sponsor retains legal responsibility.

Additionally, when IMPs are manufactured outside the EEA, a QP declaration of equivalence to EU GMP is required[4] for each IMP that is listed in the CTA application.

6.3.1   Qualified Persons

Each batch of IMP must[5] be certified by a QP as being suitable for use prior to its release for use in a clinical trial. QPs are named in the MIA(IMP) and are assessed by the competent authority upon application for a new MIA(IMP) or when a subsequent variation is submitted naming a new QP on an existing MIA(IMP).

In the UK, individuals eligible to be named as a QP on an MIA or MIA(IMP) have normally undergone an assessment process administered by one of three professional bodies: the Royal Society of Chemistry, the Society of Biology and the Royal Pharmaceutical Society. They are able to certify batches of IMP once

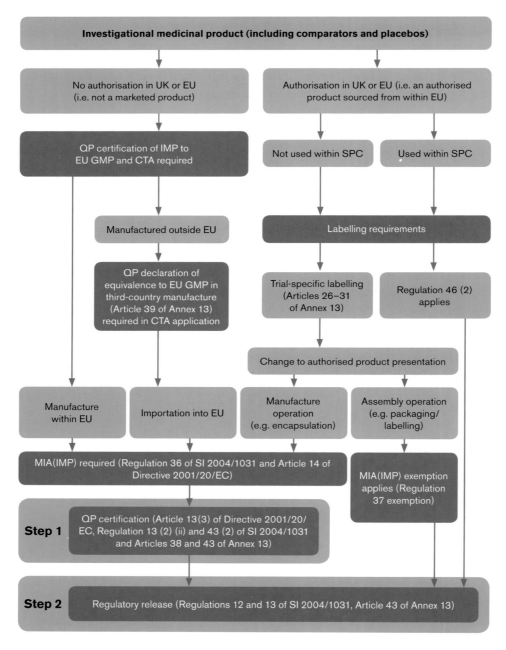

Figure 6.1 Two-step IMP release process

CTA, clinical trial authorisation; EU, European Union; GMP, Good Manufacturing Practice; IMP, investigational medicinal product; MIA(IMP), manufacturer's authorisation for investigational medicinal products; QP, Qualified Person; SPC, summary of product characteristics

they have been assessed by the competent authority and are named on an MIA(IMP). In addition, there are a number of QPs who were assessed under transitional arrangements who are named on an organisation's MIA(IMP). These arrangements are no longer available. A transitional QP can demonstrate their status by reference to their being named on an MIA(IMP).

QPs must[6] be fully aware of the requirements of GMP in general and how it pertains to IMPs and the relevant dosage forms in particular. QPs are required[5] to follow a code of practice. One of the requirements of this code is to acquire and maintain sufficient knowledge to be able to perform their duties and responsibilities adequately. An explanation of the legislative requirements relating to these duties and responsibilities, and the code of practice, can be found in the Orange Guide.

6.3.2   Importation and QP declarations

IMPs may be imported from third countries. These require[1] QP certification upon importation in a manner equivalent to IMPs manufactured within the EEA. The QP will need to know that EU GMP has been followed throughout the supply chain. If the IMP is an authorised medicine within the EEA or an ICH country (USA, Japan) then it can be expected that EU GMP or an equivalent standard has been followed during manufacture. In addition, there are mutual recognition agreements between the EEA and third countries that may apply (see European Medicines Agency (EMA) website for further details). In other cases, an audit of the manufacturer(s) should be carried out to support both the declaration and certification upon importation. Any departure from this should be justified and documented and will be subject to scrutiny during an MHRA GMP inspection. A competent authority inspection of the manufacturer should not be used unconditionally to remove the need for an audit by the organisation, as the inspection may not have reviewed the facilities or specific technical or GMP issues associated with manufacture of the IMP.

In addition, a QP declaration must[4] be submitted with the CTA application for each imported IMP, detailing the EudraCT number, the site of manufacture and the IMP details. All sites involved in the manufacturing steps should appear on the QP declaration, which should start with the conversion of the active pharmaceutical ingredient into the dosage form and include primary and secondary packing and also any contract laboratories involved with release or stability testing. The declaration must[7] be signed to confirm that EU GMP has been followed. Such a QP declaration is trial-specific and so must[3] be submitted for each new trial. There is a standard form for use in QP declarations, which is available on the MHRA website.

6.3.3 QP certification (technical release)

A QP must[7] certify that each batch of IMP has been manufactured and checked in compliance with the requirements of EU GMP (or standards at least equivalent to EU GMP in the case of an IMP manufactured in a third country), the product specification file and the CTA. This is referred to as 'technical release'.

The QP certifying the finished IMP will take final responsibility for the entire manufacturing process, even if some manufacturing steps have been conducted under a separate MIA(IMP) or in a third country. This would include an IMP packaged outside the EEA, even if the starting product was manufactured within the EEA under a marketing authorisation (MA), as well as an IMP manufactured outside the EEA and then imported and packaged within the EEA.

In these cases, the final certifying QP may receive certification from another QP that such preceding steps have been carried out in accordance with the requirements. Further information on this can be found in section 6.4.

Where an IMP that is a comparator product is being sourced from a third country and has an MA, but the documentation certifying that each production batch has been manufactured in conditions at least equivalent to the standards of EU GMP cannot be obtained, the QP needs to certify that each production batch has undergone all relevant analyses, tests and checks necessary to confirm its quality in accordance with the CTA.

If a batch is manufactured and does not meet the authorised specification, the QP cannot certify the batch. A substantial amendment to alter the specification may be submitted to the competent authority provided it is deemed that the safety, quality and efficacy are not compromised. The process for substantial amendments is discussed in section 2.3.6. However, if required, an expedited review may be requested.

As can be seen in Figure 6.1, QP certification (Step 1) is not required when unaltered licensed products are used for a clinical trial. In this case, only regulatory release (Step 2) is required, and there is no need for an MIA(IMP). However, when changes are made to the presentation of the authorised products by a manufacturing operation (for example, blinding via over-encapsulation) or by assembly operations that fall outside the Regulation 37 exemption, an MIA(IMP) and QP certification are needed.

The QP must[7] be supplied with all the relevant paperwork to perform QP certification (for example, the entire CTA as approved by the competent authority), including any conditions of approval and subsequent amendments. It has often been noted on GCP inspections that a contract QP has performed QP certification with only the CTA approval letter or perhaps with only the investigational medicinal product dossier (IMPD). Not having the entire CTA package could result in incorrect QP certification of the IMP. For example, a contract manufacturing organisation (CMO) QP could certify an IMP with an 18-month shelf life as per the IMPD they had received; however, as they had not received the authorisation letter they would be unaware that the competent authority had authorised the trial based on the condition of reducing the shelf life to 12 months.

Similarly, in the Phase I setting it is common for bulk supplies to be shipped to the unit. On occasion, they may be dispensed directly to the volunteer at the unit without the need for further assembly. However, some Phase I units hold an MIA(IMP) and where further assembly operations take place a QP would be required[5] to certify that the products have been assembled in accordance with the CTA and the protocol. These QPs are often remote from the sponsor and therefore difficulties can arise in obtaining the full information on the IMPD from the sponsor. This is essential as it is the responsibility of the QP to ensure that the product is assembled according to the correct specifications.

In very exceptional circumstances it may not be practical to perform QP certification prior to administering the IMP – for example, with an IMP that has an extremely short half-life or shelf life. Where there is clear technical justification, retrospective certification may be acceptable. The process should be formalised in a written procedure, including how this will be described in the CTA and documented in the trial master file. The retrospective QP certification will be as soon as practicable after the event, and ideally within 24 hours.

When a batch of IMP moves between Member States and is accompanied by a batch certification signed by a QP, it does not have to undergo further checks in relation to Article 13(3) of Directive 2001/20/EC. However, in order to facilitate the free movement of IMP between Member States, the content of certificates should be in accordance with the harmonised format found in Annex 13. Use of this format by an organisation may also assist in ensuring that the certificates contain all the required information. Certification statements are often found to be inadequate as they may only state that the batch of IMP complies with EU GMP. If no reference is made on the certificate to the protocol, CTA/IMPD or Article 13(3) of Directive 2001/20/EC, it is not possible to verify that Article 13(3) of Directive 2001/20/EC has been complied with.

There are circumstances where a batch of IMP may need to be re-certified. For example, if the IMP has a shelf life extension after QP certification and is consequently re-labelled with the revised expiry date by the MIA(IMP) holder (prior to shipment to the investigator site or having been returned from the investigator site), a new certification after re-labelling would be required. For product held at the investigator site, QP certification would not be required if the re-labelling activity is carried out by, or under the supervision of, a pharmacist or other healthcare professional, with appropriate documented evidence in accordance with Articles 33 and 42 of Annex 13. However, it is recommended that the documentation supplied to the investigator site(s) and the completed documentation is reviewed by a QP to ensure that it complies with Annex 13 requirements.

Technical agreements are important to ensure that all parties are aware of their responsibilities with respect to QP certification. As a result of inadequate or absent technical agreements, there have been misunderstandings between the CMO and sponsor as to which party was responsible for QP certification, which has resulted in the IMP not being QP-certified. The sponsor should also maintain oversight of the process, in particular to ensure that there are no misunderstandings regarding the difference between a certificate of conformity and QP certification, and that the QP certification contains adequate wording to verify what the IMP has been certified against.

6.3.4 Regulatory release and authorisation to start the trial

Under Article 9 of Directive 2001/20/EC and Regulation 12 of SI 2004/1031, the sponsor must not start a clinical trial until a CTA has been granted for the trial (and all conditions of that authorisation have been met), a favourable research ethics committee (REC) opinion has been granted (including verification that any conditions stipulated have been met) and each trial site has been approved. This is referred to as 'regulatory release'.

In addition to the requirements for technical and regulatory release, it is also expected that the sponsor verifies that other aspects required to comply with the Clinical Trials Regulations are in place prior to authorising the start of the trial. The documented check that all these aspects are in place is commonly referred to as the 'regulatory green light' and usually marks the sponsor's authorisation to ship IMP to the investigator sites. The regulatory green light process is covered in more detail in section 1.5.2.3.

6.4   Contracting-out activities

All activities associated with manufacture, importation, control and storage of IMPs may, in principle, be contracted out. As stated earlier, there should be a technical agreement between the sponsor or the sponsor's representative and the vendor. The number of possible permutations makes it impossible to offer more specific guidance in this area. Note that it is permissible to contract out to more than one vendor. For instance, one company may manufacture bulk IMP, another may package it and another may test it. In this case it is even more essential to clarify each party's technical responsibilities in written agreements.

The responsibility for the handling of complaints should be with the CMO (if manufacturing is contracted out); these complaints may be due to defects in the product, so the technical agreement should specify how these are to be handled and in what timeframe. When the CMO is also the supplier, it may be responsible for recalling product as necessary. Again, this should be made clear in the technical agreement.

There may well be more than one QP involved in the production chain and how they relate to each other should be clear to all concerned. Annex 16 of the EU Guidelines to GMP deals with this issue. The MHRA will grant an MIA(IMP) to sponsors for QP certification activities only; however, vendors will also need to be engaged in other manufacturing and/or importation activities to be granted an MIA(IMP). It is also strongly recommended that sponsors do not contract out only QP certification activities to a vendor, but also contract out other aspects of the IMP manufacturing and/or importation activities for which the vendor will perform QP certification.

Although it is permissible to engage a QP on a contract basis rather than having to employ one on a permanent basis, they must[7] be permanently and continuously available. Such an arrangement may permit an organisation to be involved with IMP manufacture and/or importation on a small scale that would otherwise not be economically viable. However, there is a risk that the contract QP may not devote the necessary amount of time and effort to a client company, particularly if they have contracts with numerous organisations. For example, it has been seen on inspection that the QP was not always present to perform QP certification and

6

this had routinely been performed remotely. Remote certification should not be seen as acceptable routine practice but rather to be carried out in exceptional circumstances. There is also a risk that the QP may become inappropriately isolated and lack the knowledge of ongoing relevant events that a permanent employee would become aware of (for example, updates to written procedures, process changes and staff changes).

The potential risks of engaging a QP on a contract basis should be managed and will be reviewed during any competent authority inspection. It is therefore recommended that contracts with QPs provide some guidance as to how often the organisation expects the QP to be present on site, as this is seen as important in order to maintain familiarity with the premises and procedures. There should also be a process in place to ensure that the QP is kept aware of any relevant changes to the organisation's quality system and of any relevant changes to the CTA. In addition, part of the assessment of suitability conducted by the MHRA if a contract QP is to be named on an MIA(IMP) is to check the number of authorisations on which the person is already named. If it is considered to be too many, the application or variation may be refused.

It is recommended that the section on contract QPs in the Orange Guide is read by any organisation considering using or employing a contract QP.

6.5   Active pharmaceutical ingredient

The active pharmaceutical ingredient (API) is the pure substance under test in a clinical trial. Unlike licensed medicines, it is not necessary for APIs destined for IMPs to be manufactured in full accordance with Part II of the EU Guidelines to GMP. However, the certifying QP is responsible for ensuring that the API is of a suitable quality. The steps taken to assure API quality will be an area of interest at any GMP inspection in relation to granting an MIA(IMP). An audit of the API manufacturer should take place and any departure from this should be justified and documented. If an API to be used as an IMP is a licensed medicine in its own right, it may be taken as a given that it will already have been subject to QP certification and, therefore, the API is of a suitable quality.

It is not permissible to avoid QP certification by simply claiming that it is pure API which is being administered. For example, in early development of a drug, the formulation may not be well developed and the IMP may be administered as the pure drug substance (that is, the API). However, unit doses will be weighed and put into a container and labelled prior to administration. This process is

Table 6.2 General types of blinding in a clinical trial

Term	Definition
Double-blind trial	A clinical trial in which neither the subjects nor the trial staff know which subjects are receiving the experimental medication and which are receiving a placebo (or another therapy). Double-blind trials are thought to produce objective results, since the expectations by the doctor and/or the subject regarding the experimental drug do not affect the outcome; also called double-masked trials.
Single-blind trial	A clinical trial in which one party, either the investigator or subject, is unaware of what medication the subject is taking; also called single-masked trials.
Open-label trial	A clinical trial in which the trial team and subjects know which medication is being administered.

considered to be manufacturing (not assembly, even though it is very simple and even if it is being conducted in a hospital for a non-commercially sponsored trial); therefore, the Regulation 37 exemption does not apply and QP certification is required.

6.6 Blinding

Blinding is the process that keeps one or more parties involved in a trial (for example, the sponsor, the investigator team and/or the subject) unaware of what treatment arm subjects have been randomised to. It is vital that the blind is maintained throughout the trial to ensure that no bias is introduced when making safety and efficacy assessments. The types of blinding in trial designs are provided in Table 6.2.

6.6.1 Manufacture and assembly considerations for blinding trials

Correct manufacturing and assembly processes are vital in ensuring that the blind is maintained. A common approach for tablets (should the active and comparator look different) is to over-encapsulate, that is, insert the tablets into appropriately sized capsules that are then back-filled with an inert powder, such as microcrystalline cellulose or lactose, to stop them rattling inside the capsule. These blinded capsules may be prepared manually or by semi-automatic or fully automatic equipment. It may be necessary to demonstrate that the product characteristics have not been adversely affected by the over-encapsulation.

There are many ways in which a trial can be unblinded through inadvertent clues left during manufacture. For instance:

- Tablets, capsules or other dosage forms have a different appearance (such as the test product being supplied in ampoules whereas the placebo is in plastic vials).
- Tablet embossing is different.
- Taste or smell is different.
- Labels are applied in a different position.
- Printing on labels appears different (font, typeface, printing density).
- Cartons or other packaging are constructed differently.
- Different batch numbers or other numbers appear on packs (both primary and secondary packaging).
- Over-labelling occurs that does not adequately obscure or cover underlying packaging information.
- The use of correction fluid to cover the batch numbers and identity of the IMP.
- Blinding envelopes are transparent.

These possibilities should all be taken into account when designing the trial and the IMP, including its manufacturing and assembly process. Generally, the only difference between various doses provided as part of a trial should be the subject number on the label. There should be no indication whether a given subject is receiving active drug, placebo or comparator; if this is not possible then an unblinded operator may be responsible for reconstitution and/or administering the IMP. In addition, the robustness of the blinding should also be considered. For example, the randomisation code and IMP should not simply be labelled treatment arm 'A' or treatment arm 'B', as the whole trial may then be unblinded when a single subject is unblinded in the case of a medical emergency or when the subject has a suspected unexpected serious adverse reaction (SUSAR).

In addition, it is often economical for organisations to order a bulk pack of IMP from a CMO and to re-package according to the randomisation schedule within a hospital pharmacy. Care should be taken when the batch number of the IMP and placebo are embossed on the foil pack. The batch number is essential for safety reasons to prevent accidental mixing of the two products; however, care should be taken in documenting a batch number on a label as its use would unblind the trial. For this reason it is common practice for a separate (novel) packaging batch number to be assigned that links the two products together. The actual product contained therein can then be traced by the subject or kit number and the packaging batch number. In other instances product may be dispensed directly from the pharmacy and it is important that trial teams are not in a position to be able to ascertain active drug from placebo or comparators by virtue of the lot numbers.

A vital part of IMP manufacture is the detailed instructions given on each occasion to ensure consistent manufacture between batches, as well as the checks carried out to ensure that the doses are adequately blinded. Part of the final QP certification should be a check that the steps taken to blind doses have been adequate.

6

6.6.2   Provision for unblinding

It is expected that the investigator site has the ability to unblind a subject immediately in the case of a medical emergency (see section 11.4.9). Emergency breaking of the blind may be undertaken by the use of physical code breaks (for example, envelopes or a scratch panel on the IMP supply) or via an interactive response technologies (IRT) system (Annex 4).

Code-break envelopes should be shipped before or together with the IMP in order to prevent the commencement of the treatment before the investigator has the ability to unblind. Similarly, when IRT is used, investigators or delegated individuals responsible for unblinding should have the ability to perform unblinding via the IRT system no later than when the IMP is received at the investigator site. The relevant personnel should test their username and password to the IRT system before the treatment of subjects begins to ensure that they have been granted the appropriate access to allow them to unblind. There should also be a back-up system available to the site to manage breaking the blind in the event that the IRT system is not functioning.

Reconciliation of physical code breaks (for example, envelopes) should be undertaken at the end of the trial and a check made that they have not been tampered with. When using an IRT system it should be possible to demonstrate (for example, via an audit trail) that the blinding has not been compromised.

6.6.3   Maintaining the blinding

A robust manufacturing process should be supported by equally robust processes to maintain the blinding. The processes for handling the code breaks, randomisation envelopes, master randomisation list and drug administration records are equally important to maintain the blinding. There are a number of examples where the lack of control in these areas has led to unblinding of the trial. These include:

- Opened randomisation envelopes were kept in subjects' case notes, which were accessible to those who were meant to be blinded.
- The treatment arm assigned to each subject was recorded in the subject's operation chart in the medical notes accessible to all the trial staff.
- The randomisation schedule was stored in an uncontrolled area (for example, on a free-standing computer or in the investigator site file).
- Treatment information was sent by the IRT system to a blinded sponsor and vendor team members.

In addition, there is a risk that the emergency unblinding of one subject may unblind the entire trial. For example, if there are two batch numbers, the likelihood is that one set is active and one is placebo/comparator and, therefore, if one subject is unblinded this could reveal the allocation of the treatment for all the subjects. The risk of bias due to unblinding is higher for trials with subjective efficacy end-points, such as pain scores, as if the subject thinks they are on placebo they may score differently. Therefore, extra precautions are recommended to be taken. These can include:

- Only dedicated unblinded team members to handle the supply or return of the IMP.
- When unblinding is required, where possible the trial team should not be informed (this may not be possible in the case of emergency unblinding).
- Where the principal investigator has been delegated the sponsor functions for SUSAR assessment and expedited reporting, consideration to be given to how and who will undertake this activity to ensure that there is no unnecessary unblinding of the trial team.
- Design of the packaging to allow the batch number to be cut off from the edge after dispensing. A double check of the dispensing activity should be implemented where this process is used.

In summary, it is important when designing the trial to consider how the blinding will be maintained. This will ensure that inadvertent unblinding is avoided, and that unnecessarily complex randomisation, packaging and dispensing procedures are not put in place, as involving numerous individuals carries the risk of mistakes and could lead to the administration of the incorrect treatment to a subject. Dosing errors are a common cause of serious breach reports. Careful planning,

6

communication and training are therefore necessary to ensure robust processes to maintain the blinding are in place.

6.7 Labelling

6.7.1 General labelling requirements

'Assembly' is defined within Regulation 2 (1) of SI 2004/1031 as:

'(a) enclosing the product (with or without other medicinal products of the same description) in a container which is labelled before the product is sold or supplied, or used in a clinical trial, or (b) where the product (with or without other medicinal products of the same description) is already contained in the container in which it is to be sold or supplied, or used in a clinical trial, labelling the container before the product is sold or supplied, or used in a clinical trial, in that container'.

Regulation 46 of SI 2004/1031 covers the requirement for clinical trial labelling. Under normal circumstances clinical trial labels should abide by the requirements in Articles 26 to 31 of Annex 13 and, as labelling is an assembly activity, it is required to be performed by an MIA(IMP) holder, unless the Regulation 37 exemption applies.

However, Article 14 of Directive 2001/20/EC allows for adapted provisions relating to labelling when:

- the product does not require particular manufacturing or packaging processes
- the product has an MA
- the subjects participating in the trial have the same characteristics as those covered by the indication specified in the MA.

Article 32 of Annex 13 should then apply to the clinical trial labelling requirements, provided Regulation 46 (2) of SI 2004/1031 is met, such that:

- the product is dispensed to a subject in accordance with a prescription given by a healthcare professional
- a dispensing label is applied as a minimum in accordance with Schedule 5 to The Medicines for Human Use (Marketing Authorisations Etc.) Regulations 1994.

Table 6.3 provides some examples of the labelling requirements.

Table 6.3 Labelling requirements

IMP has a marketing authorisation	Subjects have characteristics listed in authorisation	Prescribed by a healthcare professional	Trial-specific label	Hospital or health centre labelling (Regulation 37 exemption applies)	MIA(IMP) needed
Yes	Yes	Yes	No[a]	Yes	No
Yes	No	Yes	Yes	Yes	No
Yes	No	Yes	Yes	No	Yes
No	NA	Yes	Yes	Yes	No
No	NA	Yes	Yes	No	Yes

[a] Regulation 46 (2) of SI 2004/1031 applies.

IMP, investigational medicinal product; MIA(IMP), manufacturer's authorisation for investigational medicinal products

6.7.2　Post-QP certification labelling for safety purposes

An IMP is often provided and QP-certified in its final form (for example, as vials of active product and diluent). However, it may then require preparation, such as reconstitution by the pharmacy or in a ward/theatre into a syringe, giving set or infusion bag for administration.

Often, the labels used for these receptacles are compliant with Annex 13 but this is not a legal requirement. However, standard hospital practice should apply and the label should have sufficient information to identify who it is for and that the products are for clinical trial use.

Paragraphs 33 and 42 of Annex 13 allow for some packaging and labelling to take place after QP certification. This 'post-certification labelling' is primarily used for safety reasons, to ensure that the right product is given to the right person, especially if the product is to be given continuously or over a long period of time, in order to allow staff to keep updated with the situation and to act appropriately in unforeseen circumstances.

This labelling activity is usually performed prior to despatch, in the preparation area or immediately prior to administration to a subject. The circumstances in which additional labelling can be undertaken are:

Scenarios to help explain expectations and compliance with the Clinical Trials Regulations

Scenario 1

A trial has an IMP and comparator, both of which have MAs. The subjects being recruited have the indications listed in the MA. General pharmacy stock is used and is issued by a local (either community or hospital) pharmacy against a prescription. Justification for this approach is clearly documented in the risk assessment and detailed in the CTA application. Regulation 46 (2) of SI 2004/1031 will apply, as only a dispensing label will be required.

However, if the packaging of the licensed product is modified (for example, owing to a blinding process) there will be a requirement for a clinical trial label in line with Annex 13. This labelling activity will have to be conducted by an MIA(IMP) holder, unless the assembly (labelling) activity is being conducted by an organisation that meets the Regulation 37 exemption.

Scenario 2

A trial has an IMP and comparator, both of which have MAs, but the subjects to be recruited do not have any of the indications listed in the MA. A principal investigator has trial supplies issued by a community pharmacy against a private prescription and provides a clinical trial label to the pharmacy. However, as the indication is not listed in the MA, Regulation 46 (2) of SI 2004/1031 does not apply and the Regulation 37 exemption does not apply to a community pharmacy. Therefore, this is not acceptable.

Scenario 3

A commercial Phase I unit performs a 'dispensing' activity on the ward from bulk IMP/placebo supplies to avoid the need to conduct an 'assembly' activity and thus the requirement to QP-certify the individual subject dispensing pots (even though the unit holds an MIA(IMP)). However, for some of the cohorts the dose is made up by 'dispensing' a pot containing various active tablet strengths and placebo tablets. The accountability records do not adequately verify what the subjects actually receive (for example, the records show subjects have received the right number of tablets but not what strengths have been administered). The records also do not demonstrate that subsequent 'dispensing' has been performed after the previous subject's dose has been 'dispensed' and administered to ensure that there has been no confusion with the unlabelled dispensing pots. This complex activity should be performed as an assembly activity and be QP-certified.

- application of an identifier to ensure that a reconstituted IMP in its final container is administered to the correct subject
- application of expiry date labelling (or revised expiry date labelling)
- application of an investigator name
- application of a protocol number.

Post-certification labelling should, in the first instance, be performed at a site with an MIA(IMP) unless the risk to the quality of the product is unacceptably elevated by any required transportation to where the subject is being dosed. If this is not possible (as defined by the risk assessment) then there should be:

- a clear formalised procedure for the activity (including any sample labels and documentation to be completed)
- documented training and delegation of the activity to appropriate trial staff.

It is expected that the level of assurance of the quality of the final product should not be less than if this labelling were performed prior to QP certification.

If a container for reconstitution has been provided with a label already attached that contains some of these aspects and a space for completion of the relevant information during the preparation activity, this would not be considered an assembly activity and, therefore, additional QP certification is not required.

6.8   Manufacture or reconstitution

An IMP manufacturing step can only be conducted by the holder of an MIA(IMP). 'Manufacture' is defined in Regulation 2 (1) of SI 2004/1031 as:

> *'Manufacture, in relation to an investigational medicinal product, includes any process carried out in the course of making the product, but does not include dissolving or dispersing the product in, or diluting it or mixing it with, some other substance used as a vehicle for the purposes of administering it.'*

However, steps such as diluting a concentrate or reconstituting a powder to enable administration are not defined as manufacture. Therefore, an MIA(IMP) does not need to be held and QP certification of this step is not required. However, it is not always clear what activity is being carried out, as some processes lie in the grey area between manufacture and reconstitution.

The definition of 'reconstitution' can be found in Annex 13 as a simple process of:

- *dissolving or dispersing the investigational medicinal product for administration of the product to a trial subject,*
- *or, diluting or mixing the investigational medicinal product(s) with some other substance(s) used as a vehicle for the purposes of administering it.*

Reconstitution is not mixing several ingredients, including the active substance, together to produce the investigational medicinal product.

An investigational medicinal product must exist before a process can be defined as reconstitution.

The process of reconstitution has to be undertaken as soon as practicable before administration.

This process has to be defined in the clinical trial application/IMP dossier and clinical trial protocol, or related document, available at the site.'

Table 6.4 provides some examples of IMP activities and states whether they would be considered to be manufacture. The MHRA website and EU guidance on GMP FAQs can be referred to for further advice on whether a process is manufacture or reconstitution. However, it is strongly recommended that where there is any doubt, specific advice is sought from the MHRA prior to undertaking any activities.

Table 6.4 Examples of whether activities would be considered as manufacture

Activity	Manufacture
Over-encapsulation of solid dose form	Yes
Reconstitution	No
Serial dilutions	No
Reconstitution of IMP immediately prior to administration into another syringe or infusion bag which is then labelled for safety to identify the contents for transport between the preparation area and where the subject is located	No (see section 6.7.2)
Mixing two injections in one single receptacle (syringe or infusion bag)	Depends[a]
Dispersing/mixing active ingredient in aqueous cream	Depends[a]

[a] This will depend on how the activity is described in the clinical trial authorisation application. Therefore, determining this will be on a trial-specific basis. Confirmation should be sought from the MHRA where there is any ambiguity.

IMP, investigational medicinal product

6.9   The use of commercial supply in clinical trials

6.9.1   Commercial supply

When both the IMP and the comparator are authorised products within the EEA, the IMP management is relatively straightforward. The products can be dispensed from the general pharmacy stock. It is not a legal requirement for pharmacies to segregate the stock for use in a particular trial from the normal dispensing stock (that is, to 'ring-fence' the stock) when either the IMP or comparator is an authorised product. This applies to all authorised products and is not dependent on whether the product is being used to treat the authorised indication. However, some pharmacies do ring-fence stock for use in a particular trial as there are a number of benefits to this.

For example, it may be an advantage to purchase sufficient supply to last for the whole duration of the trial. This ensures that:

- the same batch and brand is used (when more than one brand and/or formulation of a drug exists), thus minimising the possibility of an incorrect brand or formulation being used for the trial
- if the NHS Trust changes suppliers or contracts during the recruitment of the trial, the IMP will not change
- the IMP is always available, especially where products are prone to a shortage in supply, so the continuity of treatment is maintained for trial subjects
- where an IMP is supplied free of charge by the marketing authorisation holder (MAH) as part of a contract with a non-commercial sponsor, the IMP is segregated from the main stock so it is not inadvertently dispensed for another trial.

However, there are disadvantages to ring-fencing stock for trials; for example, the IMP may expire before the trial has ended, or the stock occupies extra space and more resource may be required for stock checking. Also, specialised training and clear instructions for dispensing may be necessary to ensure that the correct supply is used. It has often been identified on inspection that clinical trial material has been dispensed to non-trial subjects and vice versa.

6.9.2   Use of generics and branded products

When branded products are used that have only one supplier and one standard formulation, there is no additional risk in terms of the incorrect product(s) being sourced by an investigator site. However, there may be such a risk when generics or multiple formulations are available. The issue is compounded by the fact that different regions in the UK may have their own local supply contracts that dictate which brands or makes of generics are to be used by the organisation. These contracts are usually renewed annually and, therefore, the suppliers or the brand could change during the course of a clinical trial.

It is recommended that when planning the trial the sponsor determines the risk of regional variability and decides whether the supply can be sourced centrally, whether it should provide an approved list of brands to be used, or whether any generic product is acceptable for use in the trial. This could be captured in the trial risk assessment (as described in section 4.7.1). In addition, where generics can be used it is recommended that this is clearly identified in the CTA application, as this can save a lot of time spent on amending the CTA application if a selected brand is no longer available.

6.9.3 Change in formulation

In the event of a change in the formulation by the MAH, if the product licence number is unchanged there is unlikely to be any impact on the clinical trial. However, if the change in formulation results in a new product licence number, the sponsor must[8] assess the need for a substantial amendment to the protocol. Substantial amendments are described in section 2.3.6.

European Commission 'Detailed guidance on the request to the competent authorities for authorisation of a clinical trial on a medicinal product for human use, the notification of substantial amendments and the declaration of the end of the trial' (CT-1) includes examples that would be considered as substantial amendments; these include a change of IMP, change of dosing and change to the mode of administration. Changes such as a variation in the strength of the tablets or vials would not be considered substantial, as long as the formulation and the total dose as per the protocol remains the same. However, the change from a film-coated tablet to a dispersible tablet formulation would require approval under a substantial amendment.

The exception to this is bioequivalence trials, as the reference material (the authorised product) should be clearly defined and, therefore, a substitution of the brand or formulation is unacceptable once the trial has started.

6.9.4   Withdrawal of a marketing authorisation

Occasionally, MAHs may remove a drug from the market for business reasons. When this occurs it may still be possible for a sponsor to source the supply directly from the MAH. In such circumstances, the change in MA status would not change the risk associated with the trial, and therefore a substantial amendment would not be required. There are other instances where a substantial amendment would be required – for example, where alternative formulations of the same drug are sourced from outside the EEA (these would then need to be imported and certified by a QP) and where a different formulation is used as a substitute.

6.10   Supplies for investigator-initiated trials

Pharmaceutical companies and MAHs often support investigator-initiated research by providing the IMP free of charge to the investigator. Even though the supplier of the IMP is technically not the sponsor of the trial, the commercial organisation must comply with Regulation 13 of SI 2004/1031 (that is, verify that the trial has an authorisation and that the products have been manufactured in accordance with GMP), before releasing the IMP to the investigator. It is also recommended that the supplier has sight of the favourable REC opinion. The division of responsibilities should be defined in an agreement. Key components within the agreement may include the requirement to provide CTA and REC approvals to the supplier, and responsibilities for QP certification, product recalls and defects reporting. The IMP supplier/MAH may also wish to request any safety information from the sponsor.

6.11   Product recall

The responsibility for product recalls lies with the sponsor. However, IMPs and/or comparators that are authorised products will be recalled by the MAH and the sponsor will be notified indirectly by their supplier if they are not the MAH. Before a recall for a trial is initiated by the sponsor, it is recommended that the MHRA (the Clinical Trials Unit and the Defective Medicines Report Centre) is notified, as discussions could lead to a different decision for the trial-related product (for example, the decision to continue use and keep the trial going rather than recall). In clinical trials, more than one party may be involved; in these instances the responsibilities of the different parties should be defined in, for example, technical agreements.

A system for monitoring a product recall should be in place; this is usually built into the supply agreement, which includes a stipulation that the suppliers need to inform the recipient of any relevant product recall. It is possible that counterfeit product may enter the supply chain and its use may have serious consequences in a clinical trial. There have been occasions when the commercial supply chain has been breached and counterfeit products have reached clinical trials. It is recommended that the sponsor signs up for email alerts on recalls, wherever available, as this may be another route by which they can be notified of defective product.

There are many players in a product recall, such as (for example) the sponsor, the CMO, other applicable vendors, IRT providers, and the investigator site(s) and subjects. The process for recall should be defined. The decision about whether to initiate a recall usually lies with the sponsor; however, the procedure to be followed may be a sponsor's own or that of a vendor. It is recommended that the recall process is tested to ascertain whether it is effective. Consideration could also be given to testing the effectiveness of recalling product from trial sites and, potentially, trial subjects, as the testing of product recall is often limited to just the supply depot.

A hosting site is not required to have a separate recall procedure for clinical trials. An NHS-Trust-wide medicine management policy should cover a product recall process for retrieving unused supply from wards and contacting subjects for dispensed material. This process should include clinical trial supplies. If, however, the pharmacy has been delegated the IMP management responsibilities by its NHS Trust and is responsible for distributing IMP to the other trial sites, a more detailed procedure should be implemented to manage product recall. This procedure could include the initiation of the recall, the quarantine process, the lines of communication between sponsors and the trial sites, retrieval and reconciling stock.

Recalls are not limited to IMPs and nIMPs. For example, Phase I units and non-commercial clinical trials facilities that function separately from the main hospital policies may have resuscitation trolleys which will contain medications that may be recalled.

6.12   Non-investigational medicinal products

Not all substances given to subjects during clinical trials are IMPs. Detailed guidance on these non-investigational medicinal products (nIMPs) is provided in

EU 'Rules Governing Medicinal Products in the European Union', EudraLex Volume 10. nIMPs are generally one of the following:

- rescue medication to be administered when the IMP does not produce a satisfactory response or perhaps causes too great a response (for example, subject-controlled morphine available to the subjects of a trial on an analgesic)
- challenge agent to produce a physiological response such that the IMP can be assessed (for example, triggers an allergic response to enable assessment of an antihistamine)
- medicines used to assess clinical trial end-points (for example, a radiopharmaceutical used to measure organ function after administration of an IMP)
- concomitant medication given as part of standard care for a condition that is not the indication for which the IMP is being tested (for example, cancer therapy given in a trial to test analgesic effectiveness in cancer patients)
- background treatment to treat the indication that is the object of the trial (for example, cancer therapy given to all subjects during a trial to assess a new cancer therapy against placebo).

These agents or medicines fall under general medicines legislation and GMP rather than the Clinical Trials Regulations. In this way, nIMPs that are authorised medicinal products are governed by the requirements of Directive 2001/83/EC, including Title IV, which contains the GMP requirements.

It is recommended that nIMPs with a marketing authorisation (MA) in the Member States concerned are used. When this is not possible, preference should be given to products with an MA in another Member State, then to those with an MA in an ICH country or a third country having a mutual recognition agreement with the EU, and lastly to products with an MA in another third country.

However, it is acknowledged that occasionally there may be the need to use nIMPs that are unlicensed. When this is the case, the sponsor is responsible for safeguarding the clinical trial subject, in accordance with Article 3 of Directive 2001/20/EC. Therefore, the sponsor must ensure and guarantee the quality and safety of the products and substances used in the trial (including nIMPs).

Details of any nIMPs (including any assurance and guarantee of the quality and safety of the nIMPs) and their proposed use should be included in the CTA application and identified in the protocol.

6.13   Drug accountability

Drug accountability allows the reconstruction of the trial and, put simply, documents what medication was received by the site, what medication was received by the subject and when and where, as well as what medication was returned to the sponsor or destroyed. It facilitates the reconstruction of the disposition of the IMP to demonstrate that subjects received the correct medication, in the correct form and strength according to the protocol.

6.13.1   General considerations

Drug accountability forms are usually produced to document the accountability of the IMP at each site to ensure that all supplies received have either been dispensed to the subject or destroyed/returned to the sponsor. These forms may be provided by the sponsor, in which case the site may wish to review these to ensure that they adequately cover the dispensing procedure in line with the logistics of their site set-up. Alternatively, the investigator site could design and customise the drug accountability forms in line with their own procedures (as familiarity with the forms may provide better compliance with the paperwork, especially where the site undertakes numerous trials). However, if local site procedures and forms are used, the sponsor should have oversight of this.

Design of the accountability forms, that is, capturing all the necessary information, will reduce difficulties in reconciliation. Poorly designed forms often lead to missing information and an inability to adequately reconstruct the trial. For example, it may be appropriate for some trials to have a site-level accountability form to record all medication received and used at the site, and a separate subject-level accountability form to record what was dispensed to an individual subject.

Drug accountability is an area in which issues are commonly identified on inspection, for example:

- When reconciling what medication had been dispensed from bulk supplies against what medication was recorded on each subject accountability record and against what was destroyed, there were discrepancies that could not be accounted for.
- Batch numbers of the IMP were incorrectly transcribed, such that they did not match the shipping inventory.
- Discrepancies between the main pharmacy accountability log for bulk supplies, the pharmacy manufacturing unit's batch records and the unblinded

research nurse's administration paperwork did not allow for full traceability of the IMP.

- Accountability forms were not fit for purpose, such that insufficient details were recorded on the form:
  - » A form was designed to record the number of bottles dispensed and returned, rather than tablets. Therefore, when partially used bottles were returned it was not possible to determine that the correct number of tablets had been taken.
  - » A form recorded the number of vials dispensed rather than the volume of the dilution required to be dispensed in a protocol requiring a ml/kg administration. Therefore, it was not possible to determine the volume administered.
- Forms were not completed correctly, such that there were missing entries, the forms were not signed and dated, or numerous changes were made without it being clear who made the changes and why they were made.

6.13.2 Drug accountability in line with the risk-adapted approach

Trials vary greatly in relation to the risks associated with the IMP and the trial procedures. The MRC/DH/MHRA paper 'Risk-adapted approaches to the management of clinical trials of investigational medicinal products' allows the sponsor to assess the IMP risk category of a trial (Type A, B or C; see section 2.4 for detailed information).

Once the category has been determined via the risk-adapted approach, a full risk assessment of the trial is recommended to be conducted, including the drug accountability requirements. Therefore, the level of accountability needed may vary depending on factors such as the authorisation status of the IMP, whether it is being used within its authorised indication, the trial design (such as the population, blinding and complexity of the dosing regimen), who is administering the IMP and the toxicity of the IMP. Table 6.5 gives some examples of the level of drug accountability recording within the context of the risk-adapted approach.

6.13.3 Drug accountability in relation to IMP administration

IMP may be administered by:

- one of the trial team at the trial site
- one of the trial team in the subject's home
- the subject or their carer.

Table 6.5 Risk-adapted approach to investigational medicinal product drug accountability

Type of IMP	IMP prescription/ supplies	Accountability requirement	Alternative means to determine compliance
IMP and comparator(s) used within their authorisation	NHS prescription filled by any local pharmacy (standard stock)	Low	Normal prescribing practice No requirement for: • Shipping receipt and destruction records • Drug accountability, provided the sample size is acceptable to account for the variability in drug compliance. Alternatively, if the sample size is small, subjects may be asked to complete a diary card or return the remainder of the prescription • Recording batch numbers and/or expiry dates, unless part of routine practice
IMP and comparator(s) used off-label, but use is an established practice, and supported by published evidence	Local prescribing practice and general site pharmacy stock	Low	As above
IMP and comparator(s) used within their authorisation or established for off-label use and administered at the trial site by trained staff	Local prescribing practice, but IMP supplied for trial/ ring-fenced from general stock	Low	Normal prescribing practice Requirement for: • Accountability of bulk receipt and destruction/return • Drug accountability; however, documentation can be either trial-specific or according to local practice, provided there is an ability to reconcile bulk against individual patient use • Recording batch numbers and/or expiry dates

Table continues

Table 6.5 *continued*

Type of IMP	IMP prescription/ supplies	Accountability requirement	Alternative means to determine compliance
Single-/ double-blinded trial with unblinded operator preparing IMP/ comparator/ placebo[a] (all having an MA) as per randomisation schedule	Local prescribing practice and general pharmacy stock	Medium	Normal prescribing practice or trial-specific prescribing acceptable No requirement for: • Accountability of bulk receipt and return/destruction Requirement for: • Trial-specific worksheet and dispensing log with sufficient details to verify that what was prepared was what was randomised • A second dose checker. If possible, used vials retained and reviewed by unblinded monitor • Recording batch numbers and/or expiry dates
Single-/ double-blinded trial where IMP/ comparator/ placebo require a manufacturing activity[b]	Trial-specific prescriptions and IMP supplies	High	Full accountability records of receipt, use and return/destruction
The IMP is unlicensed	Trial-specific prescriptions and IMP supplies	High	Full accountability records of receipt, use and return/destruction

[a] For example, saline product.

[b] For example, over-encapsulated product.

IMP, investigational medicinal product; MA, marketing authorisation

The level of documentation required to verify accountability will vary in each of these situations. However, it will also depend on the end-point of the trial and how the result will be used (for example, part of an MA application or a publication to support a change in prescribing practice). Therefore, documentation may range from a simple diary card completed by the subject or their carer to confirm compliance, where IMP is self-administered, to numerous records being generated to verify drug preparation and dosing, such as with intravenous chemotherapy or vaccines. Examples of documentation include full accountability records, infusion preparation worksheets (such as aseptic batch records), drug collection/return logs, administration logs and infusion charts. Based on the risk assessment, it must[9] be clear from the paperwork who was dosed with what, when and where it was dosed, and by whom.

6.13.4   Drug accountability in relation to blinded trials

6

Many trials are conducted in a blinded manner to reduce bias when analysing the results. These may be double- or single-blind. In many trials the IMP will be delivered to the site in a blinded manner; therefore only the assembly site is unblinded as this gives the highest confidence of maintaining the blinding. However, in both commercial and non-commercial trials it may occasionally be necessary for an unblinded operator at the investigator site to perform the reconstitution, dispensing and dosing of the IMP for single- and/or double-blind trials. For example:

- The IMP or comparator may have a distinct appearance, such as a distinct colour or opaque appearance, and therefore it is not possible for an operator to be blinded (unless the products are contained in an opaque syringe or giving set).
- It may not be appropriate to package the IMP for individual subjects.
- The IMP and comparator may be administered via different routes (for example, subcutaneously or through intravenous infusion).
- Administering an additional dummy drug for blinding purposes may be burdensome for subjects.

It is generally routine practice for pharmacies to keep detailed records of dispensing, which should allow trial reconstruction. However, care should be taken when the operation is performed outside pharmacy, such as by a nurse or a theatre operator selecting IMP and comparator from stock, especially when general stock is used, since records may not be routinely made. It is important to demonstrate that correct medications and doses have been prepared and that accountability records are adequately maintained, along with maintaining the blinding. Double checking may be required, but if a single operator is used there should be a clear and defined process to maintain an audit trail. This may include

Good Clinical Practice Guide

the retention of the used vials that have been labelled for each subject, where possible.

Where there are unblinded personnel there should be clear documentation (for example, in the delegation log) of who is authorised to perform the unblinded activities, to provide assurance that those performing efficacy and safety assessments remain blinded and, therefore, unbiased. In order to maintain the blinding, unblinded documentation should be retained separately from the rest of the trial documentation until the end of the trial or until the randomisation code has been broken for analysis.

There are cases where the method of administration between two arms of a trial is so different that it is not possible or convenient to blind the subjects and the investigator (for example, in a trial that compares an overnight dressing against a twice-daily application of steroid cream). In this instance, the assessor for the skin condition would need to be blinded in order to perform the assessment objectively and the subjects would need to be educated not to reveal the treatment to the assessor.

Complex blinding processes implemented at the investigator site should be defined in a formalised procedure and records must[10] be available to reconstruct who had access to the randomisation schedule, who assigned the treatment to subjects, who performed the blinding process and who released the IMP to the person who administered it. It is recommended that consideration also be given to the logistical set-up of the ward area to ensure that this is also conducive to maintaining the blinding. There have been a number of issues identified on inspection that relate to inadequate maintenance of the blinding. For example:

- An unblinded pharmacist and checker covered the unblinded cartridge label when the dosing pens were loaded prior to administration by blinded personnel. There was no record to demonstrate how this process was performed, when it was done, who performed the blinding step and who performed the quality control (QC) check before dosing.
- There was no consideration given to delegation of the unblinded activities; therefore, this activity was conducted by personnel also responsible for efficacy and safety assessments. For example, in one instance the unblinded operator was the sub-investigator who was responsible for assessing efficacy end-points.

216

- There was no separate area or location in the ward or theatre where the unblinded personnel could adequately prepare the IMP and communicate in the absence of blinded staff.

- There was no documentation of the reconstitution performed in the theatre and no evidence that this was subject to a QC check. Therefore, it could not be verified that the correct dose was administered.

6.14 Storage and distribution of investigational medicinal product

Shipment and storage of IMP is an essential part of any clinical trial, as it is imperative that the product has been stored correctly at all times to maintain its integrity. This section covers this aspect of clinical trials; however, storage and temperature monitoring are also covered in Chapter 11.

6.14.1 Storage and environmental monitoring

6.14.1.1 Shipment and data loggers

It is recommended that sponsors perform a risk assessment to determine the storage requirements (for example, temperature, humidity and protection from light) and what type and level of monitoring is required when shipping IMPs to investigator sites. An accompanying temperature monitoring device may need to be considered to ensure that the integrity of the product is maintained during transit.

Factors such as the availability of stability data, storage requirements (for example, ambient, refrigeration or frozen), transit time and the transit environment (for example, a refrigerated vehicle) may be taken into consideration when deciding what monitoring device or what validated temperature-control packaging system to use, if any. This will prevent situations where a temperature monitoring device or system is not fit for purpose (for example, a temperature range to trigger an alarm that an excursion had taken place during shipment was wider than the storage conditions specified for the IMP) or is excessive (for example, data loggers included with licensed medicines that are routinely transported with no temperature monitoring for standard use).

Sponsors are recommended to also consider the temperature monitoring requirements after the IMP has been dispensed, to ensure that these are in line with the design of the trial and not excessive. For example, transport of IMP from a pharmacy to a ward may take less than five minutes or the IMP will be taken home by the subject and thus the environmental conditions are outside the control of the investigator site and the sponsor; therefore, there would be no benefit gained from monitoring the transit after the IMP has left the pharmacy. However, in some circumstances the sponsor could impose conditions, such as limits on the transit time, and ensure that there is a mechanism to identify whether these have been breached.

When a data logger is used to monitor transit temperatures the data are reviewed either by the sponsor or by the site if this task has been delegated. In either case there should be a process and clear documentation that the data from the data logger have been reviewed and authorisation to use the IMP has been granted prior to the IMP being dispensed. This can be performed in several ways – for example, the data logger may be returned to the sponsor or the data may be downloaded by the investigator site and then transmitted (faxed/emailed) to the sponsor or printed and retained at the investigator site.

Where supplies are received in poor condition or there has been a temperature excursion during transit, the IMP should be quarantined until the sponsor (or delegate) has either assessed it as suitable for use or stipulated that it is to be returned/destroyed. Some sponsors may request the site to keep all IMP deliveries under quarantine until confirmation is provided to the investigator site that the delivery is suitable for use. In all instances, there should be a process in place to manage and document quarantining of IMP supplies at the investigator site.

6.14.1.2 On-site storage

The sponsor should ensure that all involved parties (for example, monitors, investigators and pharmacists) are aware of the storage requirements of the IMP and the actions to be taken in the event that the conditions are not met. These requirements are usually stated in the protocol or a pharmacy manual provided by the sponsor (where one has been provided). Article 26 of Annex 13 states that storage conditions should be detailed on the trial-specific label. However, when authorised products are used this may not always be apparent (for example, it may state that there are no specific storage requirements). In most circumstances the pharmacy would be familiar with how the product should be stored; however, if there is any doubt, staff should refer to any available literature (in many instances this is the summary of product characteristics) or contact the sponsor. Examples have been seen where authorised IMPs were stored under incorrect conditions, as they were not products commonly handled by the pharmacy responsible for the trials supplies and the storage requirements were not immediately apparent.

There is no legal requirement for the frequency and method of temperature monitoring; however, it is recommended that this is determined and documented in the risk assessment. A robust system should be in place to ensure appropriate storage of the product prior to dispensing to a subject, and that there is evidence to support this. Temperature monitoring can range from:

- no additional monitoring other than that required for the general stock supplies held in the pharmacy for routine care
- daily recordings using calibrated maximum/minimum thermometers (for example, where only a small amount of IMP supplies is maintained)
- continuous recordings using fully automated and alarmed electronic systems (for example, where there are large volumes of IMP supplies with varying levels of storage conditions, numerous storage locations and/or detailed monitoring requirements).

When a data logger is used as a permanent monitoring device, there should be a process to specify how the operator will be made aware of any temperature deviations prior to dispensing the IMP, if downloading of the data is only required at certain intervals. For example, if the data logger was only required to be downloaded monthly but a temperature excursion occurred on day 1, how would the excursion and the impact on the IMP be assessed and the IMP be authorised for use before the medication was dispensed to subjects? In this case, the data logger could be supplemented by a daily maximum/minimum temperature reading taken using a calibrated thermometer or by use of a calibrated and tested alarm system to show that there have been no excursions in the last 24 hours. The data logger can then be printed, reviewed, signed off and filed in the trial file as evidence of appropriate storage. The pharmacy should ensure that any data loggers used are calibrated according to the loggers' specific requirements. There are occasions where the pharmacy has been unaware that the calibration period for a device has expired or that the device has never been calibrated.

The pharmacy should have a process in place to identify and manage temperature excursions of on-site storage of IMP. This may include:

- what stock is affected (including assessment of what trials are affected, as there could be more than one)
- how the affected stock is quarantined

- how the sponsor is notified
- how the excursion will be assessed for impact on the suitability of the IMP for use (this may be done by the sponsor or investigator site, if this has been delegated)
- how the excursion will be documented, including the transfer/movement of all associated IMPs and the outcome of the impact assessment.

Failing to act on temperature excursions can have serious consequences; for example, subjects can be dosed with defective IMP without the knowledge of the sponsor. This may have an impact on subject safety in the form of toxicity of the degraded products, or may result in seriously ill subjects receiving ineffective treatment. An example has been seen where a subject died after receiving an IMP that was stored incorrectly and it could not be ascertained whether this was owing to the subject's underlying disease or whether it was attributable to the IMP. The deviations may also affect the integrity of the data/results.

6.14.2 Management of investigational medicinal product by the investigator

The investigator (or their delegate) is responsible for the management of IMP at their site. This may be a hospital (NHS/private), GP surgery, dentist or commercial facility (for example, a site management organisation (SMO) clinic or Phase I unit).

No matter where a drug is shipped to, it should be transported and stored according to the correct storage conditions. A lack of pharmacy involvement in IMP management may result in inadequate record keeping, accountability and storage. If the IMP is stored by the investigator, they and the sponsor should ensure that the storage area is secure, the storage conditions are adequate for the IMP, temperature monitoring is in place, and that accountability (including an area for returns) has met an acceptable standard, in line with the risk assessment resulting from the risk-adapted approach.

Within a hospital (and some large GP surgeries) the management of the IMP is often delegated and thus undertaken by a pharmacy; this may be covered by the hospital medicine management policy. However, there is no legal requirement for an IMP to be shipped to a pharmacy, and the drug can be shipped directly to an investigator. There are a number of examples where IMPs are managed by the investigator:

- In emergency medicine, the trial team needs to have immediate access to the IMP out of hours; therefore, it may not be practical to store it in the pharmacy (for example, emergency research in an intensive therapy unit or hospital emergency department, where the time interval between IMP administration and the diagnosis could be short).
- The pharmacy is unable to provide the service in relation to the trial requirements but these can be provided by trial staff (for example, the IMP can be stored and prepared by theatre staff).
- Out-patient visits may occur at weekends or evenings when the pharmacy is not open and it would be inconvenient for subjects to return on a separate visit for their medication.

There are a number of ways that investigators can obtain trial supplies – for example, IMPs can be shipped directly to the investigator, or bulk IMP supply can be received and maintained by the pharmacy, which then distributes the supply to the investigator at regular intervals for storage in the theatre or ward.

The Royal Pharmaceutical Society has produced 'Practice guidance on pharmacy services for clinical trials'. This guidance states that *'When a clinical trial is taking place in a hospital all IMPs should be stored and dispensed by the hospital pharmacy and managed to the same standards as licensed medicines. IMPs must not be stored in offices, clinics or ward areas unless by prior agreement with pharmacy'*. When storage areas outside the pharmacy are used, these should be assessed to ensure that they are not liable to large daily temperature fluctuations. For example, efforts must be made to ensure that the product is not stored close to radiators, boilers or other sources of heat, or alternatively that the product is not stored in refrigerators turned down too low, thereby causing the product to freeze (this may be detrimental to certain products such as vaccines).

In the hospital setting where there is no hospital policy or R&D office requirement for pharmacy to be involved, there should be a procedure in place to ensure that both the R&D office and pharmacy are aware of any trial undertaken in the hospital with IMPs and to confirm/document their agreement with arrangements for the handling of the product outside the pharmacy. In some hospitals, the storage of an IMP by the investigator needs to be approved in advance by the R&D office/pharmacy.

Therefore, where IMP is to be stored outside pharmacy, the pharmacy should have a formalised procedure for the assessment and approval of the storage area,

6

shipping arrangements (if being shipped directly) and the dispensing and record-keeping processes. The procedure may include responsibility for accountability checks and environmental monitoring of the area, recalls, quarantine, documentation and temperature excursions (including approval for use of the IMP post-excursions). It is also good practice for the pharmacy to carry out periodic environmental checks and reviews of the accountability records for storage outside pharmacy, as would occur in normal routine practice, especially if there is limited or no on-site monitoring. For commercial sponsors, the monitors should be satisfied with the storage, drug accountability and environmental monitoring arrangements.

It is a common finding at inspection that there was no assessment of external IMP storage areas and the storage conditions were found to be unsatisfactory.

6.14.3   Site-to-site transfer

Article 47 of Annex 13 allows the transfer of IMP between sites, but only in exceptional circumstances (for example, where the safety of the subject is jeopardised if supplies are not provided from another site). The circumstances surrounding the requirement to transfer material should not be due to inadequate oversight of the manufacturing or supply of the product. Where transfer does occur it should be covered by a formal process, with clearly documented records of what has been transferred, including the batch numbers and quantities of the product involved, and evidence that the storage conditions of the product at the originating site and during shipment to the receiving site were maintained. The activity should be conducted under the supervision of a person who is suitably qualified and, if required, advice from a QP should be sought. Ideally (where time permits) materials should be returned to the manufacturer for re-labelling, if necessary, and to ensure the integrity of the IMP.

It is not classified as a site-to-site transfer when a large NHS Trust with a central pharmacy stock ships medication to pharmacies in other hospitals within that same NHS Trust, or when a pharmacy of an NHS Trust dispenses IMP at one of its sites and transfers it to another of its sites where subjects are managed. However, in order to do either of these activities consideration should be given to ensuring that the quality of the product is maintained during the transit. Therefore, there should be clear formalised procedures in place to conduct these activities, with a clear audit trail of what has been transferred, when and by whom, including transfer receipts. Confirmation should also be sought, similar to that of the original shipment, that the IMP is intact and has been transferred at the appropriate temperature (if required), by a person who is appropriately qualified.

If IMP is being transferred between sites for a commercial trial, approval for this activity should be sought from the sponsor and the QP should have oversight of the procedure for assurance of the quality of the product. If transfer is being conducted for a non-commercial trial, oversight should be managed by appropriate personnel on behalf of the sponsor (this is generally delegated to the pharmacy). However, oversight could be performed by the investigator (or delegate), provided the evidence trail shows the disposition of the drug.

There have been many examples, during inspections of both commercial and non-commercial sponsors, of inadequate documentation related to the transfer of IMP between sites and confirmation of integrity of the product.

6.14.4 Returns

When subjects return used and partially used containers to the trial site, accountability of the returns may be performed by the research nurse by entering the data into the case report form (CRF); the containers may then be transferred to pharmacy. On other occasions, the pharmacy may perform the accountability check on the returns. In all cases, the monitor should ensure that there is reconciliation between the CRF and the accountability record.

Any IMP returned to the pharmacy should be segregated from available unused stock to avoid its inadvertent use, which could cause errors in drug accountability. Under no circumstances should the returns be re-used for another subject, as the storage condition of the IMP and the integrity of the product cannot always be ensured.

6.14.5 Supply of IMP by post

IMP may be posted to clinical trial subjects, when required, either as a pre-planned activity or in special circumstances. In some trials, subjects are recruited and assessed remotely, and therefore they are not physically seen by the investigator (there are a number of hurdles to cross for this type of trial, namely medical and sponsor oversight and eligibility assessment). Additionally, for some trials, certain subjects may live far away from the recruitment centres and it is therefore not easy for them to travel to the trial centre in between visits. Or the need for supply by post may arise when the IMP is lost or not available for use because of, for example, temperature excursions or the sponsor supplying drug with a short expiry date because of supply shortages. All these scenarios could result in IMP being sent directly to the subjects.

The clinical trial legislation does not currently prevent the posting of clinical trial medication to subjects; however, it is not ideal and therefore the sponsor is recommended to carefully review the storage requirements for the IMP as part of the risk assessment to ensure that its integrity will not be compromised during any such transit. Sufficient monitoring will need to be in place for products that are more liable to degrade. The following factors may be taken into consideration:

- Storage requirements:
  - » Does the medication have any specific storage requirements and, if so, can these be maintained during posting?
  - » What is the assurance that the integrity of the product is maintained during the transit? Should a temperature monitoring device be used, especially during the summer months?
  - » What is the stability of the product and the margin of safety? A product with a very stable profile at temperature extremes would require less monitoring than one with a narrow stability range. The sponsor may consider shortening the expiry of the product if the product is delivered in ambient temperature.
- Delays in posting:
  - » Is there potential to affect continuity of supply? The answer to this question is trial dependent. A few days' shortage of drug may not be detrimental for some trials but in others it may be crucial (for example, for antiretroviral therapy where resistance to the IMP may develop if treatment is interrupted).
- Drug accountability:
  - » What is the mechanism for confirming that the subjects themselves receive the IMP and that it is not delivered to someone else in error?
  - » Should the drug be signed for and therefore sent by a courier or recorded delivery?
  - » Does there need to be a follow-up telephone call to the subject?

In the event that a subject moves outside the UK while they are participating in a clinical trial and wishes to continue in the trial, the pharmacy could in theory post the medicine to the subject, provided it has been prescribed by an investigator (or delegate) in the UK. However, before this activity is undertaken it is strongly recommended that the sponsor checks with the MHRA and the local authorities of the country concerned to ensure any requirements for posting drugs to another country are met.

6.15 Administration at home

Sometimes it is not possible or is too burdensome for the subjects to visit the trial site and there may be a need for a nurse from the site to administer the IMP at the subject's home (for example, when the IMP is given regularly as an infusion over a period of time to very ill patients or is for the vaccination of babies). Alternatively, this activity may be contracted out to a home-care organisation or SMO, or the subject or their carer may administer the IMP themselves. There are a number of issues the hosting site needs to consider when any home-care arrangement is made.

6.15.1 Subject confidentiality

To comply with the Data Protection Act of 1998 regarding subject confidentiality, the subject must[11] be made aware that their personal information (such as their name, address and telephone number) may be released to third parties. This information will be necessary for service providers to contact subjects to arrange for delivery and administration of the IMP. The subject should sign an agreement to allow this information to be provided; this could be a separate agreement or part of the informed consent process (see section 3.3). There have been a number of occasions identified on inspection when subjects had not given their consent to release of their personal information to the third parties. These subjects may not even have known that the providers were not part of the investigator site organisation.

6.15.2 MIA(IMP) requirement

When assembly (packaging and labelling) of the IMP is carried out at the trial site under the Regulation 37 exemption, and the operator (for example, research nurse) obtains the reconstituted and labelled products and administers the product at a subject's home, an MIA(IMP) is not required. Likewise, if the IMP is provided in its original vials or ampoules and the operator reconstitutes the product in the subject's home prior to administration, an MIA(IMP) is not required. However, when assembly is carried out in the service provider's premises (for example, a home-care organisation) an MIA(IMP) is required.

6.15.3 GCP and protocol training

Part 2 (2) of Schedule 1 to SI 2004/1031 states that *'Each individual involved in conducting a trial shall be qualified by education, training and experience to perform his tasks'*. The operator must[6] have relevant basic GCP training to ensure they understand the record-keeping requirements. Sometimes these operators are under the supervision of the investigator. However, in some circumstances the operators are managed by an SMO, home-care provider or recruitment agency. Protocol training may be required if the administration of the IMP is significantly different from routine standard care. Personnel should be trained in:

- basic pharmacovigilance processes so that they are familiar with the adverse event/serious adverse event reporting mechanisms in place for the trial
- GCP record keeping
- reporting of protocol non-compliances and serious breaches to the trial team.

6.15.4 Contract

Where the activities are performed by a service provider (for example, an SMO, home-care organisation or recruitment agency) a contract or agreement between the NHS Trust and the service provider should define the responsibilities, standard of services and record-keeping and retention requirements (Chapter 1).

6.15.5 Self-administration by trial subjects

Subjects or, in the case of vulnerable patients, their carers may be trained to administer the IMP themselves. The trial team will need to ensure that subjects and/or carers are trained according to the requirements of the protocol in terms of storage, reconstitution, method of administration, record keeping (diary card), retention of used vials and the use of any equipment provided by the sponsor. This is usually performed at the start of the trial, when the site personnel will demonstrate and advise the subjects/carers on drug administration. However, site personnel will need to assess the subject's understanding before allowing self-administration. It is recommended that subjects have regular checks to reaffirm their understanding and assess their compliance with the protocol. This must[10] be documented to demonstrate it has been undertaken.

The following example was identified during an inspection. It illustrates both the importance of checking a subject's understanding of the instructions provided to them and of ensuring that there are safeguards in place to monitor compliance:

Subjects were given two syringes of nebulising solution to be administered together once a day via a nebuliser. However, a number of subjects nebulised one syringe twice a day. The investigator site was unable to identify the mistake, as the correct number of used syringes was returned and there was no record by the subject of when they administered the nebulisers. Therefore, the mistake was only identified retrospectively once the electronic records were downloaded from the nebulisers by the sponsor after the nebulisers had been returned.

6.16 Use of trial material after trial completion

Responsibility for IMP accountability at the trial site(s) rests with the investigator/institution. Once the trial has been concluded, the drug accountability records have been reconciled, and the used, returned or unused IMP/placebo/comparators have been accounted for, the IMP can be destroyed. However, it is good practice, where possible, to destroy the IMP only after the clinical study report has been written. This allows the IMP to be re-reviewed if there is any discrepancy with the trial (for example, in pharmacokinetic trials when there are outliers in the pharmacokinetic profile or there are unexpected drug concentrations). It is the responsibility of the sponsor to determine the most appropriate means to dispose of the drug, as long as records are maintained.

Under some circumstances it is possible to re-use IMPs in other trials and for non-trial subjects, but only if they are licensed medicinal products in that Member State.

For licensed products used in a clinical trial (provided that there is no modification to the original product, such that the product remains in its original MA primary and secondary packaging) it is relatively straightforward to transfer the stock to the pharmacy within the same site, as the pharmacy would have confidence in the storage condition of the material. Additional labelling would need to be removed from the pack (if used) without damaging the underlying package and instructions in the process.

For material manufactured as an IMP it is not possible to re-use the product unless the protocol has been amended to allow its extended use, and it may require different labelling depending on how the amendment has been made. When a clinical trial has been completed according to the protocol or a clinical trial is terminated early for ethical or other reasons, the investigator may wish to continue to treat some or all of the subjects who have benefited from the treatment (this is common for oncology trials). In these instances the medication is no longer an IMP and unless it is the subject of a MA it becomes an unlicensed relevant medicinal product and Directive 2001/83/EC therefore applies. As such it cannot be manufactured, assembled or imported under an MIA(IMP). If the manufacturer holds a manufacturer's ('special') licence, then the product may be manufactured and supplied as an unlicensed relevant medicinal product (a 'special') to meet the special needs of an individual patient under the direct personal responsibility of the prescriber.

Doses already available at the site at the time of halting the trial should be retrieved, and the appropriateness of their presentation (such as labelling and packaging) reviewed before consideration of their use for the treatment of any 'individual patients'. The MHRA website regarding importing unlicensed medicines and also guidance notes for medicines can provide further information, in particular 'Guidance Note 14: The supply of unlicensed relevant medicinal products for individual patients'.

Surplus IMP stock from one trial may be re-used for another clinical trial by the same sponsor or another sponsor. However, the sponsor must bear in mind that once an IMP has been allocated to a trial it cannot be used in another trial unless it is re-labelled and prepared for re-assessment, so it can be QP-certified against the new CTA(s) and released by the sponsor for the subsequent trial(s). A critical finding has been given to a sponsor who assumed that once the product had been QP-certified for one trial it could be used for a different trial without repeating the process in relation to the new trial. Each clinical trial for an IMP must[3] be considered in its own right and the normal process must[3] therefore apply.

6.17 Prescribing and dispensing

6.17.1 Prescription requirements

The supply of IMP and the comparator(s) to subjects falls within the remit of the Clinical Trials Regulations. It is not defined in the Clinical Trials Regulations that dispensing of IMP has to be recorded on a headed prescription form or official NHS Trust patient prescription. As long as a record is made by the investigator (or delegated medically qualified doctor) in the subject's medical notes, trial-specific prescription, clinical trial worksheets, CRF or even in a validated electronic system, this is accepted to be a valid authorisation by the investigator.

A comparator may be a prescription-only medicine in its own right; however, it is not a prescription-only medicine when used in a clinical trial. Therefore, it is not a legal requirement for the investigator to order the IMP or the comparator on a prescription to be dispensed by the pharmacy. However, the hosting site may insist on the use of a prescription because of hospital policy and it helps with tracking and providing an audit trail for the clinical trial. In addition, the sponsor should be aware that any background therapies or escape medications, when not defined as an IMP or comparator, fall outside the Clinical Trials Regulations and, as such, the standard prescription requirements apply.

When a prescription is used to order IMP from a pharmacy, this could either be on a trial-specific prescription or hospital standard prescription. The advantage of using the former is that the distinct appearance of the prescription would make it clear to pharmacy that it is for a clinical trial and not just filed according to standard pharmacy procedure. When a standard hospital prescription form is used, care must[10] be taken to ensure that it is filed in such a way that it can be tracked and retrieved for the purposes of reconstructing the trial (for example, retained in the pharmacy trial file/subject's medical notes/investigator's file). It is not uncommon for drug charts to be misplaced, especially when subjects are transferred to wards outside the investigator's control (such as an intensive therapy unit).

Chemotherapy regimens may be handled by electronic prescribing programmes that have pre-entered 'protocol regimes'. The prescribers therefore only need to select the correct arm of treatment; the doses for each treatment block will be worked out automatically against protocol-predefined criteria. These blocks can be constructed separately and re-used for different arms. These systems are used for standard prescribing as well as clinical trials and it is therefore important to ensure the correct protocol regimes are selected, as mistakes can be made such as selecting the incorrect protocol regime or block. Also, there may be trial-specific parameters that require checking for dosing/dose adjustments that differ from routine care. Therefore, when a new trial protocol is entered into the system there should be an internally documented QC process within pharmacy to ensure that the regimen is correct and authorised by the investigator (or delegate). This system should also be checked in line with any amendments to the protocol in case the amendment impacts on any of the protocol regimes. There have been examples where the QC check was not robust, resulting in subjects being dosed more frequently than specified in the protocol. On more than one occasion this has resulted in a fatality. The mistake was not identified by the medically qualified doctor, pharmacy or nurse, as there was over-reliance on the prescribing system.

The failure of the QC process for complex and highly toxic regimens is considered as high risk and, as such, a robust checking process should be in place at site level. Sponsors should satisfy themselves that the QC process at each investigator site is robust. Alternatively, the sponsor could provide sites with a centralised set-up of the trial module that would be compatible with the commonly used chemotherapy prescribing package.

6.17.2 Prescribing by a nurse or pharmacist

SI 2003/696 amends the Prescription Only Medicine (Human Use) Order 1997 to make provision for nurses and pharmacists who meet certain conditions (supplementary prescribers) to prescribe and administer prescription-only medicines in accordance with clinical management plans relating to individual patients. Article 3b(ii) of SI 2003/696 includes clinical trials, therefore allowing non-medical/supplementary prescribers to prescribe for clinical trials. In addition, it is acceptable for a research nurse or a pharmacist to act as a chief investigator. It is recommended that the NHS Trust management assesses the risk and decides whether the prescribing process is acceptable and in line with NHS Trust policy.

However, the decision for eligibility and thus trial enrolment must[12] still be made by a medically qualified doctor and there should be clear documentation of this. In addition, there must[10] be documented evidence of the medical input into the decision to prescribe (such as at subject recruitment or dose modification). The protocol may also include criteria or time points for which medical input is required to assess whether treatment can continue.

The responsibility for prescribing should be documented in the delegation log and the approval for supplementary prescribing should be maintained in the training files. All personnel involved in a clinical trial must[6] be adequately trained and qualified to perform their tasks, with the requirements increasing along with the complexity of the dispensing process.

6.18 Documentation retention

The retention requirements for IMP documentation are defined in Article 9 of Directive 2003/94/EC:

'For an investigational medicinal product, the batch documentation shall be retained for at least five years after the completion or formal discontinuation of the last clinical trial in which the batch was used. The sponsor or marketing authorisation holder, if different, shall be responsible for ensuring that records are retained as required for marketing authorisation in accordance with the Annex I to Directive 2001/83/EC, if required for a subsequent marketing authorisation.'

The sponsor of a clinical trial must[10] have access to full documentation when the manufacturing of the IMP is performed within its own facilities. These documents should include a copy of the MIA(IMP); TSE certification for the excipients, packaging components and active pharmaceutical ingredient; batch records; certificates of analysis (CoA); QP certifications for each batch; regulatory green-light release records; drug accountability for sites (at the end of the trial); and delivery notes and environmental monitoring records for each delivery.

When IMP management is contracted out to a CMO, sponsors should define their requirements for documentation retention. For example, the technical agreement may include the types of documents that are returned to the sponsor and those that are retained by the CMO, the retention period and the process to inform sponsors before record disposal. The standard retention requirements for non-IMP activities tend to be shorter than those stipulated in Directive 2003/94/ EC and sponsors should be mindful of these differences.

Pharmacies at investigator sites are often presented with a wide array of documents that they are required to maintain during the course of a trial. Often, pharmacies have requested sponsors to provide QP certification documents and TSE certification documents to be included in the site pharmacy file. It is not a legal requirement for the hosting site to maintain QP certification documents in the site pharmacy file; however, guidance requires that the CoA is present. Moreover, provision of these documents needs to be considered to ensure they do not compromise any blinding, as the CoA will contain the original lot number of the finished product(s), which could potentially link back to the supplies at the site through the delivery note, which may indicate the packaging batch number along with the original lot numbers.

There is no requirement for a hosting site pharmacy to request a copy of the MIA(IMP) and QP certification from the sponsor, as this would have been provided to the MHRA as part of the CTA.

The MIA(IMP) was not part of the clinical trial approval process prior to May 2004 and this is therefore not applicable for any batches of IMP manufactured or imported prior to May 2004. However, the sponsor is responsible for ensuring that, for those trials started prior to May 2004 under a clinical trial exemption (CTX) or that had been notified under the doctors and dentists exemption (DDX) scheme, any batches of IMP manufactured or imported after May 2004 are compliant with the regulations.

6.19   Chapter legislative references

Throughout this chapter, specific terminology – 'must', 'required' or 'requirement' – has been used to interpret activities that are legislative requirements. These terms have been number-coded in the text where used, and the corresponding reference in the legislation can be found below.

1. Regulation 36 of SI 2004/1031
2. Regulation 37 (2) of SI 2004/1031
3. Schedule 3, Part 2 (7) of SI 2004/1031
4. Schedule 3, Part 2 (8) of SI 2004/1031
5. Regulation 43 of SI 2004/1031
6. Schedule 1, Part 2 (2) of SI 2004/1031
7. Article 13 of Directive 2001/20 EC
8. Regulation 24 of SI 2004/1031
9. Schedule 1, Part 2 (9) of SI 2004/1031
10. Regulation 31A (4) of SI 2004/1031
11. Schedule 1, Part 2 (13) of SI 2004/1031
12. Schedule 1, Part 2 (11) of SI 2004/1031

CHAPTER 7

Monitoring

Editor's note

ICH Topic E6 (R1) – 'Guideline for Good Clinical Practice' (hereinafter 'ICH GCP') defines monitoring as the act of overseeing the progress of a clinical trial, and of ensuring that it is conducted, recorded and reported in accordance with the protocol and any amendments, written procedures, Good Clinical Practice (GCP), and the applicable regulatory requirement(s).

The sponsor may perform such monitoring directly or may use the services of a vendor (for example, a contract research organisation (CRO) or freelance monitor). It is the responsibility of the sponsor to ensure that trials are adequately monitored. Therefore, the sponsor must determine the appropriate extent and nature of monitoring; this should be based on the objective, purpose, design, complexity, size, blinding and end-points of the trial as well as the risks posed by the investigational medicinal product (IMP) and trial-related activities, and the experience of the investigator sites. It is recommended that this is identified via the trial risk assessment and clearly documented (for example, in the form of a monitoring plan).

There are a number of different approaches to monitoring; the type and combination of monitoring activities can be adapted and tailored to suit a particular trial. Examples include traditional on-site monitoring, central and statistical monitoring, trial steering committees and data monitoring committees. This chapter discusses the different approaches to monitoring, the activities involved in monitoring and how a risk-adapted approach can be used to ensure that available monitoring resources are used in an effective and proportionate manner.

7.1 Introduction to monitoring

Monitoring is one of the key mechanisms whereby the sponsor can be assured that it is in compliance with the legislation[1, 2] and the trial protocol/procedures. Effective monitoring may also provide useful feedback to the sponsor for continuous process improvement. The general approach to monitoring must[3] form part of the protocol, although the detail can be in the form of written procedures and monitoring plans. The specific approach to monitoring can be determined following a risk assessment, ensuring that the approach is proportionate and directed to critical areas.

There should be clear written procedures explaining how and when monitoring will be conducted and reported. The level of monitoring will vary significantly depending on the outcome of the risk assessment, which can take into account the type and complexity of the clinical trial being conducted. There may also be trial-specific procedures, such as a monitoring plan, detailing the monitoring activities in line with the mitigating actions identified in the risk assessment.

The personnel responsible for monitoring activities must[1, 4] follow the designated written procedures (either the sponsor's or vendor's procedures) and/or any trial-specific procedures for monitoring a specific trial.

7.2 Monitoring overview

An overview of clinical trial monitoring is provided in Figure 7.1. In summary, the purpose of monitoring clinical trials is to verify that:

- the safety, rights and well-being of trial subjects are protected
- investigators are appropriately selected, trained and supported to complete the proposed clinical trial
- processes are consistently followed and activities are consistently documented to ensure high-quality trial conduct and protocol compliance
- the reported trial data are accurate, complete and verifiable against the source documents
- the conduct of the trial is in compliance with the currently approved protocol/ amendment(s), with GCP and with the applicable regulatory requirement(s).

The monitoring personnel act as a point of contact for the investigator site and have a key role to play in the communication between the sponsor and the site,

Clinical trial monitoring

Approvals
Ensuring trial is conducted according to current competent authority authorisation and favourable REC opinion that are in place (including implementation of protocol amendments)

Communication
Open and effective communication between the monitoring personnel, sponsor and investigator site

IMP management
Checks on receipt, storage area and conditions, accountability and destruction

Documentation
Ensuring that all the documents required to reconstruct the trial are filed in the investigator site file and support ancillary department file(s)

Protocol compliance
Ensuring subjects are eligible, the protocol is followed and non-compliance is captured and reported to sponsor

Consent
Ensuring subjects have given their initial informed consent prior to trial participation and ongoing consent for any updates

Training
Ensuring staff are appropriately trained before and during the trial

GCP compliance
Ensuring principles of GCP are complied with and any non-compliance is captured and reported to sponsor

Data integrity
CRF review and source data verification

Delegation of duties
Checks that staff undertaking trial duties have been appropriately delegated by principal investigator

Safety
Checks on recording data and reporting SAEs to sponsor and receipt of safety information

Facilities and equipment
Ensuring that the facilities and equipment are and remain suitable for conducting the trial

CRF, case report form; GCP, Good Clinical Practice; IMP, investigational medicinal product; REC, research ethics committee; SAE, serious adverse event

Figure 7.1 *Overview of clinical trial monitoring (see Table 7.1 for further details)*

the support for the investigator site and the resolution of any issues that may affect the trial conduct.

Monitoring can include:

- **On-site monitoring** Monitoring activities are primarily undertaken during a physical visit to the investigator site by one or more monitoring personnel
- **Central or remote monitoring** Monitoring activities are undertaken by the monitoring personnel in a location remote from the investigator site (for example, a data centre).

7.2.1 Trial steering committees and data monitoring committees

The use of data monitoring committees (DMCs) (also known as data monitoring boards or data safety monitoring boards (DSMBs)) and trial steering committees (TSC) can also be considered as part of the monitoring strategy to mitigate other risk factors in clinical trials as identified by conducting a risk assessment. Guidance on these committees can be found on the Health Research Authority website and in the EMA 'Guideline on data monitoring committees' (EMEA/CHMP/EWP/5872/03).

7.2.1.1 Data monitoring committees/data safety monitoring boards

Clinical trials may extend over a long period of time. Thus, for ethical reasons it is desirable to ensure that for subjects participating in such trials there are no unnecessary increased risks. However, it is also important to ensure that a trial continues for an adequate period of time and is not stopped too early to answer its scientific questions. A DMC/DSMB is a group of experts that may be put in place to review accumulating data from ongoing trials (particularly in relation to the safety and efficacy end-points of the trial) and to advise the TSC or trial team of any important information (for example, whether there are any safety issues that should be brought to the subjects' attention) and the continuation of the trial (that is, whether there are any reasons for the trial not to continue). A DMC/DSMB is not needed for all clinical trials. More information on DMCs/DSMBs and when they should be put in place can be found in section 5.9.

7.2.1.2 Trial steering committees – role and formation

The role of the TSC is usually to provide overall supervision of the trial to ensure that it is conducted to rigorous standards. The TSC will concentrate on the progress of the trial at a top level, including adherence to the protocol, subject safety and considerations for new information (this can include a review of and decisions on the recommendations made by the DMC/DSMB, if there is one for the trial). A TSC may be made up of personnel directly involved in the trial and/or individuals who are independent of the trial. An independent committee can provide a non-biased oversight of the management of the trial, ensuring activities and key decisions are made objectively.

The need for a TSC will depend on the complexity of the trial and could be considered as part of the risk assessment. For example, a risk assessment would be likely to identify that a TSC is not necessary for a very small, investigator-initiated pilot trial of a topical product.

When deciding on forming a TSC it is recommended that consideration be given to:

- risks associated with the IMP, such as whether it is a well-known authorised drug, commonly used and easily administered, or whether there are aspects that require more intense scrutiny, such as availability and distribution
- any safety implications or unusual assessments being conducted that need additional review and may inform subsequent key decisions
- size of the trial – trials with a single site or a small number of sites are less likely to require a TSC, whereas large multinational, multi-centre trials may need such a committee to provide a greater level of oversight
- complexity of the trial protocol – that is, where procedural aspects potentially add a level of risk or complexity that requires close monitoring.

Where it has been decided that a TSC is required there should be formalised procedures in place detailing its formation, remit and membership. The requirements of the committee should then be described in a formal trial document, such as the protocol or a TSC charter. It is recommended that this document clearly identifies:

- the members and core quorum of the TSC
- the responsibilities of the TSC, including any key decisions it will have to make
- how meetings and decisions will be formally documented and to whom these outputs will be circulated
- who is responsible for maintaining the TSC documentation during the course of the trial and the requirement[5] for it to be maintained as part of the trial master file (TMF).

Where a committee is not set up with a charter prior to the trial commencing and therefore its responsibilities are not agreed, issues can arise, for example, with respect to the decisions taken and the documentation of the activities of the committee. Other issues often seen on inspection relate to the retention of TSC documentation, such as the following:

- There was no assignment of responsibility for maintaining the TSC documentation when it was held separately from the TMF, and as a result the documentation could not be located when requested during an inspection.
- There was no consideration of the archiving of the TSC documentation at the end of the trial, and as a result it was not amalgamated with the TMF at the point of archiving.

7.3 Monitoring strategy

7.3.1 Risk assessment and monitoring approach

It is recommended that a risk assessment is conducted at the start of a new trial to identify the risks associated with the trial that have an impact on the safety and rights of the subject or the integrity of the trial results (see sections 2.4 and 4.7.1). The risk assessment will identify any vulnerabilities in the trial that need to be mitigated by monitoring and management activities, potentially indicating whether either on-site or central methods would be suitable (or a combination of both) and these should be considered in developing the monitoring strategy and plan for the trial. The risk assessment should be considered in formulating the monitoring strategy for the trial, ensuring that monitoring approaches are targeted and justified.

Table 7.1 outlines in more detail the aspects and objectives of monitoring a clinical trial before, during and afterwards, and details can also be found in ICH GCP. The monitoring strategy should target these objectives; some of them may be achieved using remote processes but some may only be achieved by undertaking on-site visits.

Table 7.1 Details of suggested monitoring activities before, during and at the end of the trial

Monitoring		
Before	**During**	**End/After**
Case report forms and source data		
Determine what will be the source data and how the data will be collected	Ensure all data recorded in case report form are legible and entered in a timely manner	Ensure all case report forms (including any data queries) are complete and filed in investigator site file
Ensure direct access to subjects' notes (paper and/ or electronic) and other source data	Confirm all subjects exist	Ensure all source data are filed in the subjects' notes or investigator site file (as necessary)
Preparation of monitoring plan, to include: Protocol considerations: • trial population • eligibility criteria • identification • recording and reporting adverse events Internal procedures: • non-compliance handling • escalation process Risk assessment: • priorities • risk mitigation	Check that: • all assessments have been conducted correctly • medical decisions have been clearly documented • no confidential identifiers are on any documents that have left investigator site • protocol and GCP non-compliances have been identified and recorded • all data queries have been resolved and returned	
	Confirm data have been initially recorded in subjects' notes or source worksheet and case report form as per protocol and expectations for source data	

Table continues

Table 7.1 *continued*

Monitoring		
Before	**During**	**End/After**
Facilities and equipment		
Ensure all ancillary supplies have been received (such as case report forms, laboratory supplies, investigator site files)	Confirm that clinical samples have been handled and processed correctly according to laboratory procedures	Check retained samples have been sent to laboratory or destroyed
Ensure all equipment required is available, maintained and calibrated (as required)	Verify any ongoing maintenance and calibrate equipment being used in the trial	Verify any supplied equipment has been returned
Check the facilities are suitable for conducting the trial	Assess any new or altered facilities	
Train/notify all support departments (for example, pharmacy, laboratories, radiology)	Visit any clinical areas and support departments (as needed)	
Documentation		
Ensure investigator site has investigator site file with all pre-trial documentation	Ensure investigator site file is up to date with all current documentation (including implementing approved amendments etc.)	Complete and archive the investigator site file
Ensure investigator site has support department files with all pre-trial documentation (for example, pharmacy, imaging, laboratories)	Ensure support department files are up to date	All support department files are present, complete and archived with the investigator site file
Training of investigator site staff		
Obtain and assess qualification and experience of staff (curricula vitae)	Ensure curricula vitae are present for any new staff joining investigator team	Confirm all curricula vitae are present
Document investigator responsibilities and delegation of duties to staff	Verify updates to the delegation log are completed	Confirm delegation log is complete
Complete signature log	Ensure signature logs completed for any new staff joining investigator team	Confirm all signature logs are present

Monitoring		
Before	**During**	**End/After**
Training of investigator site staff *continued*		
Initiation visit training: complete and document GCP, protocol and trial-specific training (for example, electronic systems and portals for investigational product management or data capture, assessments, procedures)	Train new staff and current staff to correct/prevent non-compliance	Ensure training evidence filed
Investigational medicinal product		
Train site staff on investigational medicinal product handling	Verify ongoing receipt, accountability, return	Confirm accountability completed
Visit to pharmacy/IMP store to assess facilities and obtain requirements	Check randomisation (where appropriate) and treatment compliance	Destroy or return IMP
Check suitability of storage area/storage conditions	Ensure blinding has been maintained (where appropriate)	Make evidence of storage conditions available (or indicate location of these data)
Organise dispatch of investigational medicinal product	Review storage conditions and manage any temperature excursions appropriately	
Informed consent		
Ensure approved versions of documents available for use	Ensure correct versions of documentation are being used	Ensure all consents present and complete and filed

Table continues

7

Table 7.1 *continued*

Monitoring		
Before	**During**	**End/After**
Informed consent *continued*		
Ensure appropriate procedures are in place and that local arrangements with consent processes are in accordance with favourable research ethics committee opinion	Check that consent was: • appropriately undertaken • taken by an authorised delegated person • prior to participation/trial assessments • personally signed and dated by subject • signed by an appropriate witness or legal representative (as required) • assented to (if required)	
	Check any re-consent has been conducted (where appropriate)	
Subject safety		
Train site staff in procedures for identification, recording and reporting adverse events	Ensure all adverse events are identified and recorded and reported to sponsor as required	Confirm the investigator site file contains all adverse event documentation
	Confirm all safety updates received by investigator (for example, investigator's brochure)	
Protocol compliance		
	Confirm subjects are eligible for the trial (meet protocol inclusion/exclusion criteria and have been reviewed by a medic prior to entry)	
	Identify potential serious breaches of GCP and trial protocol or fraud/misconduct	

Monitoring		
Before	**During**	**End/After**
Protocol compliance *continued*		
	Confirm compliance with trial protocol and ensure non-compliances are documented	
General		
	Review recruitment rate against agreed target	Document and collect all protocol and GCP non-compliances
	Ensure case report form completion rate corresponds to an agreed timeline	Provide the investigator with a copy of the final trial summary report and/or clinical study report
	Ensure regular contact with the principal investigator and check principal investigator's trial oversight	

GCP, Good Clinical Practice; IMP, investigational medicinal product

On-site monitoring is the traditional commercial approach to monitoring, which most organisations are familiar with. Although this form of monitoring has many advantages, other forms of monitoring could potentially replace some aspects of on-site monitoring and also identify issues that would not readily be identifiable using on-site monitoring. For example, owing to the increased availability of electronic case report forms (eCRFs), central monitoring can, using reports from the database and statistical analysis, identify signals from metrics that may suggest non-compliances at sites or compare data across sites. This could identify a site that is significantly different from the others, such as from a metric measuring the ratio of serious adverse events (SAEs) reported between sites, and can identify a site appearing to be an outlier.

On-site monitoring can be resource intensive in relation to the resources and funding available. Therefore, it is recommended that sponsors consider how on-site monitoring can be achieved by making the best use of the resources available without compromising subject safety and data integrity. For example:

- Could the R&D office of the sponsor support full on-site monitoring of all host sites?
- Could research staff at one site be used to monitor another site?

- Could the monitoring aspects be delegated to the R&D office of the host site (provided they have adequate systems for monitoring)?
- Is there sufficient funding to outsource monitoring to an external organisation or contractor?
- Could the on-site monitoring be reduced or targeted?

Table 7.2 provides a summary of what can be achieved by central and on-site monitoring that may help when considering the need to address the trial

Table 7.2 Aspects of central and on-site monitoring

Criteria	Central monitoring	On-site monitoring
Face-to-face interaction with the site personnel to build rapport	✗	✓
Travel burden (for example, time away from office and not contactable)	✗	✓
Allows ongoing training and motivation of the site	✗[a]	✓
More remote contact with sites (for example, by telephone or email), as not out on the road	✓	✗
Access to and assessment of information not captured on case report forms (source data verification)	✗[a]	✓
Ability to verify subjects' existence (for example, review consents and identification)	✗[a]	✓
Identification of unreported adverse events	✗	✓
Identification of non-case report form protocol deviations/violations	✗[a]	✓
Statistical monitoring to identify site outliers, and obvious data patterns and trends across the trial	✓	✗
Automatic data checks to identify issues with plausibility or consistency	✓	✗
Early safety signal detection (for example, increase of values close to defined limits)	✓	✗
Early identification of sites not completing or submitting case report forms or other data	✓	✗[a]
Direct viewing of facilities and equipment (for example, the location of investigational medicinal products, trial records)	✗	✓
Identification of new staff and hands-on mentoring/support for new staff/sites	✗	✓

[a] No or limited.

vulnerabilities by central or on-site monitoring, or a combination of both. It is acknowledged that monitors' remote access to data such as electronic health records and registries may be possible for non-commercial sponsors (dependent on subject consent) and remote monitoring may therefore be more appropriate. Trials may use any type of monitoring or a hybrid of them all. A combination of central and on-site monitoring can be a means of directing visits to sites as and when the sites most need them, thereby making the best use of the resources available without compromising subject safety and data integrity.

7.3.2 Intensity and focus of monitoring

In defining the monitoring strategy, based on the vulnerabilities identified by the risk assessment, the intensity and focus of the monitoring could vary. The following examples illustrate this concept by providing details of activities that would necessitate different levels of monitoring intensity or focus as dictated by the risks associated with subject safety and reliability of the trial results.

7.3.2.1 Sample processing/handling

A high intensity of monitoring would be necessary when the sensitivity of sample analysis is very dependent on how the samples are taken, processed, stored and transported (for example, pharmacokinetic or pharmacodynamic samples that are linked to the primary objective of the trial). It may be important to be able to verify when samples are taken, centrifuged, refrigerated/frozen and shipped to ensure samples are handled in accordance with the protocol or other relevant instructions.

Conversely, low intensity or no monitoring may be appropriate where no samples are being taken or, if they are taken, their handling will have no impact on the reliability of the results of the analysis – for example, where the samples may be related to exploratory objectives of the trial protocol or where minor errors in processing will not affect the results.

7.3.2.2 Investigational medicinal product

A high intensity of monitoring would be appropriate when compliance or storage of the IMP is critical to the end-points of the trial. Here, there needs to be close management to verify what was shipped and when, when it was received, and then exactly which subject had what and when; also that the trial material was maintained under the appropriate storage conditions and that adequate temperature excursion and quarantine procedures were followed, if needed. A high intensity of monitoring may need to be implemented for IMPs that:

- pose a higher risk to the trial results or subject safety (for example, unlicensed medications and advanced therapies)
- are considered 'higher risk molecules' (that is, as defined for review by the Clinical Trials Expert Advisory Group (CTEAG); see section 2.5)
- require refrigerated or frozen transit
- are blinded (may require use of an unblinded monitor – see below)
- have a short expiry date or result in a short expiry date once reconstituted.

Conversely, a low intensity of monitoring may be appropriate in a situation where a licensed product is being used within its licensed indication from general stock, particularly (though not exclusively) those stored at ambient temperatures.

Monitoring for blinded trials can be more complicated, especially if the IMP is unblinded to some of the staff at the investigator site (for example, the pharmacist). If the monitor is unblinded, there could potentially be bias introduced into the queries raised by monitors when conducting data verification on adverse events or SAEs, and they may risk unblinding the investigator's team. In these circumstances the allocation of unblinded monitors for the IMP aspects will need to be considered along with how any visits and communication will be documented, reviewed and approved during the trial without compromising the blinding.

7.3.2.3   Equipment

A high intensity of monitoring would be needed to verify that equipment used to make primary end-point assessments or to calculate doses or dose adjustments is suitable for use and being used correctly (for example, spirometers, treadmills or special equipment supplied specifically for the trial).

No monitoring or a low intensity of monitoring may be implemented where no equipment is being utilised or, if equipment is used, it is being maintained under standard contracts as per the hospital's or site's normal procedures, or it will not affect the credibility of data or results.

7.3.2.4   Data and source data verification

A high intensity of monitoring would be needed in trials where a large proportion of the data collected need to be verified for reliability because they are considered to be 'critical data' such as safety data, primary and secondary end-point assessments, and eligibility verification. This is particularly important in early phase trials, pivotal trials to be included in marketing authorisation applications, or where publications could result in a major change in standard clinical practice. In some exceptional cases it may be that close to 100% of all the data collected need to be verified.

The intensity could be reduced where not all of the data are considered to be critical, but it is still necessary to ensure that the data are accurate and that minor discrepancies will not affect the safety profile of the IMP or the statistical power of the analysis. Source data verification (SDV) may then range from certain data requiring 100% SDV for all subjects to a percentage of data per subject or a percentage of the number of subjects recruited.

Finally, a low level of monitoring or no monitoring could be used when the accuracy of the data collected may not have a significant impact on the results or there are adequate quality control procedures in place providing assurance that the data are reliable. For example, the investigator site may have some quality control on data entry or the eligibility criteria are minimal (for example, to be eligible for a trial of a topical coagulant applied to a surgical wound, subjects are only required to have had a particular type of surgery) or the primary efficacy end-point is easy to assess (for example, post-surgical blood loss, survival or viral load). Alternatively the equipment may be capturing data directly and sending them to the sponsor by electronic data transfer so SDV is not required.

7.3.2.5 Investigator site experience

The risk assessment may identify that some sites have more inexperienced investigators or staff and therefore a higher intensity of monitoring at these sites is recommended than for those with more experienced staff. For example, this may mean undertaking on-site visits for less experienced sites, with other sites being monitored centrally. Alternatively, the on-site monitoring activities at inexperienced sites may need to be more frequent and longer at the start of the trial, but could then be reduced once the monitor is satisfied that the site is performing well.

7.3.3 Flexible and adaptive approach

Irrespective of which type and intensity of monitoring is identified and selected for a clinical trial, flexibility can be inbuilt in order to adapt the requirements during the course of the trial; for example, if the protocol is amended, new risks may be identified or issues may arise that require additional monitoring. Also, there may be a certain amount of flexibility allowed in the frequency and focus between sites, depending on the experience and performance of the sites throughout the course of the trial. No matter what methods of monitoring are implemented, it is always worth noting that where there are issues and non-compliances in one area it suggests there may be more in other areas not identified. Therefore, escalation procedures should be incorporated to allow the triggering of additional heightened monitoring to identify, assess and correct non-compliances early on in the trial. Monitoring requirements could be adjusted during the course of the trial to focus more on those sites where poor performance or non-compliances have been identified. Such flexibility also enables monitoring resources, particularly where they are limited, to be focused where they are most needed. Conversely, the monitoring strategy could also consider a reduction or revision in monitoring during the course of the trial.

This flexibility would be based on the outcome of the monitoring activities (reports) as detailed in section 7.6. There should be a clearly documented process containing 'triggers' (those that can be predetermined and those that are ad hoc) to ensure that where issues are identified the escalation of these issues is prompted and actions taken to address them. This is particularly relevant for central monitoring activities. Actions may vary from a telephone call in the first instance or additional data queries, to conducting a 'for-cause' on-site monitoring visit or an audit to investigate the issues and implement a corrective and preventative action plan to ensure future compliance. Evidence of the subsequent visit or actions based on the trigger must[5] be documented and available in the TMF. It is recommended that responsibility for this process is defined to ensure it occurs, as failure to adhere strictly to the plan can result in ineffective monitoring and potentially compromised data. Examples have been seen on inspections where central monitoring procedures contained well-defined thresholds but when these thresholds were met during a trial the escalation process was not triggered, as the responsibility for this part of the process was not clearly defined.

7.3.4 Monitoring plan

It is recommended that the monitoring strategy for a clinical trial is formalised by the sponsor. This usually takes the form of a monitoring plan (the terminology may differ depending on the organisation) and often supplements the written general monitoring procedures as it is trial-specific. It is recommended that this plan clearly identifies the elements of monitoring to be covered and how these are to be conducted, including the adaptive and escalation aspects.

The following are some examples of what could be considered for inclusion in the monitoring plan:

- type of monitoring to be used (central and/or on-site)
- standards and written procedures to be followed
- frequency of monitoring
- monitor site capacity (that is, maximum number of sites per monitor)
- ancillary departments to be visited (such as pharmacy, laboratories, imaging)
- data to be reviewed (percentage of SDV required and on what data)
- considerations for unblinded monitors and reviewers (if required)
- expectations for availability of the principal investigator during monitoring visits
- how non-compliances will be recorded and circulated
- oversight of the investigator and ancillary department site files
- escalation processes:
  - » for central monitoring, what triggers will be used for escalating to on-site monitoring
  - » for both central and on-site monitoring, how unresolved issues or serious non-compliances are handled
  - » how corrective and preventative action will be implemented
- management of supplies (IMP and ancillary materials)
- SAE reporting and associated monitoring responsibilities
- query management:
  - » data queries
  - » protocol queries to medical monitor
  - » IMP (including temperature excursion management)
- documentation and review of monitoring activities:
  - » types and formats of reports (such as monitoring visit reports, central monitoring metrics, statistical monitoring)
  - » responsibility and timelines for preparing and reviewing the reports
- training of monitors
  - » specific protocol or therapeutic area training
  - » co-monitoring considerations
  - » handover of monitors.

It is recommended that this monitoring plan is prepared in accordance with the instructions referred to in Chapter 4 and is prepared with consideration of the risk assessment, data management and data validation plans, where appropriate.

7.4 Monitoring personnel

All monitoring personnel must[6] be thoroughly familiar with the IMPs, the protocol, written informed consent form and any other written information to be provided to subjects, the sponsor's or vendor's written procedures, GCP and the applicable regulatory requirement(s). There must[5] be clear documented evidence of the qualifications, training and experience of monitoring personnel. Monitors, typically on-site monitors (also referred to as clinical research associates or CRAs), will be appointed by the sponsor and/or vendor and must[6] be appropriately trained, with adequate scientific and/or clinical knowledge as needed. For further details on training, see section 14.2.

For non-commercial sponsors the models can vary – for example, the monitoring may be undertaken by staff who are part of the R&D office, part of a clinical research facility/unit or may be selected and managed by the chief investigator as part of the trial team, particularly where the trial is multi-centre. The role of monitor can be divided between several members of the trial team, including the data manager, trial statistician and trial manager. In some cases, the trial risk assessment may determine that little if any monitoring is required (for example, for a very small, investigator-led non-commercial trial, particularly one of an exploratory nature), and it may be sufficient to use self-assessment reports that are completed by the investigator and then assessed by the R&D office. On the other hand, commercial sponsors, particularly for a global trial, may have a large monitoring team reporting into lead monitors in a region, who then report into a global trial manager. In all cases, it is recommended that the monitoring team structure is clearly defined and documented, with clear lines of communication.

When contracting out monitoring, sponsors must[7] consider how they will maintain oversight of the monitoring team. Lack of continuity of monitoring caused by a high turnover of on-site monitors can lead to issues at site with respect to communication, building rapport and protocol compliance. It is therefore useful to ensure there are formalised handover procedures for when the monitoring of sites changes hands. Sponsors may also wish to review and approve contracted on-site monitors (for example, by a review of CVs). It is recommended that these aspects are considered when drawing up contracts with vendors (see Chapter 1 for more methods to maintain sponsor oversight).

7.5 Monitoring activities

7.5.1 Investigator site selection

During the set-up of the trial, investigator sites will need to be selected. This activity is usually undertaken by the sponsor's clinical group or may be outsourced to a vendor. However, this may be done by the chief investigator or research networks for some non-commercial trials. The site evaluation will, as a minimum, include a feasibility assessment or questionnaire that has been prepared by taking into account the specific aspects of the clinical trial.

Sponsors have many means of identifying potential investigator sites; these can include:

* investigator sites with which they have previous experience/knowledge
* identifying specialist sites/experts in the therapeutic area
* identifying investigators with previous experience of the IMP or similar products
* asking other investigators for recommendations
* using research networks.

How this evaluation and selection of investigator sites is conducted may vary. It can range from site visit(s) (for example, in situations where there is little knowledge about the site and staff, the trial is complex and/or requires specific equipment) to remote assessments (for example, where there is already an in-depth knowledge of the site/staff or the trial has a very simple design).

However, for those sites used in the trial there should be clear documentation of the assessment of the site and the eventual decision on whether to use the site, including the rationale for that decision demonstrating that the site was suitable for the trial.

7.5.2 Site initiation and training

Once the sites have been selected there may be an investigators' meeting. This is where all the sites meet to be trained by the sponsor and any vendors on the trial protocol, any equipment to be used, specific procedures and other data collection tools. This may be achieved using face-to-face meetings but could also be via teleconference or videoconference.

In addition, there is usually an initiation visit when the monitor will meet the site staff to ensure they are adequately trained and ready to start the trial.

There may be occasions where either an investigators' meeting and/or the initiation visit can be more limited in scope – for example, conducted via telephone between the monitor and the site, and/or consist of an initiation pack sent to the site containing information and instructions with forms/checklist to complete and return. Alternatively, the meeting(s) may not be conducted at all – for example, where there is familiarity with the site, the site has previously received training in similar trials, or the simplicity of the trial is such that training is considered unnecessary. However, any such decisions should be clearly documented and justified in the risk assessment and/or monitoring plan.

7.5.3   Monitoring during the trial

Once the trial is underway, compliance with the protocol is principally ensured through the investigator's supervision at the site and through the sponsor's monitoring of the trial. The purposes of trial monitoring at this stage include verifying that the conduct of the trial is in compliance with the currently approved protocol/amendment(s), with GCP, and with applicable regulatory requirement(s) (see Table 7.1). Each trial will have its own specific requirements and the actual monitoring to be performed for a particular clinical trial must[2, 4] be undertaken according to the monitoring plan, protocol or other procedures. Where on-site monitoring is taking place such procedures must[4] be followed to ensure the on-site monitors are addressing the monitoring activities consistently across each site.

7.5.3.1   On-site visits

An on-site visit can allow a detailed review of the conduct of the trial. The monitor can ensure this occurs by discussing the trial with the investigator and the trial team to understand exactly how the trial is being conducted, and not relying on assumption. Asking staff about the trial conduct during inspections has revealed activities that the monitor was unaware of; for example, safety reports not being reviewed by the investigator, additional IMP storage areas, lack of checks on IMP receipt, the process for source data collection and who is doing what (for example, completing subject diaries, taking consent). The monitor can also easily undertake training activities at site, and face-to-face meetings can assist in building the relationship between the sponsor and the investigator site. Therefore, the role of the monitor is much more than undertaking SDV and data queries. The sponsor is responsible for ensuring that adequate time is allowed for effective monitoring, and that the monitor's time is not solely devoted to SDV and resolving data queries.

7.5.3.2 Central or remote monitoring

Central monitoring, or remote monitoring as it is sometimes called, has been widely used by non-commercial sponsors. However, increasing numbers of commercial vendors and sponsors are now adopting this monitoring approach as part of their monitoring strategy.

Central monitoring can be particularly useful in large trials with many sites and large numbers of subjects. Central monitoring does, however, rely on extensive communication with and cooperation of the site (for example, to provide documentation and reports). Typically, monitoring personnel are based at a remote data centre that receives information from the investigator sites and they do not make routine on-site visits. Even where on-site visits are taking place it is perfectly feasible to apply some central monitoring techniques; for example, data management query processes are effectively a form of central monitoring. Figure 7.2 provides an overview of the typical central monitoring model.

Documentation such as consent forms or laboratory reports provided may be reviewed as it would be during an on-site visit. This review will, however, not be as extensive as that undertaken during an on-site visit where the subject's full medical records are available for review. Additionally, the central monitoring group may elicit compliance information and checks by sending instructions, questionnaires and checklists to the investigator site for completion and return, such as a checklist of the contents of documentation in the investigator site file.

When using central monitoring, other legislative requirements must be considered. For example, when collecting signed consent forms, laboratory results with subject identifiers or contact details for follow-up telephone calls/questionnaires, a formal system should be in place that complies with the Data Protection Act 1998 to ensure access to the confidential information is restricted and that the subjects of the clinical trial are aware that a sponsor or third party may have access to their data. This may be explicitly detailed in the subject information sheet or consent form approved by the research ethics committee (REC).

Central monitoring relies on the use of data: clinical data in the CRFs, data from operational activities, or data and documentation provided from investigator sites in addition to the clinical data in CRFs. These are used by the central monitoring team to produce metrics and queries and undertake analyses (see section 8.5.1).

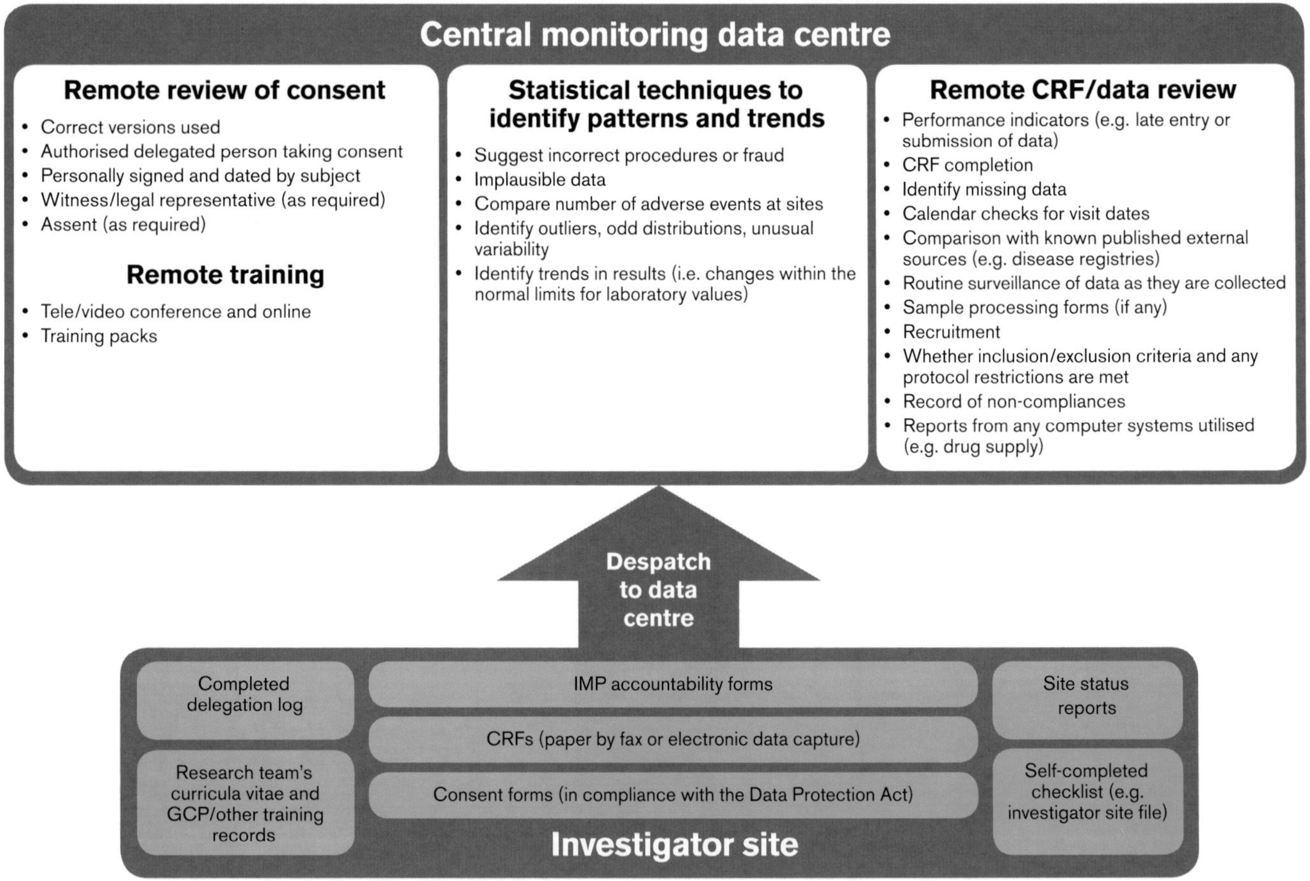

Central monitoring data centre

Remote review of consent

- Correct versions used
- Authorised delegated person taking consent
- Personally signed and dated by subject
- Witness/legal representative (as required)
- Assent (as required)

Remote training

- Tele/video conference and online
- Training packs

Statistical techniques to identify patterns and trends

- Suggest incorrect procedures or fraud
- Implausible data
- Compare number of adverse events at sites
- Identify outliers, odd distributions, unusual variability
- Identify trends in results (i.e. changes within the normal limits for laboratory values)

Remote CRF/data review

- Performance indicators (e.g. late entry or submission of data)
- CRF completion
- Identify missing data
- Calendar checks for visit dates
- Comparison with known published external sources (e.g. disease registries)
- Routine surveillance of data as they are collected
- Sample processing forms (if any)
- Recruitment
- Whether inclusion/exclusion criteria and any protocol restrictions are met
- Record of non-compliances
- Reports from any computer systems utilised (e.g. drug supply)

Despatch to data centre

Investigator site

- Completed delegation log
- Research team's curricula vitae and GCP/other training records
- IMP accountability forms
- CRFs (paper by fax or electronic data capture)
- Consent forms (in compliance with the Data Protection Act)
- Site status reports
- Self-completed checklist (e.g. investigator site file)

Figure 7.2 Examples of central monitoring methods

CRF, case report form; GCP, Good Clinical Practice; IMP, investigational medicinal product

Metrics can then be evaluated across sites and used as indicators to adapt the monitoring or trigger escalation procedures.

The submitted paper CRFs (by fax) and eCRFs can be used to assess subject progress and review site compliance to ensure the site has performed tests and taken actions in accordance with the protocol. This can be part of the data validation activities and could include checks on:

- CRF submission times to ensure they are in accordance with trial instructions (late completion and submission could be a metric)
- the quality of the data (legibility, missing data, number of data queries could be a metric)
- the investigator's response to the queries assessed (response time could be a metric)
- out-of-range laboratory data to check for any unreported SAEs, that any repeat samples have been taken or that the subject has been withdrawn as defined by the protocol
- visit date compliance
- concomitant medications to find prohibited medications.

Statistical monitoring can be achieved using both paper CRFs and eCRFs, provided there is a robust mechanism for submitting the CRFs to the sponsor for analysis regularly and promptly throughout the trial. When this mechanism is implemented, the sponsor may want to incorporate statistical aspects into central monitoring to detect outlier sites or repeat data patterns within a single site. The sponsor may want to examine outliers by manual inspection of graphical data or statistical analyses throughout the trial. These could include complex multivariate techniques to identify outlier sites. There is likely to be a need to set tolerance limits to identify the outliers and when to trigger additional monitoring activities. Statistical monitoring of data collected in the CRF during the conduct of the trial can enable a sponsor to identify irregularities and investigate them promptly.

Common assessments that can identify compliance issues at a site can include:

- unexpected data distributions/variability (for example, lack of/low variability, non-normal distributions, digit preferences)
- the ratio of AEs/SAEs to recruitment (to reveal any sites with significantly more/fewer than the majority of sites)
- the results from assessments being too similar or irregular in terms of expectations of the IMP or disease

- dose changes (reductions or increments) not being in accordance with the protocol
- assessment of demographics (this could highlight duplicate information to identify possible repeated inclusion of subjects to the same trial or copying of the data)
- review of subjects assigned to treatment against the randomisation allocation (if known)
- review of audit trails on eCRFs/subject diaries for consistency with visit dates
- visit days at site being plausible (for example, not bank holidays/weekends, where appropriate).

The effectiveness of central and statistical monitoring may depend on how quickly and accurately the data are captured, transmitted to the sponsor and validated by the sponsor. For example, a sponsor could detect via central monitoring that subjects have been given the incorrect chemotherapy treatment regimen; however, if the data are not assessed by the sponsor until several months after the subjects have been treated, the subjects' safety can be seriously jeopardised.

7.5.3.3 Other remote forms of monitoring

There are other methods of maintaining oversight of a site, which could be considered part of monitoring, whether on-site visits are taking place or not. These include, but are not limited to, the following:

- regular status, self-assessment or progress reports sent to the data centre by the site regarding recruitment and any operational issues (for example, staff changes, key document amendments, deviations and non-compliances, checklist of investigator site file contents)
- regular communication with sites (for example, by telephone and email)
- regular status reports and summaries from third parties, if involved (for example, reports from interactive response technologies, laboratory summaries).

7.5.4 Closure of investigator sites

Once the trial has been completed or a site closed prematurely it is important to ensure the investigator has a complete and independent record of the trial at their site and that this will be kept securely for the required[8] time period under control of the investigator (see Table 7.1 for details of other close-out activities). Close-out activities can be achieved by an on-site visit, which may include review of the documentation and archiving facilities. Alternatively, this can be achieved centrally via discussion and documentation (for example, using questionnaires and checklists completed by the site).

7.6   Output from monitoring

For any monitoring performed, there should be a formal output to document what was actually done and to verify that the monitoring plan and escalation procedures that were put in place were followed. There may be occasions when a checklist can be used to ensure all the required activities have been undertaken; however, on other occasions this may not be detailed enough. The following are examples of documentation that may need to be retained:

- Central monitoring of a consent form or accountability log may be acceptable as a checklist, which is signed and dated by the person undertaking the check (for example, verifying signatures, dates and the correct version of the document).

- An on-site monitoring visit should be documented in the form of a written report and may contain a checklist. It should also document what activities were performed during the visit and it is recommended that this includes a summary of site staff present, what was reviewed and verified, any significant findings/facts, non-compliances and deficiencies, conclusions, actions taken and issues closed out. There should also be evidence of adequate follow-up of any actions by the sponsor/vendor.

- Output reports from central monitoring reviews of the clinical trial data that are run regularly (for example, SAE reporting rates, CRF completion rates and data query tallies) could be filed as evidence of these central monitoring activities having taken place.

- Documented review of any status updates or questionnaires returned from sites as part of central monitoring activities to demonstrate that the sponsor has assessed the information and taken appropriate action.

- Documented receipt and review by the sponsor of documentation provided by the site (for example, delegation logs and accountability logs).

- Documented review of any reports from third parties (such as central laboratories, interactive response technologies).

- Evidence of the statistical monitoring analysis conducted (that is, retention of the statistical outputs and their review).

Inadequate monitoring procedures have led to a number of issues with the outputs of monitoring being identified on inspection. For example:

- There was insufficient information in the on-site monitoring visit report so it could not be established what activities the monitor had actually performed during the visit (what subjects/visits were reviewed, what consents were checked or which SAEs were reviewed) and whether any issues and actions identified at previous visits had been resolved and closed. This may happen if the report template only allows boxes to be ticked and a summary of issues to be recorded.
- Owing to poorly designed central monitoring documentation, triggers to conduct for-cause on-site monitoring visits, as per the monitoring plan, were not identified. As a result, the on-site visits were not conducted and serious non-compliances continued unnecessarily.
- Production and review of the monitoring visit reports were not done in a timely manner to ensure that any issues identified could be actioned or escalated and subsequently closed.

Non-compliance with the protocol, written procedures, GCP guidelines and/or applicable regulatory requirement(s) by an investigator/institution or by member(s) of the sponsor's staff must[5] be documented and retained, and lead to prompt action by the sponsor to secure compliance. Therefore, if the monitoring identifies serious and/or persistent non-compliance on the part of an investigator/institution, then the sponsor should ensure that there is an escalation process, which may include consideration of the following actions:

- Address the non-compliance through an investigation and resulting corrective and preventative action plan.
- Assess the non-compliances in terms of identifying and reporting them as a serious breach.
- Escalate issues with the investigators via management (for example, the R&D office), as they may be able to facilitate future compliance.
- Trigger a for-cause on-site monitoring visit or audit.
- Terminate the investigator's/institution's participation in the trial and notify the competent authority and/or REC as required.

Any escalation, investigation and resulting decisions must[5] be clearly documented in the TMF.

7.7 Source data verification and case report form management

7.7.1 Source data

ICH GCP defines source data as:

> *'All information in original records and certified copies of original records of clinical findings, observations, or other activities in a clinical trial necessary for the reconstruction and evaluation of the trial'.*

In essence, it is where the data are first captured (either written or electronically). Further details on source data can be found in Chapter 11.

Source data will always be required.[9] Good documentation of trial activities and results in subjects' source notes (that is, source worksheet, medical records) is not only essential for the clinical management of the subject, but allows the accurate reconstruction of the trial. Depending on the complexity of the trial design and the number of data points required, the source data requirements are likely to vary. The source notes will vary depending on the investigator site organisation. For example:

- **Hospital or GP setting** Medical records typically include subject case notes (paper and/or electronic), laboratory reports, ECGs, X-rays, CT scans, radiology reports, drug and infusion charts (paper or electronic), pharmacy aseptic preparation worksheets, referral letters.
- **Large NHS centre** There may be multiple sets of notes for a single subject from different departments or hospitals, depending on the various treatments at different locations. All of these should be considered in terms of available information recorded and assessed or checked during the subject's participation in the trial – for example, to identify adverse events or SAEs.
- **Phase I unit** There may be direct electronic data capture, source workbooks or direct entry into the CRF plus laboratory reports, X-rays, spirometer print-outs.

It is therefore not possible to have a standardised method of recording clinical source data, especially in an international multi-centre trial. There will be variations between sites due to a number of factors, such as how clinical data are reported through the local hospital laboratory system, how drug charts are laid out, the use of different monitoring tools, and differences in standard of care and hospital policy. Because of this variability it is recommended that the sponsor reviews the type of data that are required for the trial and how such data will be recorded at each site (whether as part of routine practice or by a method specific for the trial).

In order to conduct SDV the monitor must be aware of what constitutes source data at a particular site and so it is recommended that there is an agreement with the investigator covering how, when and where source data are recorded. This is usually in the form of a source data agreement. However, this could be detailed in the protocol. Inspections have repeatedly revealed problems with the identity of the source data, such as whether they consist of the electronic notes system, the signed print-out of the data or a worksheet.

Data can be entered directly into the CRF. However, for subjects in a hospital setting this information may also need to be in the medical records, as they may be vital for management of the subject by different medical specialities outside the trial team. Where it is agreed that data can be recorded directly into the CRF, these data should be clearly identified and detailed in the protocol.

7.7.2   Source data verification

Source data verification (SDV) is the act of checking the accuracy and completeness of the CRF entries against the source documents in accordance with the protocol requirements, ensuring that:

- All assessments have been conducted and completed in accordance with the protocol and within the specified timeframe.
- The data from those assessments have been recorded in the source documents.
- The source data have been accurately transcribed into the CRF.
- Any deviations have been identified and recorded.
- All adverse events, concomitant medications and intercurrent illnesses are recorded and reported in the CRF in accordance with the protocol.
- Assessments have been made by an appropriately qualified person who has been delegated that activity.

It is recommended that the monitoring plan specifies the level of SDV required (that is, what percentage of subjects and what percentage of data are to be verified). This will vary from trial to trial based on the risk assessment that would identify the data that are critical to the reliability of the results and subject safety.

For example:

- A first in human Phase I trial may require 100% of the data from all subjects to be verified.
- A non-commercial trial with an authorised product being used within its authorised indication and having simple eligibility criteria and end-points may require only a small percentage of the subjects/data to be verified (that is, only consent, eligibility and primary end-point for a small percentage of the subjects).

For trials where only a percentage of the data require SDV, there are often pre-specified rules (determined by the sponsor) about what SDV will be undertaken. For example, there may be full SDV of all data for the first subject recruited and then only full SDV of certain data (for example, primary end-points) for a percentage of the following subjects. These subjects and data could be chosen at random without the investigator having prior knowledge of which subjects will have full SDV. A statistician may be called upon to produce a random sample for SDV purposes.

When conducting SDV, there are numerous factors to consider in ensuring the relevant data are recorded initially as well as transcribed correctly. The following are examples of issues in relation to source documents that have been seen on inspection:

- There was no documented review of laboratory reports, imaging reports and X-rays, which were required as eligibility criteria, prior to inclusion of the subject in the trial.
- There was no clear evidence that the eligibility decision had been made by a medically qualified doctor (that is, eligibility was assessed and documented by a nurse).
- The relevant details associated with any adverse events or SAEs were not recorded in the source documents (for example, the event was recorded, but the start or stop dates were not).
- Lack of awareness of what the source data consisted of, especially when calculating end-point data or reviewing for adverse events or SAEs. For example:
  » There was no verification by the monitor of any manometry (primary efficacy) data generated at the investigator site. The monitor was unaware that the source data were generated electronically and that an average value was calculated manually by the investigator and transcribed into CRF.

» A monitor at a GP practice was unaware that the source data were a mixture of both paper and electronic records and therefore failed to look at the electronic notes system. The electronic notes contained details of adverse events that were not on the paper records.

» A research nurse had a notebook that was used to record trial assessments (such as vital signs), which were then transcribed into the medical notes and CRF. The monitor was unaware of this practice and therefore did not review the source data in the nurse's notebook, assuming that the medical notes were the source.

» The monitor failed to notice a protocol deviation whereby repeat laboratory tests were analysed locally rather than by the central laboratory. These repeat tests were not transcribed into the CRF and therefore did not prompt the monitor to look for the corresponding entry in the medical notes to verify them.

» The trial subjects' departmental notes were used for SDV but other hospital notes were not reviewed by the trial monitor, who failed to see other visits (for example, to the hospital emergency department), and therefore adverse events were missed.

7.7.3   CRF management

Once SDV has been completed and the CRFs have been approved by the principal investigator (or delegate) and assessed as complete by the monitor (as defined by the monitoring plan), the CRFs or pages of CRFs will be sent to the sponsor. This may differ depending on the format of the CRFs – that is, whether they are electronic or paper and whether on-site monitoring visits are taking place.

It is recommended that when CRFs are retrieved from site for submission to the sponsor, the monitor (or member of the investigator's trial team) ensures any copies are legible and that the movement of the CRF is tracked (that is, the use of a transmittal form). There have been many instances where CRFs have gone missing and there was no tracking mechanism to be able to identify where they went astray. See section 8.4.2 for further details on handling CRFs and data queries.

7.8   Chapter legislative references

Throughout this chapter, specific terminology – 'must', 'required' or 'requirement' – has been used to interpret activities that are legislative requirements. These terms have been number-coded in the text where used, and the corresponding reference in the legislation can be found below.

1. Regulation 28 (1) of SI 2004/1031
2. Regulation 29 of SI 2004/1031
3. Schedule 1, Part 2 (7) of SI 2004/1031
4. Schedule 1, Part 2 (4) of SI 2004/1031
5. Regulation 31A (4) of SI 2004/1031
6. Schedule 1, Part 2 (2) of SI 2004/1031
7. Regulation 3 (12) of SI 2004/1031
8. Regulation 31A of SI 2004/1031
9. Schedule 1, Part 2 (9) of SI 2004/1031

7

Data management

8

8.1   Overview of the data management process

The data management process typically covers the design and production of the data capture tool (whether paper or electronic) for collection of subject data at the investigator site, the design and construction of the database to maintain the data electronically, the processing of the data (entry/uploading, cleaning and query management) and the production of the final dataset(s) ready for analysis. Figure 8.1 gives an overview of the key activities of data management. In many non-commercial data management operations, it has often been observed during GCP inspections that there is no clear differential between data management and statistical analysis. This is often as a result of the statistician undertaking some data management activities, typically data validation, and liaising extensively with data management to produce a clean database. Although there is no particular concern about the activity being undertaken by a statistician, data validation should not be an ongoing process throughout the analysis. There should be a clear boundary in the process, with a final data release, as illustrated in Figure 8.1. This is particularly important in blinded trials to avoid accusations of bias.

During the data management process there are many appropriate points for quality control checks (QC), computer system validation (CSV) and validation of applications created in validated computer systems as highlighted in Figure 8.1. These will be covered in this chapter; however, further detail on QC, CSV and validation activities can be found in Chapter 14. The data management processes should be formalised and all operational activities should be adequately documented; for example, signed and dated documentation/quality records must be retained in the trial master file (TMF) in order to comply with Regulation 31A (4) of SI 2004/1031.

Data management is a key function of the clinical trial process, and data management personnel will interface with a number of clinical trial disciplines within a typical clinical trial team in order for a successful outcome. For example:

- investigators
- trial site coordinators/research nurses
- medical monitors
- pharmacovigilance personnel
- laboratories and specialist services personnel
- trial monitors
- statisticians
- statistical programmers
- medical writers
- project/trial managers.

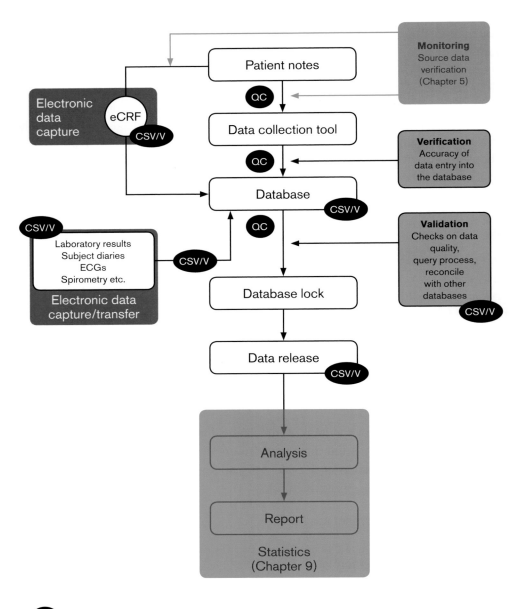

Figure 8.1 Simple overview of data management process

Data management personnel must[1] be appropriately trained in the data management procedures, the trial protocol and aspects of GCP relevant to their role (see section 14.2).

Data management can be a complex activity. The trial risk assessment will identify the level of risk to the integrity of the data and therefore the results. The proposed mitigations are likely to recommend that for large and complex trials a data management plan (DMP) is produced. This provides an overview of the data management process to be applied to the trial to assure data quality and is recommended to be in place prior to the start of the trial. The DMP would typically reference the written procedures to be used, the data flow (sources and how they will be integrated), systems to be used, validation, the query process, QC, protocol non-compliance definitions and handling, pharmacovigilance reconciliation, training, personnel, data location and archiving (or return of trial data and documentation to the sponsor). Where there is no written procedure available to cover the detail (for example, a sponsor may be sponsoring only one trial or the trial could involve processes not completely covered by the written procedure), then the DMP can be used for documenting the trial-specific data management processes, such as the interaction between the sponsor's and vendor's systems for pharmacovigilance activities. A DMP can be particularly useful when the data management is contracted out by the sponsor.

When data management is contracted out, the sponsor must[2] have oversight of the process and it is recommended that the sponsor confirms and agrees with the vendor which specific data management documents the sponsor wishes to review and/or approve. This may be done by review of the vendor's procedures to confirm the documents the vendor will send or by the sponsor having their expectations documented in their own procedures or within the DMP. How the documents are reviewed and approved is for the sponsor to decide, but this should be able to be demonstrated. Typically, the documentation that the sponsor may want to review and/or approve as part of the oversight includes the following:

- case report form (CRF)
- plans (for example, DMP, validation plan, QC plan)
- agreements (that the vendor puts in place with its subcontractors)
- specifications for systems (for example, the electronic CRF, database, validation/edit checks)
- validation/release reports for key systems (for example, the electronic CRF)

- self-evident corrections
- medical coding
- database lock/unlock.

In all cases, procedures should be in place to ensure that the data management group is fully aware of any protocol amendments as these may affect the data management processes.

This chapter will cover the process from the design of the data capture tool to the provision of the data for analysis.

8.2 Case report forms and data collection tools

Capture of much of the clinical data begins with a data collection tool or case report form (CRF), which will need to be finalised prior to the conduct of the trial. This may be a paper CRF (pCRF) which can be a very simple paper document of a few sheets to a folder of pages. It may also be a computer application, where the data are entered into an electronic case report form (eCRF), commonly in a web-based portal system or, less frequently, on a stand-alone computer/laptop. This type of system can be referred to as remote data entry or capture but is more usually known as electronic data capture (EDC). Data are transcribed into the tool from the source documents, although EDC can be used directly for source data recording if identified in the trial protocol. Additionally, data may need to be provided by trial subjects directly, for example by a trial diary. This may again be on paper or an electronic device. Finally, some data may not need a data collection tool or CRF at all, as the data are captured electronically at source with no manual human input (for example, central laboratory data) and then submitted to the data management centre directly by electronic data transfer (see section 8.4.3).

In some situations, although likely to be few, the sponsor may decide that a bespoke trial CRF is not necessary – for example, in a single-centre trial for which the investigator is also the chief investigator and has been intimately involved in the development of the protocol, and for which the design is so simple that the outcome measures are captured as part of routine clinical practice. In this case a CRF may be considered unnecessary as the data can easily be captured retrospectively from the source (that is, the case notes and laboratory results) and entered directly into a spreadsheet (with essentially the spreadsheet acting as a very simple eCRF and database). The sponsor may decide, however, that the resource required to extract data months after a subject's visit, as opposed to the resource required for the trial team to enter the data into a CRF shortly after each visit, is not beneficial.

Other factors to be considered are whether key data could be missing from the source records, as some could be time-dependent (such as data that must be captured at a certain time point of the trial), the frequency and variability of activities between visits, the data intensity (amount and frequency of data collection) and the trial data requirements compared with the standard of care. For multi-centre or multinational trials there could be variability in the standard of care both within and between countries, which could impact upon the data to be recorded in the source documents. In all multi-centre trials, this complexity will necessitate the use of a CRF or data collection tool to ensure consistency of the data collected and allow it to be combined. In such circumstances, care should be taken to avoid 'country-specific' amendments that could compromise the ability to combine the data.

8.2.1 CRF design

CRF design will be based on the requirements of the protocol and the statistical analysis of the trial data; this principle remains the same whether the CRF is in paper or electronic format. The CRF will also be appropriately structured, with each visit clearly defined. Examples of key elements that would be considered for the CRF include the following, and further details for some of these are in subsequent sections:

- field for an unambiguous subject identity code and visit date on each page
- screening and baseline visit(s) (see section 8.2.1.3):
  » subject demography
  » disease characteristics of the subject
  » medical and medication history and physical examination
  » data used to assess eligibility (list of inclusion and exclusion criteria)
  » confirmation of eligibility
  » initial data for the primary and secondary end-points
- subject randomisation (may be incorporated in baseline visit)
- trial visits:
  » during and post-treatment data for the primary and secondary end-points (see section 8.2.1.4)

» data to assess compliance with the protocol and the investigational medicinal product treatment regimen, particularly where central monitoring is being used (see sections 8.2.1.5 and 8.2.1.6)

» exploratory or health outcome data not related to the main end-points

» safety data (such as vital signs)

- final visit (trial completion/withdrawal)
- adverse events (see section 8.2.1.7)
- concomitant medications and other interventions (see section 8.2.1.7)
- serious adverse event forms (see section 8.2.1.7)
- field for the approval of the data by the principal investigator or authorised delegates.

Where central monitoring is used, the CRF may have to be expanded to collect more confirmatory or trial conduct information than if site visits were taking place – for example, to capture protocol deviations, consent confirmation, eligibility, randomisation and dispensing/dosing.

8.2.1.1 CRF design based on protocol

Excessive data capture that is surplus to data analysis only increases the resources required for data input and verification. Conversely, if too little data are requested this could result in some essential data not being captured or protocol non-compliances going unnoticed. Therefore the CRF should be designed with detailed reference to the trial protocol and there should be a documented review of consistency of the CRF with the trial protocol requirements.

CRF design can be performed simultaneously with the development of the protocol. An advantage of this approach is that it helps to identify problems with the protocol prior to its finalisation. The disadvantage is that there could be numerous versions of the CRF produced compared with designing it after protocol finalisation. Whichever approach is chosen, there should be a process in place for adequate version control of the CRF once released and version control is also recommended during the drafting process. For pCRFs it is recommended that each page contains the version control information. It should be possible to match a version of the CRF to the version of the protocol upon which it is based; this could be achieved for pCRFs by maintaining a simple log of pCRF versions with details of the protocol version used, whereas for eCRFs it would be part of the system specification.

The CRF development process should be robust and is usually demonstrated by evidence of input into, review of and approval of the CRF by appropriate personnel, including those within clinical operations, pharmacovigilance, statistics, medical writing, data management and quality assurance as well as the medical monitor, chief/principal investigator and sponsor (if the service has been contracted out to a vendor). On some GCP inspections it has been found that the review process has not involved the appropriate personnel listed above and this has caused problems. For example, if the review does not involve a medically qualified doctor or investigator then the CRF may be difficult to use because it does not flow in an appropriate clinically sequential way; or if the statistician is not involved, all the data required for the planned analysis may not be collected. For eCRFs, the review could be of the specification of the system with the individuals previously referred to included in the user acceptance testing (UAT). It may also be possible to pilot the draft pCRF or eCRF (perhaps during UAT) with investigators, as this will identify any problems and, as these are the users of the document, this approach is recommended.

Further information on the principles of document development can be found in Chapter 4.

8.2.1.2   CRF templates and modules

In many large organisations, templates and standard modules have been developed that are used as a starting point for CRF design, which can then be customised to some extent to meet the needs of the trial protocol. It is recommended that sponsors which conduct a large number of trials consider developing a library of CRF components and other standards that can then be re-used across similar protocols in the same therapeutic area. Some components could also be standardised across therapeutic areas (for example, pages for conventional baseline assessments and measurements). This approach of requesting the data in the same way and assigning the same attributes to the same pieces of data each time (see section 8.3.1) can promote consistency of data across trials, projects and clinical development programmes. This has a positive effect on the resource requirements for data management, statistics and monitoring as processes can remain the same and much standardisation can be achieved, which can improve quality and compliance yet save time and resources. It also facilitates the combining of trial data to undertake meta-analyses, which may be useful for the marketing authorisation common technical document.

8.2.1.3 CRF data for eligibility, screening and baseline visit

The CRF may contain a checklist of the eligibility criteria to be completed (either overall or for each criterion from the protocol) to confirm that these have been met and the subject can participate in the trial. Consideration may be given to collecting the actual data that relate to a particular eligibility criterion in the CRF (or via electronic data transfer, such as laboratory data). Data validation can then be used to confirm that a subject is eligible from the actual data, rather than reliance on a tick box alone. This could be particularly helpful when central monitoring is being used and there is no source data verification (SDV) taking place. Additionally, there may be a section to confirm that the subject has consented to participate in the trial and the date consent was given. Some trials also require completion of a registration form that includes data related to eligibility, which is sent to a central data centre in order for the investigator to be provided with subject identity and randomisation codes. Interactive response technologies (IRT) systems may also use forms in order to assign subjects to treatment (see Annex 4).

Where any eligibility criteria are confirmed, there must[3] be evidence of who performed this confirmation to verify that the final decision to enter a subject into the trial was made by a medically qualified doctor. Consideration may therefore be given to designing the CRF to record and confirm who has undertaken these activities (such as signatures and dates). Similarly, the trial may require specific assessments to be undertaken by appropriately qualified staff; for example, the physical examination and dosing decision should be undertaken by a medically qualified doctor, and an eyesight test should be conducted by an ophthalmologist. The CRF can again be used for this purpose if suitably designed.

8.2.1.4 CRF data for end-points

The CRF should capture the data that have been determined by the protocol to be the end-points of the trial. Additionally, if the planned protocol analysis includes the use of covariates in the analysis (for example, relating to subject, disease and demographic factors, including age groups, gender, disease staging and prior exposure to certain treatment), the CRF should be designed to capture these data.

The key to data management is to ensure that all data relating to the end-points are captured at predefined time points. Sometimes, the primary end-points are relatively straightforward – for example, clinical end-points such as time to death and time to relapse, or surrogate end-points such as CD4 levels and viral load.

In these cases the data may be transcribed from the source to the CRF. Alternatively, these data can be imported directly into the database from, for example, a central laboratory.

Sometimes the efficacy end-points are less straightforward, such as those based on a composite score. For example, the Mini Mental State Examination (MMSE), Response Evaluation Criteria in Solid Tumours (RECIST) and Psoriasis Area and Severity Index (PASI) overall scores are calculated by adding the scores for individual components. For example, the PASI score is often derived from a combined score rating the redness, scaliness and thickness of the skin. It is recommended that the CRF captures all the component data. If the composite score is required during the trial for the clinical management of the subject, how the composite score was calculated should be documented or an automated calculation can be used for an eCRF.

A visual analogue scale (VAS) may be used to capture data for end-points, such as pain score. There are validated methods for capturing this data, and they should be used when available. Problems can arise when VAS diagrams are used (such as a line that the subject has to mark to indicate pain levels); if the line is not printed to the correct length or a non-calibrated ruler is used for measurement, inaccuracies can result. It is also important to decide whether these measurements will be undertaken at the investigator site and recorded in the CRF or centrally by the sponsor or vendor. Again, this may be dependent upon whether this information is required during the trial for the clinical management of the subject.

Consideration may also be given to ensuring that the CRF captures the times of time-dependent events, so that confounding factors are recorded and assessed. For example, the timing of blood sampling is key to pharmacokinetic (PK) analysis and this information needs to be captured, ideally in the CRF. Additionally, the protocol may impose certain conditions on the timing of blood sampling (such as breakfast should be taken not more than six hours before sampling) or sampling may be timed in relation to the dosing of the investigational medicinal product (IMP). If the food intake has a significant impact on the analysis of the sample, a direct relationship with the sample or interaction with the IMP, then it may be important to capture the timing of these events in the CRF.

8.2.1.5　CRF data for drug compliance

Sometimes it may be necessary for the CRF to contain fields to capture information on compliance with the trial treatment. Examples of such fields include the following:

- a question asking for the investigator's judgement of subject compliance
- data taken from the pharmacy accountability log (for example, tablet counts to work out the percentage compliance or weights/volumes of IMPs formulated as creams and topical agents to confirm usage per subject application)
- the start and stop times (including interruptions) of an IMP infusion to ensure compliance with the protocol or to ensure that the drug has not been given above a certain rate; this is particularly important for first in human trials
- the date/time of reconstitution of an IMP (to confirm that it was used within a limited shelf life or short half-life – for example, a radiolabelled IMP)
- dosing time for an IMP (for PK analysis or where there is a requirement for a limited period of time between the onset of the disease and the start of the therapy, such as emergency research in head injury)
- subject diaries (see section 8.2.7).

It is recommended that superfluous data recording is avoided. For example, on inspection a trial was reviewed in which the IMP (an authorised product) was given over 15 minutes once a week for 24 weeks, resulting in 48 data points. The sponsor indicated that the data were being collected for safety reasons; however, adverse event data were required to be captured in addition to the infusion times. This is over-recording of data as the chance of infusion interruption was low, the reconstituted IMP was stable and the adverse event data had already been captured elsewhere.

8.2.1.6   CRF data for protocol non-compliance

The process for capturing and documenting protocol and GCP non-compliances should be well defined (see section 1.3.5). Non-compliance may be noted by the monitor or site personnel and may be documented in the monitoring visit reports, in the file notes or in a log. If the method of documentation is unstructured, the sponsor is taking the risk that some non-compliance may be omitted. It is recommended that non-compliance is collated centrally and must[4, 5] be documented and also eventually provided to the statistician and medical writer. Non-compliance can also be captured through the data validation process (see section 8.5), when computer edit checks or contemporaneous validation of eCRFs can highlight departures from the protocol.

Non-compliance checks are not easily built into the CRF design but consideration may be given to including a dedicated CRF field for non-compliance due to predefined reasons plus a comments field for site staff to record other, unclassified, non-compliance. Unstructured data recorded in the comment fields are, however, difficult to categorise and therefore it is recommended that an alternative method (such as logs) is used to capture non-compliance data, although this could be located in the CRF to record non-compliance for that subject. The log would include all the non-compliance data in the database and therefore make it available to the statistician. Here, the data can be reviewed and possibly coded or labelled according to different categories, such as inclusion and exclusion criteria, drug compliance, visit windows and prohibited medication (see section 9.7.1).

8.2.1.7   CRF data for concomitant medications and adverse events

It is recommended that the CRF contains a log for adverse events that allows the investigator to record the adverse events, assess their relationship to the IMP, and assess their severity and seriousness as per the requirements of the protocol and the legislation. Where an adverse event is judged as serious by the investigator it is usual practice to then complete a serious adverse event (SAE) form that is separate from the CRF; this is quite often a standard and non-trial-specific form. These forms are often used to report to the sponsor and the data are placed in a pharmacovigilance database rather than the clinical database; however, the log in the CRF would be a record of summary information about the SAE. The original SAE form can be retained with the CRF or more usually kept in the investigator site file. At each visit throughout the CRF there should be a prompt to ask the person completing the CRF whether any adverse events have occurred and, if so, to complete the next record on the adverse event log in the CRF. The protocol should give the timescale for the collection of adverse event data. For example, some trials may not require collection in the CRF of adverse events in a follow-up phase of the trial and any such requirements should be designed into the CRF. For further information on pharmacovigilance in clinical trials, see Chapter 5.

Concomitant medications can often be quite difficult to capture adequately in the CRF because they can change frequently and be numerous. It is therefore recommended that an appropriate collection tool is designed. It is also recommended that a log is created in the CRF where each medication is a separate record; this can then be updated with indication, dose, start and stop dates following a prompt for completion at each visit in the CRF (for example, using the question 'Has there been any change in concomitant medication?'). It is important that there is clarity on where concomitant medications to treat SAEs are recorded, as it is often necessary to record this in both the concomitant medication log and the SAE form.

8.2.2   Paper CRFs

Paper CRFs (pCRFs) are usually produced with at least one 'no carbon required' (NCR) copy included. It is recommended that they are suitably constructed to segregate the separate forms, and instruction pages can also be included to assist investigators. The incorporation of wallets to file loose-leaf results, data query forms or subject diaries should also be considered as this keeps all the subject's data together in one place. Checks should be performed to ensure that the correct version of the pCRF is sent to the printer and that the printed version matches the final approved version.

As the original wet-ink CRF pages are completed, they are taken by the trial monitor or faxed/posted from the trial sites to the data management centre for data entry. pCRF systems should, and typically do, ensure that either a contemporaneous copy or, in some cases (for example, when CRFs are transmitted via fax) the original CRF pages are retained at the investigator site. When fax-based systems are used, there is no need for the CRF to be on NCR paper.

8.2.3   Electronic CRFs

More recently, eCRFs have been used to allow investigator sites to enter data via a website portal or, less commonly now, a stand-alone computer/laptop. In this situation the investigator site staff are undertaking remote data entry into the clinical database and the trial is an EDC trial. In the second scenario there is usually is a need to upload the data from the computer/laptop on a regular basis. There are advantages and disadvantages to both approaches. Design and implementation decisions should be made after considering the protocol and operational requirements.

8.2.4   Comparison of paper and electronic CRFs

The sponsor has an option for which CRF system to use, paper or electronic, and Table 8.1 lists the differences between the two systems against a range of non-business-related criteria. The sponsor will need to decide which system is most suitable for the trial that it is undertaking and its circumstances. Either system is acceptable, as both can result in high-quality data and reliable trial results.

Table 8.1 Comparison of paper and electronic case report forms

Criteria	pCRF	eCRF
Can see who at site completed the data entry (including amendments to data)	✓ [a]	✓
Straightforward to set up; limited information technology skills required at investigator sites	✓	✗
No computer system validation of case report form (though needed for database)	✓	✗
Legibility of handwriting of personnel entering data can be problematic	✓	✗
Contemporaneous copy held by investigator at all times	✓	✗ [b]
Easy to manage and low risk of losing data	✗	✓
No data entry into computer database by sponsor (no verification)	✗	✓
Additional resources (for example, computers, internet access) and training required at investigator site	✗	✓
Facilitates central monitoring	✗ [c]	✓
Data validation can occur at point of data entry at investigator site	✗	✓
Ability to monitor remotely	✗	✓
Ability to build in workflow through the case report form (screens to enter detailed data appear following a question answered in a particular way, such as concomitant medications or adverse events)	✗	✓
Version control can be managed centrally and more easily	✗	✓

[a] This can be problematic if entries are not signed and dated.

[b] This can be problematic (see note c).

[c] Depending on the speed of submission.

eCRF, electronic case report form; pCRF, paper case report form

The processes and mechanisms of data input, data clarification and data flow have changed with advancing computer system technology. The functionality of an eCRF offers the potential for improving data quality by incorporating work flows (for example, appropriate screens that open based on the data entered) and by the ability to perform some data validation during the entry of data at the investigator site, which is not possible with pCRFs. The eCRF is a computer system (interface) and therefore should be validated whether it is a trial-specific build using a commercial off-the-shelf system or a bespoke system for the trial requiring full computer system validation. The CRF design is part of the specification process for the system build. There have been failures seen on inspection to fully document the validation of the eCRF, in particular the UAT and ensuring the system is fully validated and therefore fit for purpose, prior to use. The principles of validation for computer systems and usage outlined in section 8.3.2 and section 14.5 can be consulted for further information.

An eCRF cannot accommodate an investigator's wet-ink signature; the investigator must[4] instead be given their own user account and password to facilitate an audit trail. The eCRF may require electronic or digital signatures for various sections or may have the functionality to allow role-based access to particular areas. This can be useful, for example, to confirm the eligibility of a trial subject, where only users registered as medically qualified doctors would have access. Unfortunately, there is the possibility that site personnel will share their passwords. Examples have been seen on inspection where investigators have granted access by providing their personal password to trial nurses, without the knowledge of the sponsor. This is clearly not an acceptable practice.

When a pCRF system is used, data from source documents are transcribed onto the CRF and a duplicate copy made at the same time using NCR paper or photocopies (unless the originals are retained at the site owing to the CRF being faxed to the sponsor/vendor). With eCRFs, however, such contemporaneous copies may not be produced. It is not acceptable for the sponsor to have exclusive control of the data, for instance when the data are held on the sponsor's servers and no contemporaneous copy of the data is maintained by the investigator. This is of particular concern if the CRF has any source data entered (see section 8.2.5), as there is potential for unauthorised changes to be made to the data. Often, the sponsor's solution is to provide a copy of the entered data to the investigator at the end of the trial, for example on a disk (CD or DVD). For transcribed data, the investigator must[4] have the source data at site and be able to compare the provided data with the source to confirm its accuracy. On inspection, however, it has often been noted that this has not been done, even when the investigator has signed to certify that the provided data are accurate. Additionally, there is often no consideration given to the long-term access to the data on the disk (for example, if software becomes obsolete) or to backing up the data.

The sponsor should therefore ensure the CRF data are available both during and after the end of the trial; that is, the investigator should at all times maintain an independent copy of the data provided to the sponsor. Examples of methods used to address this issue include:

- The investigator completes worksheets (shadow CRF) to capture the data. An advantage of this method is that site staff do not need to check against the database to confirm what is needed for a visit. The disadvantage is that it creates an additional set of documentation, which could lead to discrepancies, especially when changes need to be made. It is therefore recommended that there is a mechanism to change these worksheets to reflect the database if the database is changed by a data query, particularly if the data query is undertaken and authorised electronically in the eCRF and there is no paper record to file with the worksheet. Also, the CRF would no longer contain any source data, as the source document is the worksheet. Careful consideration would need to be given to this approach to ensure integrity of the data.

- The independent vendor (a separate legal entity from the sponsor) hosts the data when the trial is live, retains a copy of the database after the trial has been completed and provides the data to the investigator, with access during and after the trial (such as on a disk). It is recommended that the contract between the sponsor and vendor confirms that the sponsor does not have access to the data, but could be provided with a copy.

- An eCRF system facilitates the download of an independent certified copy of the data onto the investigator's computer or other electronic storage device (CD or memory stick) during or after each input of the data into the system. The investigator should verify that this is readable and that the data are adequately stored, protected and backed up.

For further information on this subject, the EMA GCP Inspectors Working Group paper, 'Reflection paper on expectations for electronic source data and data transcribed to electronic data collection tools in clinical trials' (EMA/INS/GCP/454280/2010) should be consulted.

8.2.5 Paper and electronic CRFs used for source data

While the CRF is normally used for transcribing data from the source data at the investigator site, there may be circumstances where the CRF has data directly recorded into it, meaning that at least part of the CRF is a source document. For example, as discussed in section 8.2.7, subject questionnaires may be included in the CRF. In these circumstances such data should be listed as source data in the trial protocol. The sponsor should never have sole control of the CRF when it has become a source document at any time. For pCRFs and diaries, for example, this is usually achieved by using NCR paper or, alternatively, the paper can be photocopied prior to sending to the sponsor.

8.2.6   Amendments to the CRF post-finalisation

Often during a trial a protocol amendment may be required and, when the documented assessment of the impact of the amendment has been made, changes to the CRF design may be required. There should be a procedure in place to control this, in particular how the change would be implemented at the investigator sites (such as issue of replacement pages in line with approval of the amendment at that site and collection of old versions). With an eCRF this would be managed by a change control process, but there would still be issues of control of implementation at each investigator site, as with a pCRF. In one inspection it was observed that, when there were country-specific amendments made to the protocol, changes were made to the eCRF, but the validation did not sufficiently address whether the correct version of the eCRF was available to the correct sites, so there was a risk that the approved protocol would not be followed.

8.2.7   Data recording tools for trial subjects

Occasionally, data are entered by trial subjects themselves (or the subjects' carers) into paper or electronic subject diaries/self-assessment questionnaires. These enable the subjects to record their symptoms, side effects, well-being and IMP usage. The recorded data may have a high level of importance – for example, they may be an end-point for a trial for pain recording or asthma symptoms. When subjects are requested to complete paper diaries, the data will either be transcribed to the dedicated CRF pages or collected by the monitor for return to data management for data entry. In the latter case, diaries must[5, 6] be checked prior to removal from the investigator site to ensure there are no subject identifiers present and a copy should be retained by the investigator. Diaries are recommended to be designed to facilitate data collection, for example by taking into consideration possible infirmities of the subjects, such as difficulty in writing or eyesight problems that may require large font sizes and/or boxes to be used.

Some self-assessment questionnaires may form part of the CRF. In some cases, investigator site staff have admitted completing these questionnaires for the subject, contrary to the protocol requirements. When quality-of-life data are a key component of the efficacy end-point, a more robust system of demonstrating data integrity could be implemented (for example, by having dedicated CRF pages that include a serial number, are barcoded, pre-printed and contain subject identifiers, or by using ring-bound booklets to prevent loose-leaf questionnaires from dropping out or being replaced in the wrong order in the CRF). Additionally, consideration could be given to the subject signing and dating the diary.

Data from electronic diaries may periodically be transmitted and imported directly to the database of the sponsor. The set-up of the electronic device in relation to the requirements of the trial protocol should be subject to validation to ensure that it is fit for purpose (see section 14.5), and documentation of this must[5] be retained. The devices are usually required to be used by subjects at set time points, for example each morning and evening. It is recommended that the device has a 'window of opportunity' to complete the questions to prevent retrospective completion by the subject (for example, on the way to the visit or in the car park) or by any staff at the investigator site. This is an advantage over paper diaries. Additionally, if the device has the functionality of a hidden date/time stamp to provide an audit trail, this would assist in demonstrating the robustness of the data. There has been an example seen on inspection where the investigator was completing the pre-screening diaries for subjects to ensure their eligibility for the trial. This was detected from the IRT data, which showed entries being made on the same day, in consecutive order, minutes apart and with no overlapping calls, which would be unlikely if subjects were making the calls at home themselves. If the devices are for repeated use in other trials or by other subjects in the same trial, it is recommended that there is a formalised process to delete any data before and after use.

When electronic devices are used to capture subject self-administered questionnaires, care should be taken to ensure that the source data are available to the site. This is to confirm that the data have not been changed after leaving the investigator site (for example, once the device is attached to the docking station and the data have been electronically transferred to an external database). In such situations there are the same issues with sole sponsor control of the data referred to above with eCRFs (see section 8.2.5). It is important that the subjects, with support of the site staff, have the ability to amend any errors in the diary data independently of the sponsor. It was found at a sponsor organisation during a GCP inspection that the sponsor had to authorise any requested changes. This is not acceptable. There must[4] be an audit trail to record any changes to the diary data. Finally, the subject should have the ability to set up their own secure access to the device to prevent unauthorised use. The ability to demonstrate that the subject had completed the diary themselves is more difficult with paper diaries, as there is no ability to implement the control processes that are available within electronic diaries.

The issues described above will have much greater importance where the diary data provide the data for the primary or important secondary end-point. This would be highlighted during the bespoke risk assessment for the trial and the above considerations should inform any potential mitigating activities.

8.3   Clinical database

8.3.1   Annotated CRF

When using a pCRF it is common practice for data management personnel to annotate or mark up the pages to facilitate data management processes, including database system design. This annotation process is completed by making notes on each field, such as the table and field names, as well as, where appropriate, the variable type or length, the variable name and the format of the variable. This facilitates the process of providing a clear link between the data source and its location within the clinical trial database. In some circumstances there will be standards for the naming and formatting of the data in order to facilitate the use of standard modules, programs and meta-analyses as discussed earlier.

For eCRFs, the annotated CRF is from part of the trial-specific system specification for the eCRF, as these requirements will have been necessary in order to design and validate the system. This may involve the use of screen shots of the system.

8.3.2   Database system build

8.3.2.1   Validation requirements

Database systems for clinical trials can use commercial off-the-shelf software or bespoke software developed in-house. The system itself will need an appropriate level of validation and details of these principles can be found in section 14.5.

The database system is used to create a trial-specific database and data entry system with fields and tables created to reflect the CRF, using the annotated CRF as the design specification. This should be validated to confirm that the database system is fit for purpose specifically for the trial. For eCRFs, the eCRF system may be the database itself or be a separate web-based system, which will then map onto the clinical database. In these circumstances there will still need to be database design, and the validation should confirm that the eCRF data are mapped to the appropriate locations in the database and that the eCRF/database system is fit for purpose specifically for the trial.

For small, simple trials, the database system specification may be relatively straightforward, particularly in the non-commercial setting, where the results are not to be used in a marketing authorisation application. In these cases, MS Excel may be considered appropriate to be used for the data management and analysis. The choice of MS Excel, as opposed to a formal clinical trial database, will have been guided by the sponsor's risk assessment for the trial because it was considered proportionate to the potential risks to the data integrity and trial results. Validation of such spreadsheets is also discussed in section 14.5 and has often not been considered by the sponsor when the spreadsheets have been reviewed on inspection.

Standardisation of CRF design (templates and modules) facilitates the database system build as the construction of screens or tables has already been undertaken and the developer can select the appropriate component. It is usual that standard components of the database system have been validated previously, thus reducing the level of testing required of the final database system build.

8.3.2.2   Database system specification

The final annotated pCRF is used for database design and forms part of the specification. For an eCRF the database structure/screens may be built directly from the protocol design, a database design specification, or a mock-up of the required database screens. Additional features to consider in the database system specification include:

- screen layout to reflect the pCRF page
- use of drop-down lists or menus (expected values)
- on-entry validation
- pop-up help function

- dictionary help, if required (for example, Medical Dictionary for Regulatory Activities – MedDRA)
- comment fields
- flow of information (for example, if adverse event is ticked, the screens lead the user to the adverse event form)
- protocol non-compliances.

8.3.2.3 Database system testing

Once the database system is built, testing will need to be undertaken according to a pre-specified plan. The testing will normally consist of the system developer testing against the design specifications, which would include technical checks of mapping the data to the correct tables, formats, lengths, variable types etc. UAT will also be required, with the users in this context being those personnel who would enter the trial data, although sponsor staff will usually do the testing for eCRFs (rather than investigator site staff). This is often done by the creation of dummy data, whereby CRFs are completed with deliberate errors to test the robustness of the database system with 'test scripts', known as 'stress testing'. There should be a formal process to either delete the test data or use subject identifiers to clearly identify the test data so that they can be excluded from subsequent data management activities. Inspectors have also seen UAT being undertaken with real trial subjects' data. This is not recommended as it does not specifically test the database system's attributes (such as designing 'bad' data to test edit checks on data entry) and results in real data being used in the database that should still be in a test environment.

It is recommended that database testing considers at least the items listed below:

- The database system flows correctly and is presented in a way that is consistent with the pCRF.
- The links between screens function correctly.
- Fields accept the correct type of data (for example, if designed to hold numerical data, it should reject entry of letters or symbols).
- Field lengths are appropriate (for example, comment fields have the ability to input many characters).
- On-entry validation edit checks are functional (field accepts only valid answers or ranges and warning flags appear if the value appears to be unexpected).
- All data fields required for any calculation of a score or other derived value (for example, body mass index) are present.

- The system to enter and manage ambiguous values is functional (for example, when data entry staff cannot decipher handwriting on the CRF).
- Where double data entry is used and comparison is contemporaneous, that this is functioning correctly and identifying discrepancies.
- The audit trail is functional (an audit trail should be on the database).
- Database imports/exports function correctly.

These tests are recommended to be thorough to avoid repeated change control requests to amend database fields during the live phase of the trial. An example was seen where the clinical database did not collect all the assessments of pain in a subject paper diary, an error that was not detected on testing, but was identified when the GCP inspectors performed SDV of the clinical study report (CSR) listings. This resulted in a considerable effort after reporting of the trial to assess the impact of the error. Finally, the testing evidence and corrective actions must[5] be retained in order to demonstrate, for example during audit or inspection, that the process has been undertaken.

8.3.2.4   Database system activation

Any bugs and issues identified from testing should be resolved and there should be a formal activation or movement of the database system (or modules thereof) from the test to the production environment. It should be possible to track in the documentation any test failures and their rectification. Inspectors have seen that this can sometimes lack control; for example, the database is activated before all the errors have been eradicated, any work-arounds have been documented in the user manual or prior to the system owner having reviewed all the necessary documentation and authorised its release to the live environment (that is, before the validation report has been completed). Once the database is activated, any further changes would be dealt with according to the validation principles of change control.

8.3.2.5   Optical recognition

In some trials, the pCRFs contain shaded boxes or even handwritten text that can be scanned and recognised by a software system. These systems are not extensively used. The system should be appropriately validated (see section 14.5) to give assurance that the system is reading the data accurately. A QC check of the resultant database is highly recommended.

8.4 Data capture

8.4.1 CRF completion guidelines

The investigator should ensure the accuracy, completeness, legibility and timeliness of the data reported to the sponsor in the CRFs. In large, complex and multi-centre trials, it may be useful to compile a CRF completion guideline or build one into the online help/structure of the eCRF (as part of the specification and build). CRF completion guidelines typically include advice on:

- date format and partial dates
- time format and unknown times
- rounding conventions
- trial-specific interpretation of data fields
- entry requirements for concomitant medications (generic or brand names)
- which forms to complete when
- what to do in certain scenarios, for example when a subject withdraws from the trial
- missing/incomplete data
- completing SAE forms and reporting SAEs
- repeat laboratory tests
- protocol and GCP non-compliances.

8.4.2 CRFs, data entry and verification

8.4.2.1 pCRF handling

The top copies of pCRFs are removed from the investigator site, leaving the duplicate copies behind. Alternatively, if NCR copy paper is not used, the CRF original should be copied prior to removal from the investigator site. Occasionally, the investigator site may fax the CRF page and retain the original; however, this can have an impact on how the resolution of the data queries can be documented (see section 8.5.7). Use of a tracking system is recommended to ensure the correct pages are received by the data entry site. Any discrepancies should be identified in a timely fashion so the missing pages can be located.

If the CRF pages are scanned or faxed (to become a digital copy), for example to avoid transit of paper across the world, the transfer process should be validated to ensure the scanned or faxed CRF is a certified copy of the original (see section 10.5.4 for more information on scanning documents). The pCRFs, as part of the TMF, must[5] be managed as essential trial documents with respect to storage.

8.4.2.2 Quality control of data entry into the CRF or database (data verification)

QC should be applied at each stage of data handling to ensure that all data are reliable and have been processed correctly.

Where pCRFs are used there would normally be a need to manually transcribe the data into an electronic clinical database. It may be appropriate for QC to confirm that this has been done accurately. Similarly, transcribing data from the source into the eCRF at the investigator site presents the same opportunity – although this QC is usually done with SDV by the trial monitor, and extensive contemporaneous on-entry data validation can reduce errors. There may be circumstances where there is no routine on-site monitoring; however, QC activities may be undertaken by investigator site staff. General requirements for QC are contained in section 14.3. The options for the QC process of establishing the accuracy of the data entry from pCRFs into the database are detailed in Table 8.2. The trial risk assessment can determine the data that should be subject to 100% QC (for example that relate to primary end-points) and those data that require QC of a sample, or require no QC. In complex arrangements it may be appropriate to describe the QC process in a QC or monitoring plan if it has not been covered in a formal procedure.

8.4.3 Electronic data transfer

The transfer of data electronically between service providers and data management is routinely performed and involves no manual entry of data. The type of data that can be transferred electronically can include that from central laboratories, IRT, electronic subject diaries, ECGs and spirometry. Although the transfer of such data may be electronic, there may also be paper records of the results at the investigator site that are necessary for management of the trial subject. Where this is the case, the paper results are the source data and are not returned to the central data management function. Sometimes the results may be reviewed by the investigator but interpreted centrally, and this central review is the data submitted to the sponsor.

Table 8.2 Options for quality control of data entry from paper case report forms (verification)

QC level	Methodology	Comment
As required, but often 100% for small datasets	Print-out of entered data and direct comparison with case report form. If same individual, it is appropriate to include a time delay prior to undertaking the check. Print-out annotated, signed and dated to confirm check.	Applicable particularly to small non-commercial trials, where investigator or research fellow is undertaking data management and analysis activities.
100%	Double data entry by independent operators.[a] This can be by the comparison taking place as the second entry is done, thus flagging discrepancies immediately (contemporaneous checking model), or by producing two separate databases that are then compared using a computer program (for example, PROC COMPARE in SAS®) at a later date (retrospective checking model). Records maintained (usually in database audit trail) of who did the entry and any comparison output retained (all copies until comparison completed).	Used extensively by commercial sponsors. Although not 100% accurate (for example, the two operators could enter the same data incorrectly, which is of higher risk in the contemporaneous checking model), it typically results in high levels of accuracy.
Sample checking – data entry operator competency-based	Data entry operators have high level of training and experience. After entering data, accuracy rate is assessed and judged as competent to continue with data entry, with further checking at the end of the trial when assessing database quality.	Used by some commercial companies. It is important that statistical sampling is applied to the data selected for the competency assessment to minimise bias from the case report forms visits used. For example, if all the case report forms assessed were for visits 1, 2 and 3, a later visit with potentially a more difficult dataset to enter (resulting in more errors) may be missed giving an inaccurate competency rating.

QC level	Methodology	Comment
Sample checking	A statistical sampling process is used to select data for checking. This may be targeted to certain data or the percentage check may vary dependent upon which data are used – this would be informed by the trial risk assessment. The actual checking could be done by print-out and manual comparison or double entry and contemporaneous or retrospective comparison of the required data (although the latter may be logistically difficult – entering odd data points from across the case report form visits). Records of who did what and what was checked would be required to be maintained.	This is a proportionate approach to the data quality issue. It may be in a quality control plan or other document (for example, a written procedure) and there would be an expectation of an escalation process if error levels were above a predefined limit. This process is often used for calculation of an error rate for the final quality check of the database (see section 8.5.10).

ᵃ A variation may be that the same person does the second entry at a later date.

8.4.3.1   Agreements

There should be an agreement between the data management function and the vendor responsible for the provision of the data to cover the detailed technical requirements, such as:

- the format to be provided (for example, SAS®, ASCII or MS Excel)
- how it will be provided (for example, by portal or email)
- data security arrangements (including maintaining the blinding)
- the number of datasets, how they are named and their structure (variables/ observations layout)
- formats and codes applied to the data observations (for example, 1 = High and 2 = Low)
- the process for the transfer/mapping
- validation requirements
- the process for resolving issues/queries during data validation.

8.4.3.2   Validation requirements

Ideally, tests of the mapping process and transfers between the parties will be carried out before live data are migrated between the systems. If real trial data are

8

used for the validation process, there will be a mechanism to remove the data prior to using the approved process for the trial. Testing would include transfers of test data from the source dataset into any new format (for example, ASCII or MS Excel into SAS datasets). As part of the validation of the programming utilised, input and output datasets would be reconciled to confirm that the programming runs successfully.

Merging or uploading of any non-CRF electronic data (such as central laboratory data) with/to the CRF clinical data would also be subject to testing as part of the validation of the process. This would also include the security aspects of the transfer, for example the use of passwords or encryption techniques. This would involve verification that each data item is populated correctly in the data field with the correct subject identifier and date. When errors are identified during validation testing these would be resolved and documented in a validation report. Changes to the manner in which data are collected, structured and transferred may be required during the trial and these should be captured as part of a change control process.

Mapping errors that have not been picked up at the test transfer or validation stages have been observed during inspection. For example, in one trial, the coding standard for subsets of fields was assigned an incorrect meaning/format, such that when the data were transferred, mismatched data were left out and were therefore missing from the final dataset (that is, the data field was labelled as numerical but alphanumerical data were transferred instead and the mismatched data were left out).

Once all the data are amalgamated with the CRF clinical data, data validation can take place as discussed in the following section.

8.5   Data validation

Data validation is the process of checking the data for such elements as logical consistency, protocol deviations (for example, subject ineligibility) and missing/incorrect/implausible data. This is achieved by setting up formalised validation or edit checks on the data. The process can be manual, electronic or a mixture of both. These processes identify data issues that can then be resolved by clarification with investigator sites and vendors/holders of related databases (for example, laboratory analysis vendors, pharmacovigilance database). The aim of validation is to generate a database/dataset that is of appropriate quality, as decided as part of the risk assessment and defined in written procedures, DMP

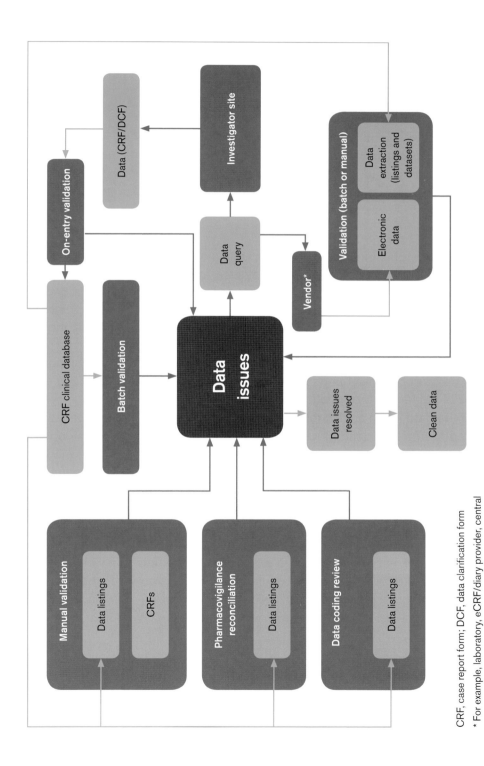

CRF, case report form; DCF, data clarification form

* For example, laboratory, eCRF/diary provider, central
assessment centre for reading scan/images

Figure 8.2 Simple summary of data validation and cleaning

or protocol. An overview is shown in Figure 8.2 and the following sections will discuss each aspect in more detail.

8.5.1 Data validation and central monitoring

Validation that occurs at the time of data entry (for example, in eCRFs) or done centrally in a timely manner can allow real-time actions to prevent harm to the trial subject and/or loss of data integrity. For example, ineligibility identified early on may prevent ineligible subjects from progressing further or avoid systematic protocol deviations. As such, data validation is a key component of central monitoring activities.

Undertaking thorough checks on the data in real time (for example, with eCRFs, EDC or pCRF faxing) can detect problems at sites, in particular by comparing particular metrics between sites, which may lead to an escalation in monitoring. It is reliant on data being provided promptly (a site failing to do this is an indicator of a potential problem in itself) and the validation being applied in a timely manner. Standard reports and metrics will need to be routinely produced from the database as part of the monitoring plan. These must[5] be retained to demonstrate that the monitoring plan has been followed. Additionally, there may be a need for extractions of data to be provided for the statistician to undertake more complex analysis of the data (such as distribution comparisons, identification of outliers) to produce reports/metrics used for central monitoring. It is strongly recommended that, where central monitoring is used, staff from the involved disciplines review the monitoring plan, DMP, validation plan and validation specification to ensure that there is consistency among the documents and that they meet the requirements of the mitigations identified in the risk assessment. This may include staff from the data management and statistics department, monitoring staff, investigators or medical monitors and the project manager. Reference could be made to the trial risk assessment, as this would identify the data that would be subject to the most detailed validation requirements, compared with other less important data, where a predetermined level of error or missing data may be acceptable. Such decisions and their rationale would be documented in the validation plan.

8.5.2 Validation plan and specification

A plan for how the data will be validated is usually prepared and may be a separate document or part of the DMP. The plan may cover roles and responsibilities, the types of check and how they will be chosen and documented, the processes used for implementing the checks and how any problems will be resolved (for example, via a data query process). The plan(s) may make reference to existing formal procedures.

The description of checks to be performed (sometimes called the validation specification) is usually prepared by data management and reviewed and approved by responsible personnel. These would include those within clinical development, statistics and quality assurance as well as the medical monitor and sponsor (if the service has been contracted out to a vendor) and, often in non-commercial trials, the chief investigator. It is recommended that the validation specification is written in plain English to enable all reviewers to understand the requirements without having to learn programming languages. The data managers and reviewers will need to be familiar with the risk assessment, protocol, CRF and key data (for example, end-points or covariates) for the trial. It is essential that those performing statistical analysis of the data are involved in defining the validation and consulted on aspects of defining the quality of the data. It is recommended that all the proposed checks are listed in the specification together with the methodology by which they will be undertaken. These include checks that are:

- performed manually by reviewing print-outs with possible reference back to actual CRFs (such as for complicated cross-form checks, where data must be compared across several visits or logs – for example, adverse events, concomitant medication, end-of-trial data)
- programmed into an eCRF or data entry system (on entry)
- done on a batch or continual validation basis.

Often, unfortunately, only the latter category appears in the specification. The specification for on-entry validation checks in the eCRF/data entry system will also form part of the specification for the eCRF/database system build.

In very small non-commercial trials, the data validation is likely to be fairly minimal and conducted manually (checks of print-outs and CRFs). Where any checks on the data's validity are being done, however, these must[5] be documented and retained, so it is evident from the TMF what was checked, when and by whom.

The validation specification should be version-controlled and updated in line with the change control procedure. Often, when examined during a GCP inspection, the document is a live version, with continual uncontrolled edits taking place. As the document is the specification for subsequent programming, this lack of control is unacceptable from a validation perspective. The validation specification should be reviewed when there are amendments to the protocol and CRF.

8

Examples of areas to consider and checks to undertake are in the following three subsections.

8.5.2.1 Data validation: inclusion and exclusion criteria

An important ability of data validation is the facility to verify subject eligibility by comparing the appropriate actual clinical data against the inclusion and exclusion criteria for the trial. It may be decided to do this rather than rely solely on a tick box for each criterion or an overall assessment that all eligibility criteria have been met. To do this validation check, however, it is necessary that the appropriate eligibility data are collected in the CRF. An inspection finding had previously been given for an ineligible subject being in the per-protocol dataset, as the edit checks had not included a check on eligibility even though the data were available to do so. Examples of such validation checks include the following:

- **Physical measurements** Body mass index calculated from weight and height is within the required range.
- **Demographics** Subject age calculated from date of birth and visit date is within the required range.
- **Screening tests** Haematology/biochemistry laboratory values or tumour size are within the required range.
- **Pregnancy test** Result is negative (for females of child-bearing potential).
- **Onset of symptoms** When onset of symptoms to time of treatment is included as an eligibility criterion, such as time of onset of heart attack, aneurysm or severe septicaemia.
- **Disease characteristics** Staging in oncology trials.
- **Disallowed medications** Use of medical history and concomitant medications data.

Another inspection revealed that trial-specific screening laboratory samples had been retained by a site in error (that is, they were not sent for analysis) and subsequently found not to be analysable. All the subjects screened were dosed and enrolled in the trial and the error was only identified by the monitor several months after trial initiation. A simple validation check could have identified the absence of the screening results, which would have triggered a query or monitoring visit to address the issue.

8.5.2.2 Data validation: protocol compliance

Data validation is a useful tool for ongoing monitoring of the site and subject compliance with the protocol when the data are analysed in real time (for example, when EDC or central monitoring is used), as well as for retrospectively identifying non-compliance with the protocol and GCP, which may prove important for data analysis. Adhering to the visit window is important in terms of protocol compliance as, if not followed, the subject may run out of medication, certain observations or tests (efficacy end-points) may not be performed at predefined time points, or safety checks may not be performed, which could compromise subject safety. Examples of such validation checks include:

- laboratory data tie up with the sample date/time in CRF
- correct dose of IMP has been given to subjects when the trial includes a complex IMP regimen
- trial time points, such as dates of screening, baseline visits, trial visits, are within the predefined window
- use of disallowed concomitant medication (to check for protocol violations)
- IV infusion start and end times (compliance check)
- pharmacokinetic sample time points.

8.5.2.3 Data validation: other checks

Validation is used to detect and rectify data entry errors and logical inconsistencies within the data. It can be done in real time to assist monitoring and compliance, and some errors can even be prevented by on-entry contemporaneous validation checks. These can be simple within-form checks or quite extensive cross-form checks. For example:

- missing values are detected
- visits are chronological
- test results are available and entered before decisions on dosing are made
- out-of-range or implausible values
- values that suddenly deviate from trend (as assessed by a statistician)
- adverse event log completed if adverse event confirmed at a visit
- concomitant medications updated if a change is confirmed at a visit
- concomitant medications and adverse event treatments are consistent
- trial discontinuation reason consistent with a reported event (for example, an SAE).

8.5.3   Validation programs/routines and release

Depending on the systems being used, some edit checks in the validation specification can be set up within the database build, but others may need specific programs/routines to be written. Any programming not included in the database build would need to be validated in its own right. This would need to be formally released prior to the first run on the real clinical data. Examples have been seen on inspection where 'draft' programming has been used on the real data, contrary to CSV principles. This would mean that there is no guarantee the validation is functioning correctly, which may result in unnecessary queries and/or missed data issues that have to be addressed once the finalised programs are run. Testing the programming of the validation checks would follow the validation principles in section 14.5.

Common issues on inspection include a lack of documentation on how the validation of the edit check programming was carried out and of a change control process for amendments to the validation programming (that would correlate with changes to the specification; also uncontrolled). It is also possible for previously validated standard routines to be used, which saves resources. During testing it is recommended that dummy data are entered in order to challenge the system and ensure an edit check 'fires' (detects an inconsistency) and produces an output for assessment as a potential data query when the appropriate criteria have been met. The simple example in Figure 8.3 illustrates the principle.

The example illustrates checks of logic, chronology and missing data; in reality the laboratory data would likely be an electronic data transfer, so a type of cross-forms check and a range check would be undertaken. It is clear that a number of combinations would need to be programmed in this example to detect all the potential problems with the data. Generally, validation is assisted with good CRF design (in this case, the simple addition of DD/MM/YY above the date boxes could help prevent data errors).

There is a benefit of targeting the validation to the data of primary importance to the trial results identified in the trial risk assessment, as this could save a substantial amount of programming and testing. This would be realised by ensuring a review of the specification is undertaken to eliminate any unnecessary validation. Additionally, it can be seen that, in small datasets, manual validation of a data listing or the CRF could easily pick up many inconsistencies.

It is important to note that the data validation is only as good as the systems used to detect the inconsistencies, and it is advised that sufficient time is devoted to

Case report form

1. Blood sample taken:	☐☐/☐☐/☐☐ Date	☐☐:☐☐ Time
2. Blood results received:	☐☐/☐☐/☐☐ Date	☐☐:☐☐ Time
3. Results:	Cholesterol	☐.☐ mmol/L

Edit check test data	Edit check fires
Cholesterol value missing; date and time present for 1 and/or 2	Yes
Cholesterol value present; date and time missing for 1 and/or 2	Yes
Date and time present for 1 and 2; cholesterol value out of specified range	Yes
Date and time of 2 previous to the date and time of 1	Yes

Figure 8.3 Data validation example

developing the scripts to ensure they test all the requirements defined in the validation specification to avoid extensive work at a later point.

8.5.4 Data validation process

The first type of validation process consists of on-entry validation, where data are checked contemporaneously as they are entered, either into an eCRF by the investigator team or into the database by data management staff. This is a useful way to prevent errors, in particular with the eCRF. With on-entry systems, consideration needs to be given to whether the system will either not allow invalid data to be entered at all or allow it to be entered and attach a 'flag' or alert to the observation so that it can be detected in the query management process for attention. A similar alert is useful to have in place for double data entry when it is unclear exactly what the real value should be. Contemporaneous validation may also run quite complex validation checks on entry of a variable value, negating the need for batch validation.

The second type of validation is batch validation, where the edit check programs are applied to large quantities of data in a 'validation run' and all the edit check 'fires' are output for assessment and action. The validation runs are undertaken repeatedly as more data are entered into the system. Also, the rectification of one query may result in another one being generated.

If data validation generates output, there should be a process to assess it and decide whether a data query needs to be raised, and whether it is a self-evident correction or a validation edit check error. Sponsors should ensure that where there may be several members of staff undertaking this task on the same trial there is a process to ensure consistency.

Finally, there is usually some validation that by choice is undertaken manually. This might be the entire trial, if it is small simple dataset, or it can be specific checks that are difficult to program. These would usually involve producing data listings for review. Any listings that are annotated must[5] be retained as a record of the validation check.

For all methods the validation process can become quite extensive as it essentially involves keeping track of many issues within the database and their status (for example, queries, resolved, error, disregard). While some data management systems will have a process within the system to track all the issues, simpler systems may require specific and separate tracking to be set up, either paper based or via spreadsheets. The tracking system needs to be robust and is essential in order to reach a conclusion that the database is sufficiently clean. Inspections have seen data management systems and databases that have essentially become out of control, such that it was not possible to see what had been checked when, what issues had been detected and how they had been addressed, in particular what data queries had been raised and what were outstanding, essentially rendering the database unreliable.

8.5.5   Non-CRF data validation

While much of the validation is focused on the CRF data and subsequent queries with the investigator site, the electronic data that have been provided from vendors also need to be validated. These data often take the form of observations at various time points for a specific measurement for each subject or could be the data from IRT regarding allocation of treatment kits. It is necessary to validate these data against the related data in the CRF (effectively a cross-forms check); for example, that the dates of blood sampling in the CRF correspond to samples analysed in the laboratory data, or the dates of dispensing IMP kits in the CRF corresponded to allocations in the IRT data. Internal consistency validation is also necessary. Details of the proposed validation checks involving non-CRF data will be included in the validation specification along with the method for amalgamating the non-CRF data with the CRF data, and the validation applied to this process.

The validation may highlight the need to raise a query with the investigator site (as described in section 8.5.10) and/or the vendor. There should be a documented, robust, controlled and clear process for this. Unfortunately, GCP inspections have shown that this is not always the case. For example, situations have been seen where no formal process was in place and all that was available was a series of emails with replacement datasets supplied by the vendor. It was impossible to reconstruct the process and follow an audit trail from data issue detection to data validation activities and the resolution of the issues by the vendor. In one inspection there was no validation of the data at all, nor any evidence of the interaction to clean the data, so it was not clear whether these data were in fact appropriately clean.

8.5.6   Self-evident corrections

Sometimes the sponsor may have a 'self-evident corrections' or 'assumptions' document. This lists changes that can be made to the data by data management personnel without specific referral to the investigator with a data query. An example would be the correction of the common error that occurs in early January when dates are written using the previous year. Such an agreement can reduce the effort to correct obvious mistakes and therefore the time that both data management and the investigators spend on data corrections. This document should be approved by the investigator prior to the data management activities taking place. Any changes to the document should be approved by the investigator prior to implementation.

At the end of the trial, the investigator should be provided with details of the actual changes made using the process, which is often not done. It would therefore be clear in the database which data edits had been made as a result of self-evident corrections. The use of self-evident corrections is expected to be limited and is certainly not a substitute for a formal data query process, particularly when under time pressure.

8.5.7   CRF data query process

Any change or correction to the data in a pCRF should be initialled, dated and explained (if necessary) and should not obscure the original entry. If the changes are in an eCRF system an electronic audit trail should be maintained. In both cases the change should be authorised by the investigator or delegated team member. Sponsors should have written procedures in place to ensure that changes or corrections to CRFs made by the sponsor's designated representatives are documented, necessary and endorsed by the investigator.

In data management, data queries are usually generated from the following sources:

- inability to read information on the pCRF at data entry
- data validation (on-entry validation when a value cannot be entered or data are inconsistent or contrary to agreed data handling guidelines, or from output of validation runs or manual checks on listings/CRFs)
- data reconciliation (for example, with the pharmacovigilance database)
- QC of the database
- the statistical analysis, although this should be rare, as data validation should have been effective and dry runs of the analysis programs undertaken.

Data queries are normally documented on a data clarification form (DCF) and these are authorised by the investigator. For paper DCFs the original is signed and returned to data management and a copy remains with the CRF copies at site. Where NCR pCRFs are used there should not be any amendments to the pCRF copies at site, but this has been a finding on some GCP inspections. This can lead to issues such as the research nurse making changes to the severity assessment of adverse events after the investigator has signed off the top copy of the pCRF, with no corresponding DCF.

In the situation where the original pCRFs remain at the investigator site (having been faxed to data management, with the originals remaining at the investigator site), changes can be made to the original pCRF rather than the DCF, and the page re-faxed. The systems of data query resolution should be in a formalised procedure. Queries in eCRFs are resolved within the eCRF system and the audit trail should show that these were made by an authorised person.

Some systems will produce the DCFs (paper or electronic) directly and contain an ability to make text edits to automated queries. If this occurs it may mean a change control initiation to amend the system. It is common practice to add any manual queries to the automated queries and to send the whole package to site. It is acceptable for the trial monitor to facilitate resolution of the query, but it is not acceptable for the monitor to write in the CRF or authorise the DCF.

If data queries are routed to the site and back via the trial monitor, the monitor will know whether the DCF has been changed by unauthorised personnel because they have access to the delegation log. In situations where the DCF is routed directly to the site and back by data management, without access to the signatures and initials of the investigators at each site (or previous knowledge of them by DCFs handled by the trial monitor), it is impossible for data management to check that only authorised personnel have endorsed the changes in the CRF. This has been a finding on several inspections and can be avoided by data management personnel holding a copy of the site delegation and signature log, when appropriate, or only using the trial monitor conduit for query resolution.

Once the DCF is returned to data management there should be an amendment to the database if this is required by the DCF. The audit trail of the database should confirm when changes were made and by whom, and there should be records of receipt of the DCF (as with the original CRF) to complete the trail fully. A list of who is authorised to make changes to the data will need to be maintained. In most cases, with pCRFs, the edit is not done as double data entry (even if the original data entry was); it is, however, recommended that database edits are subject to QC – for example, specifically sampled as part of the quality assessment of the whole database.

8.5.8 Reconciliation of pharmacovigilance and clinical trial databases

A sponsor may hold both the pharmacovigilance and clinical trial database in-house, or one or both of the databases may be maintained by the same or separate service providers. The process of regular reconciliation between the pharmacovigilance and clinical database should be clearly defined in an agreement (this may require a tripartite agreement in some circumstances or in a written procedure for in-house databases), and can detail the responsibility of each party, the process of reconciliation, appropriate periodicity and type of reconciliation and the audit trail of data changes. In some short-duration trials that generate few SAEs it may be acceptable to perform reconciliation at the end of the trial only. For long-term trials, however, reconciliation would need to be undertaken during the trial; for example, it would be appropriate to ensure it was undertaken as part of the preparation for production of the development safety update report. It should also be clear which party has responsibility for overseeing the reconciliation. Even within the same organisation it has been seen on inspections that the data management and pharmacovigilance departments both believed it was the other party's responsibility.

The reconciliation process should be documented in a formal procedure, which should clarify which data points will be reconciled (if less than 100%) and how. Any omissions noted in either of the databases need to be addressed and the data updated accordingly. This may necessitate a DCF being generated for the investigator to action, for instance where the definition and detail of adverse events are inconsistent (for example, the symptom is reported in the clinical database but the diagnosis is in the pharmacovigilance database). Records of the database reconciliation process should be produced and must[5] be retained.

Two scenarios that may occur during the reconciliation of pharmacovigilance and clinical trial databases

An SAE is identified in the clinical database but is not in the pharmacovigilance database

Actions to take:

- The case should be assessed to determine whether it is required to be expedited. If it is reportable, day 0 should be the date when the CRF was first received by the sponsor (or a contractor acting on behalf of the sponsor). The case must[7] be reported to the competent authority and research ethics committee without further delay, and to concerned investigators as per the organisation's process.

- The normal timescale for SAE reporting by the investigator to the sponsor is immediate (that is, within 24 hours) unless specified otherwise in the protocol (see section 5.4.1).

- The root cause of the failure should be investigated and corrective and preventative actions taken.

An SAE is in the pharmacovigilance database but not in the clinical database

Actions to take:

- The case will need to be added to the adverse event log in the clinical database. A DCF should be raised with the investigator to rectify this.

- Investigate that the case has been appropriately assessed and expedited if required.

- The root cause of the failure to record the SAE in the CRF should be investigated and corrective and preventative actions taken.

8.5.9　Data coding

In large trials there is usually a need to apply standard coding to the verbatim terms that have been given by investigators in the free text fields, primarily within the adverse events and concomitant medication data. This is because there can be ambiguity in the adverse event descriptions given or brand names could be used for medicines. The coding facilitates the presentation and comparison of the safety data. Dictionaries are available that can be used to apply coding to the clinical trial data, for example WHO Adverse Reaction Terminology (WHO-ART) and MedDRA. There should be a process to decide how updates to the dictionary are handled in terms of applying the new dictionary to previously coded data.

The systems can be used automatically to assign codes when run on the appropriate data, but this is not usually 100% successful and some manual coding is usually required. It is recommended that there is the ability to demonstrate which terms have been applied using which of the two methods. It is recommended that there is a review by an appropriately trained person of any automatic coding, and where the dictionary terms are applied manually it is beneficial that this is undertaken or at least reviewed by a medically qualified doctor. It is also recommended that this medical review is documented and there is traceability of any actions taken as a result of the review. There has been at least one example where the sponsor's medical advisor did not like the term that MedDRA applied, as it sounded too serious, and a data query was raised to the investigator to change their description in the free text field so that it was then coded as a more favourable term. Additionally, an example was seen where the coding was not applied consistently, so that a significant safety signal was not identified. Coding should be completed as part of the database cleaning and prior to locking of the database.

8.5.10　Data quality

For pCRF trials it is usual practice to examine the quality of the database as part of its final acceptance prior to database lock. An error rate often chosen by organisations is 0.05%, but this standard is not defined in any official guidance or clinical trial regulations. The quality assessment process should be documented in a formal procedure, the DMP or a specific QC plan. Following the assessment of quality, a formal report or statement is often issued. The quality check is essentially a check of a proportion of the data in the database against the pCRF. The proportion of data to check is usually predefined and is not necessarily a random sample of CRFs – sponsors are recommended to apply a risk-proportionate approach to the level of QC performed, based on the complexity and risk of a trial on a case-by-case basis. A decision may be made, based on the trial risk assessment, that it is highly important that particular aspects of the trial data are accurate in order to ensure the reliability of the trial results. As an example, 100% of the data related to the primary objectives of the trial may be checked whereas other data, predefined variables or pCRFs may be checked at lower, varying percentage levels. It is good practice that where less than 100% checks are being done, the sample of the data is chosen by a genuinely random process.

QC activities must[4] be appropriately documented to ensure that errors and resolutions are traceable. It is often observed at inspection that sponsors do not define what should happen to QC documentation after the end of the trial. It is not possible to reconstruct the QC that has been carried out if the QC is not documented or the QC records are not retained. It is recommended that the QC plan also covers an escalation process for root cause analysis and additional checks where the error rate is not consistent with the sponsor's predefined level.

For eCRFs the quality of the data is influenced in two key ways: firstly, by the accuracy of the site staff completing the eCRF and whether there is QC of the source data against the eCRF, perhaps by SDV being undertaken during on-site monitoring visits or by QC processes being implemented by the site staff; and secondly, by the level of data validation that is taking place, in particular the on-entry validation in the eCRF. It would be difficult to determine an error rate in eCRF trials where no on-site monitoring is taking place and, where it is occurring, the SDV queries give an indication of the quality of the data being entered. It is recommended that the trial risk assessment identifies the key data that affect the reliability of the results and that appropriate mitigations have been taken to ensure that the appropriate level of quality of these data is assured. See section 4.7 for further details on the generation of a risk assessment.

8.6   Database/dataset lock

8.6.1   Principle of a final database/dataset

The aim of any data management process, no matter what size, is to provide a high-quality and appropriately clean final database/dataset suitable for statistical analysis, no matter what format the database/dataset takes (for example, Oracle,

MS Excel spreadsheet(s), ASCII file(s), SAS or SPSS® dataset(s)). There should be a process for controlling this, but most importantly it should be clear when the database/dataset is declared as final, what is checked in order to make the decision, how the final database is made available, where the final database is stored and how it is accessed and protected. This principle applies irrespective of the size and type of clinical trial. There have been many GCP inspection findings related to failures to adequately control this process and follow these expectations.

Although the end of the trial implies the final database, there may be other occasions when a clean database/dataset is required (all or part of it) – for example, at the time of an interim analysis or for data monitoring committee meetings. The same principles apply to interim databases/datasets as the final database, especially where this may be in relation to dose escalation decisions. It might also be appropriate, however, dependent upon the purpose of the analysis of the data, to provide 'un-cleaned' databases/datasets, often referred to as 'snapshots'. These are often used for the development activities (for example, programming tables/figures/listings) and blinded dry runs of the statistical analysis programs.

8.6.2 Completion of data cleaning/validation

The previous section has described processes concerned with cleaning or validation of the data in the database. When all these processes are completed, that is, all the data issues have been resolved, the data can be declared appropriately clean. Sometimes an organisation may decide not to resolve all the queries on specific data in large clinical trials (for example, minor secondary end-point data). The decision and rationale for the decision should be documented; however, this need should be avoided if the validation specification is thoroughly reviewed so that queries are not raised on data issues that have no impact on the reliability of the trial results. Again, this is linked to the risk assessment of the trial. In some cases, the data management system allows parts of the data to be declared clean, for example particular visits or trial subject's data, so that the final cleaning may concern just a handful of subjects or visits.

In some organisations there is a two-step process to finalising the database, although the terminology is not consistent across organisations. There is typically a provisional or 'soft' lock, where there is some further activity to be undertaken (for example, when all the known data issues have been resolved but there may be a requirement to finalise the statistical analysis plan or undertake the final QC of the database) and then a final or 'hard' lock when no further changes to the data can be made without further formal approval. It should be clearly documented how the provision of further data after database lock is to be handled. This may happen with PK data, for example, because its provision unblinds the trial. If validation is to be undertaken on the new data, this could require unlocking of the database to rectify a query.

Most organisations that are undertaking complex data management processes will use a form/checklist to confirm what activities have been completed; this approach is recommended. Examples of activities that may be included on the list are:

- All the data queries have been closed.
- Pharmacovigilance reconciliation has been completed.
- Coding and coding review have been completed.
- All electronic data have been received, uploaded and validated.
- Statistical analysis plan has been approved.

The form is then signed and dated and the activity (provisional/soft or final/hard) lock is undertaken. Problems seen on inspection relate to such systems being in place but not being followed, so that the form has not been used or is incomplete. One inspection revealed that the form, though used, was not retained as it was not considered by the sponsor to be an essential document, although this is clearly not the case (see Chapter 10 for further information on essential documents). Inspectors will review this form, where used, as part of establishing the sequential flow of events (see Figure 9.1). It is appropriate to have documented checks, akin to those of the final lock, of the interim lock of the data that are provided for interim analysis.

For a simple situation, perhaps involving a simple spreadsheet, a file note signed by the person responsible, together with the properties of the MS Excel file (for example, date/time stamped, file location), would be sufficient to confirm that the data are final. If it is a very small dataset then this could be printed and stored (either to paper or PDF). In such situations seen at non-commercial sponsors on inspection, there is often a failure to provide documentation to confirm what checks have been done on the data, by whom, when, and that the data are considered final.

8.6.3   Locking the final database/dataset

How the database is 'physically' locked is hugely dependent upon how large the data management function is, the systems being used and whether it is a one- or two-step process.

In a two-step process in a large organisation, at soft lock, edit rights to the database are taken away from the operational data management group and only a limited number of individuals retain the right to add, modify or delete data as required for the remaining activities. In the case of hard lock, edit rights should be removed from all personnel as no changes should be made to the database after this point. The list of people who have access to change the data should be amended to reflect the impact of locking the database.

Large data management databases may have functionality allowing them to be locked in terms of access rights to particular trial data within it. This could be controlled by a senior data manager or head of department, or by the IT department. It is recommended that the staff controlling the lock are independent from the operational staff.

Alternatively, the final database could consist of files in the general operating system of the organisation, for example SAS datasets (potentially extracted from a large relational database such as Oracle), or the database may be an MS Excel spreadsheet file. Locking these may mean resetting the protection rights of the file or the folder containing the files by someone independent of operations, such as the IT department. The files should be protected from editing and deleting. Usually, system-level access properties need to be changed rather than password-protecting the file by using the software in which it was created, although this level of protection may be justified in very small, open trials managed by an investigator. Essentially, the decision on the level of security of the final data would be made on a risk-based approach.

Whatever the situation, the lock procedure must[4] be appropriately robust to protect the final data and there should be documentation and an ability to demonstrate how and when the physical lock was done. There have been instances seen on inspection where the lock involved the removal of a handful of people with access to the database, leaving more than 50 people with full access. Often files are not fully protected either; in one inspection the final dataset files could be deleted.

8.6.4   Release of and access to the database/dataset

There should be a process for how the final data are provided for statistical analysis. This is typically done by the provision of datasets (for example, SAS), rather than direct access to a large relational database. The tool used to extract the datasets from the database should be validated. Often, test extractions are done for this purpose or for the development of the analysis programs (for example, blinded dry runs of the analysis programs).

Extractions from the database for final analysis should be undertaken after the database is locked and this should be clear from the properties of the files and the documentation surrounding the lock checks and physical lock. Where appropriate, it is recommended that the naming and control of the files makes it clear that it is the final dataset. On inspection, it has been found that the test extractions and the final data are all present in the final dataset file; it is recommended that any test data are removed prior to the final extraction. It has also been seen that not all the datasets have been extracted as some data are not yet ready for locking, but the documentation surrounding the lock does not clearly state the separation of the database into subsets. Finally, one inspection revealed that the extracted datasets used in the analysis and published in the CSR predated the finalisation of the database. In this case, pharmacovigilance reconciliation activities had not been completed and further changes to the database were made after the 'final' datasets had been extracted. This was a failure to appropriately follow the database locking procedures.

Some organisations copy the files that have been created by data management to another location, potentially losing some of the security aspects. It is recommended that this is not done and the statistical software reads the data directly from the files in the final dataset location. Often seen on inspections is that the data released by data management end up in a completely uncontrolled environment, negating all the controls that have been in place up until that point. All datasets used for interim analysis must[4, 5] be retained to provide an audit trail.

8.6.5   Unlocking the final database/dataset

Occasionally, it may be necessary to correct previously missed data errors or inconsistencies after the data have been released for analysis (whether the analysis has been carried out yet or not). There should therefore be a process in place to resolve this by unlocking the database, correcting the data and providing new extracted datasets after the query has been resolved. However, unlocking a final locked database or dataset should be limited to important corrections (that is, if the data to be changed will have a significant impact on the reliability of the results) and the CSR should include details of all changes made to the database while it is unlocked.

The risk of bias ranges from high in a blinded, comparative trial to low for an open, non-comparative, pilot trial. This risk assessment, together with whether there is truly a need to unlock in relation to the impact on the integrity of the trial results, is considered in the decision to unlock. For example, in a trial with hundreds of subjects included in the primary analysis set, an error in the primary variable for one subject is unlikely to have any important effect. However, if the trial has a cross-over design with only 24 subjects, one data point could make a difference. In some cases it is possible to unlock only part of the database, thereby ensuring that only a limited number of variables may be changed; this is to be encouraged.

The expectation is that a higher level of authorisation is required to unlock the database, to ensure that this only occurs under extraordinary conditions, and should be undertaken in consultation with the statistician. Extensive unlocking that is being undertaken for issues that should have been resolved prior to database lock may indicate a quality issue with the data management process. There is also the potential for bias if, for example, the investigator is asked to change adverse event data (after the data have been unblinded).

The justification for requesting the unlock, the written approval and the effect on the statistical outcome should be documented and must[5] be filed in the TMF prior to unlocking. If a database is unlocked, only the agreed changes should be made. Only those individuals required to implement the required changes should be granted access to the database again. The database should be re-locked as soon as reasonably appropriate to prevent other data changes being made. A check of the audit trail should be made at the point of re-locking to show all that was changed. When re-locked, the new final database should not overwrite any analysis datasets that were created at the original database lock. Inspectors and assessors view with concern trials that have been subject to repeated locking and unlocking because this will have a serious impact on the integrity of the trial.

8.7   Chapter legislative references

Throughout this chapter, specific terminology – 'must', 'required' or 'requirement' – has been used to interpret activities that are legislative requirements. These terms have been number-coded in the text where used, and the corresponding reference in the legislation can be found below.

1. Schedule 1, Part 2 (2) of SI 2004/1031
2. Regulation 3 (12) of SI 2004/1031
3. Schedule 1, Part 2 (11) of SI 2004/1031
4. Schedule 1, Part 2 (9) of SI 2004/1031
5. Regulation 31A (4) of SI 2004/1031
6. Schedule 1, Part 2 (13) of SI 2004/1031
7. Regulation 32 of SI 2004/1031

CHAPTER 9

Statistics

Editor's note

Clinical trials are scientific experiments, with the experimental unit, the human subjects, being affected by between-subject biological variability. As such, it is essential that the design of the trial (experiment) and analysis of the resultant data are scientifically sound, so that the appropriate design and pre-specified statistical methodology are used to ensure that the results are meaningful, free from bias and answer the research question. Statistics is therefore a fundamental component of clinical trials.

Good Clinical Practice (GCP) impacts on statistics in terms of the processes being followed, rather than on technical or methodological aspects. The application of statistical concepts and methodology is instead addressed by peer review, and may be reviewed by research ethics committees and, for trials that are part of a marketing authorisation application, by statistical assessors.

Many of the familiar requirements for quality systems, such as documentation, quality control (QC) and computer system validation (CSV), impact on the area of statistics. These and other aspects specific to GCP are discussed in this chapter.

9.1   Statistical processes, procedures and records

A suitable quality system should be implemented for conducting clinical trials and this extends to statistical processes (see Chapter 14 for further information on quality systems). This is of particular importance where multiple trials and numerous members of staff are involved, as it ensures consistency of the process. In single trials, the protocol, provided it is sufficiently detailed, may suffice without the need for many written procedures to be produced, or the written procedures could be trial-specific. Where written procedures have been produced these must[1] be followed. As a result of compliance with written procedures many records may be generated, and these must[2] be retained where they meet the definition of essential documents. The legislation requires[2] that these records are retained in the trial master file (TMF) as these are documents which enable the conduct of the trial and the quality of the data to be evaluated. Although statistics records, particularly electronic ones, are often not regarded as being part of the TMF, all the processes used in statistics may be subject to inspection and there should be adequate documentation for inspectors to verify that data have been accurately handled and reported in accordance with GCP principles which state that *'All clinical information shall be recorded, handled and stored in such a way that it can be accurately reported, interpreted and verified, while the confidentiality of records of the trial subjects remain respected'* (Part 2 (9) of Schedule 1 to SI 2004/1031).

The statistical analysis process relies extensively on computer systems and therefore suitably documented processes and controls should be in place to enable security of data, in terms of access limitations and back-up.

9.2   Statistics personnel

Those advising on trial design and statistical methodology and analysing clinical trial data, who should be appointed by the sponsor, must[3] be able to demonstrate relevant statistical qualifications and experience. Additionally, they must[3] have received relevant GCP training and should have awareness of and/or training in relevant guidance (for example, ICH Topic E9 – 'Statistical principles for clinical trials'), and any specific therapeutic area trial design guidance and specific guidance on, for example, including missing data, choice of non-inferiority margin, switching between superiority and non-inferiority, small populations and adjustment with baseline covariates. Finally, where an organisation has formal procedures, there must[3] be documented training in those that are relevant to the statistical role.

9.3   Trial and protocol design

Trained statisticians should have extensive knowledge of different experimental design techniques. They should also be aware of new and evolving statistical methodology and designs used in clinical trials. The sponsor should ensure that there is an appropriate level of statistical input into the trial. It is usual practice for a qualified and experienced statistician to be involved in designing the clinical trial, and the more complex the trial, the greater this requirement would be. A small trial using simple summary statistics and significance tests may not require a qualified statistician as, for example, the chief investigator in a non-commercial sponsored trial may themselves have sufficient knowledge and experience. It is highly recommended that a qualified statistician is consulted as early as possible in the trial design process – that is, before protocol development. This has been a weakness of many trials in the past. Examples have even been seen where in a non-commercial sponsored trial the chief investigator's first contact with the statistician was with the final trial dataset.

Statisticians can advise on formulating the trial objectives, suitability of the end-point(s) and their measurement, potential sources of bias, sample size, randomisation and blinding and the methods of analysis (including use of interim analysis) as required to be included in the protocol. Statistical input to the trial can also be invaluable to advise on the appropriateness of the design (for example, sequential, adaptive, crossover and other within-subject or parallel group designs). The statistician can also advise on the hypotheses within the trial; for example, the trial may be powered to answer the question asked in the primary objective. However, the secondary objectives may all be exploratory as the trial may not be powered to meet the secondary objective. There may also be a statistical reason for stopping the trial early after an interim analysis (for example, superiority, inferiority, futility), which should be included in the protocol.

The statistical assessors at the MHRA can be involved in discussions of clinical development programmes including giving advice on particular trial designs prior to submission of the clinical trial authorisation (CTA) application. The assessors review and provide a statistical assessment on pivotal trials contained in the application for a marketing authorisation application or variation. However, it should be noted that not all marketing authorisation applications are reviewed by a statistical assessor, and a statistical assessor does not review the clinical trial authorisation application.

Statistical input into the trial design and protocol development is recommended; evidence and/or procedures should be in place to accomplish this. Therefore, the role of the statistician in designing the trial and writing sections of the protocol will be examined during GCP inspections at the sponsor site. It is recommended that, where the statistician is not editing the protocol directly, the statistical input to the protocol (that is, the statistician may supply a 'statistical considerations document'), is version-controlled with the ability to link it to the version of the protocol upon which it is based. The statistical aspects of the trial design and analyses contained in the protocol are required,[4] by legislation, to be followed and thus the statistician should be familiar with the final protocol. It is recommended that they approve and sign the protocol. It is also advised that a second check of the statistical section of the trial protocol is performed; for example, to ensure that the calculation of the sample size was correct. Where the sponsor has the resources available to do this (that is, access to a second statistician) this should be undertaken and must[2] be documented.

In general, including a statistician in a trial team is to be recommended and will almost always add value to the design and analysis of the trial. In some very simple studies, such as early pilot studies, little statistical input may be required where only descriptive statistics are used to report the findings. In such cases the sponsor's risk assessment may consider that the statistical methods are well established and straightforward and the use of a qualified statistician is not required. For trials undertaken to support marketing authorisation applications, or large non-commercial trials where their publication may change prescribing practice or the standard of care, an appropriately qualified and experienced statistician should take responsibility for the statistical methods.

When protocol amendments are proposed these should be reviewed by a statistician (or investigator, as appropriate, depending on the complexity of the trial) to assess the impact on the design and analysis of the trial, as this may also require an update to the statistical analysis plan. A process should be in place to ensure that this occurs.

9.4 Statistical input to case report form design and data management activities

The person analysing the data, who is usually a statistician and is referred to as such in this section, but may well be another person – for example, the investigator in the situations as outlined above – will have an obvious interest in the data collection for the trial. The data type (for example, continuous, categorical scales or alphanumeric) may be discussed with and be agreed by the statistician as this will have a great effect on the statistical methods chosen. The number and scale of measurement of the variables will also have an impact on the statistical technique used for the trial. Additionally, the analysis may require baselines and adjustments for covariates and, where more complex analysis is planned, the statistician can ensure that the appropriate data are collected. A statistician who is part of the trial team can also take part responsibility (together with data management personnel) for ensuring that the data captured are consistent with the trial protocol. The case report form (CRF) should be reviewed and formally approved by the trial statistician (when considered appropriate by the sponsor), primarily because this tool is the basis of obtaining the dataset for analysis (see section 8.1). There should be procedures for and evidence of this review.

As part of the data management processes, an annotated CRF is often produced. This would usually be made available to the statistician as this document becomes the specification for the database and thus defines the type and format of data that the statistician will eventually be analysing (see section 8.3.1).

The statistician may be involved in data validation and should at the very least review the validation specification (see section 8.5). The statistician will be able to assist the data manager in deciding which data are of primary importance to be 'clean' and which validations could be omitted. This approach is particularly important in applying the MRC/DH/MHRA paper 'Risk-adapted approaches to the management of clinical trials of investigational medicinal products' to trials as it involves assessing which data present vulnerabilities to the trial in terms of the risk of obtaining inaccurate results. Additionally, the trial may be subject to central monitoring and the statistician would then have a role to play in specifying which analyses are to be conducted, conducting these analyses and reviewing numerous reports on the data to identify outlying data (for example, centres with very low or very high serious adverse event (SAE) reporting) and other metrics used to trigger on-site monitoring visits. With increasing use of electronic data capture (EDC) and central monitoring techniques, statisticians may have an increasing involvement in statistical monitoring of trials. Statisticians should provide considerable input into data validation and central monitoring plans.

For further details on monitoring and data management activities, refer to Chapter 7 and Chapter 8 respectively.

9.5 Randomisation and blinding

Randomisation is a key feature of many clinical trials. It can be a very simple process or more complex algorithms may be used (for example, complex stratification techniques).

9.5.1 Randomisation specification

The protocol should describe the method of randomisation and any stratification factors. It is recommended that a 'randomisation specification' is developed that contains the key features of the randomisation (for example, treatments, stratification factors and number of sites to allow the randomisation schedule to be produced). A specification may not be required if the protocol contains sufficient information and the trial has a straightforward design.

9.5.2 Randomisation methodology

The methods of preparing the randomisation schedule (or randomisation list) can be quite varied; these include the use of random number tables, online randomisation programs and bespoke programs/macros (for example, in SAS). For the latter situation and for complex algorithms, where computer programs are used, there should be some method of QC or validation of the program (see section 14.5). Documentation to demonstrate this must[2] be retained. The method of generating the randomisation schedule should be clearly documented and should include who was responsible for its generation and who had access to the schedule before database lock.

The randomisation schedule should be version-controlled so that it is clear which is the final version. Many examples have been seen on inspection where a piece of paper found in a pharmacy file, containing only treatments and subject numbers, serves as the randomisation list, but it is not clear from the document who produced it, when it was produced, what trial it was applicable to and whether it was the official final version.

Methods of randomisation that cannot be verified at a later date and reconstructed must[5] be avoided. Therefore, for schedules produced using software based on a random number generator the seed used for the randomisation should be documented, but stored securely. The same principle applies if a simpler method is used. For example, in a non-commercial trial that was inspected, the trial was randomised by individual treatment paper slips being placed in an envelope and then all the envelopes being shuffled. Each envelope was then numbered sequentially with the subject number. In this case, there was no way of checking, after the trial had been completed, that a pre-specified randomisation had been followed (not least because the paper slips and envelopes had been discarded). In this trial, there was also unequal allocation of subjects (there should have been a 1:1 allocation when all subjects had been recruited) and it was not possible to determine why this had occurred.

Where an interactive response technologies (IRT) system is used (Annex 4), a statistician should be involved in any specification and programming of the system to undertake complex randomisation (for example, with multiple stratification). This would not be needed if the statistician was just providing a randomisation schedule (that the system uses as a 'look-up' table).

9.5.3 Distribution and storage of the randomisation schedule and maintenance of the blinding

The randomisation schedule may consist of a paper record only, or in many cases, also an electronic version. The latter may simply be a representation of the paper version, but more usefully could be a data file. Additionally, the schedule may be used, for blinded trials, to generate physical code-break methods (for example, envelopes containing a treatment slip or scratch cards) and will probably be used to prepare documentation for assembling trial medication. There should be adequate control of all electronic versions of the randomisation schedule, both as it appears on the computer system and on the document, if printed. It should also be apparent which version is the final one.

The randomisation schedule can be used for numerous purposes; therefore its recipients can vary. It is recommended that the distribution requirements are documented on the specification. Recipients could include pharmacovigilance, pharmacy, IRT providers, clinical trial supplies departments, laboratories and Phase I units. There has been a serious breach reported to the MHRA where the randomisation schedule used to prepare the code breaks was different from that used to prepare and label the investigational medicinal products (IMPs) as a result of a failure to appropriately control the final randomisation schedule. This issue could have impacted on subject safety as, in the event of an emergency, a subject could have been unblinded using the code breaks; however, this might not have reflected the actual treatment received by the subject and they might have received inappropriate medical care.

The sponsor should implement procedures to control the randomisation schedule, or documents containing treatment information, to prevent accidental or deliberate unblinding. This must[1, 4] be strictly enforced for blinded protocols. It is advised that the procedures include consideration of documented access restrictions for electronic schedules, so it is clear who had access, and when, to the code throughout the conduct of the trial. Tamper-proof procedures should also be considered for when paper or electronic codes are moved to mobile media (computer disk, memory stick/card) and then stored in an envelope in a safe. As part of an inspection for a marketing authorisation application, inspectors have been asked by the assessors to specifically investigate who had access to the randomisation schedule and when.

Many examples have been seen on inspection where, in trials designed to be double-blind, access to the randomisation schedule or ability to break the code was easily undertaken by the trial team, as in the following examples:

* The randomised treatment cards were contained in envelopes, but once the cards were removed, they were stapled into the subject notes so that the investigator, and anyone else, was able to view them.
* The randomisation schedule was created by the investigator and retained on their computer.
* The randomisation schedule was in the investigator site file.
* The font of the active treatment on the paper slip in the envelope was such that it could be seen through the envelope when it was held up to a light source.
* Treatment codes were sent from the IRT system to blinded trial managers.

In addition to controlling the code itself, the statistician can provide input to assessing the robustness of the IMP blinding process in a trial. For example, labelling the IMP as 'A' and 'B' is not robust, as an emergency unblinding of one subject unblinds the entire trial. Also, knowledge of two or more subjects being on the same treatment, even if the treatment is not known, compromises the blinding. See section 6.6.1 for considerations for blinding trials.

In cases where data monitoring committees require interim unblinded analysis reports, there should be robust procedures in place to protect the trial team from gaining access to unblinded data or the randomisation schedule. It is recommended, therefore, that all interim unblinded analysis reports are produced by a separate team of statisticians and programmers from those who undertake the final analysis.

9.5.4   Unblinding the trial for analysis purposes

Although there should be a robust process in place for emergency unblinding of an individual subject (see sections 6.6 and 11.4.9), there should also be a formal process to control the unblinding of the trial for analysis purposes and this should be recorded. There should be documentation available to confirm when the randomisation code was requested or provided and when the randomisation data were applied to the analysis datasets or database at final analysis (and controls in place for any interim analyses). It is recommended that this information includes the time as well as the date. To ensure that there is an accurate record of the time the documentation was produced, and that sequential reconstruction can take place, caution is advised particularly where emails are used and staff are located in different time zones.

9.6   Statistical analysis plan

There should always be pre-specified statistical methodology documented for a trial, either directly in the protocol or in a separate document such as the statistical analysis plan (SAP). This document may not be required where the trial protocol contains all the necessary information on the analysis, including important details such as adjusting for multiple testing and handling missing data, as required. Commercial organisations often prepare lengthy SAPs that also include templates for tables, figures and data listings, thus clearly demonstrating the output of the statistical methodology. This can be a useful process and it is recommended that the SAP is reviewed by those responsible for preparing the clinical study report (CSR) to ensure that the tabulations, figures and listings provided are suitable. It is recommended that sufficient time is spent on this as it can reduce the number of manually created tables in the CSR that require extensive QC against the statistical output used to create them; that is, it is beneficial to have many of the required tables and figures created directly by the analysis software.

The SAP should be based on the trial protocol statistical considerations section. The SAP is usually produced during the conduct of the trial and may go through several versions. For blinded trials, additions and changes to details of the statistical methodology in the SAP are often made based on the results of blinded interim data review. For open-label trials, full details of the statistical methods for the analysis of the trial data, in particular for the primary end-point(s), should be included in the protocol. Changes to the pre-specified analysis for open-label trials once the trial has commenced should be avoided to prevent potential accusations of bias because of availability of the unblinded data.

The SAP should be finalised following review by appropriate personnel and approved by the statistician; the final version should be in place prior to the release of the randomisation code for blinded trials. The SAP should also be finalised prior to any interim analysis for blinded trials. This should be clear within the organisation's written procedures. Most organisations would stipulate that the SAP should be finalised prior to database lock. The SAP should be version-controlled during its production and it should be clear which version is the final one. Usually only the final version is included in the CSR.

Changes to the SAP should be appropriately controlled. As it is a legal requirement[4] to comply with the trial protocol, the SAP should be consistent with the protocol and any analyses in the SAP that are not supported by the protocol should lead to an assessment by the sponsor of whether a protocol amendment is required. For example, changing the primary end-point(s) of the trial or the definitions to the analysis population datasets would be considered substantial amendments to the protocol (if an end-of-trial notification has not been submitted) and would need clear and complete justification. If these changes are in relation to a marketing authorisation application, this may result in an inspection being performed. For example, an inspection was requested by the Committee for Medicinal Products for Human Use (CHMP) on behalf of the European Medicines Agency (EMA) for a marketing authorisation application that contained two identically designed trials, but the primary end-point of the second trial was subsequently changed to give a more favourable outcome once the first trial had been analysed and the results had been found to be not statistically significant.

The SAP (and the analysis specified in the protocol for open-label trials) should be followed and any changes to the planned analysis (post-unblinding for blinded trials) should be fully justified and communicated in the report of the results of the trial. This is particularly important if the change is not consistent with the protocol. Any such changes to the SAP following the unblinding of a trial should result in a formal amendment of the SAP.

9.7 Statistical programming and analysis

9.7.1 Protocol compliance and analysis datasets

The SAP or the protocol will normally include the definition of datasets for analysis, usually a safety population, an intention to treat (ITT) population (or full analysis set) and a per-protocol population. The ITT and safety populations usually have a very straightforward assessment of whether a subject should be included. However, defining whether a trial subject will be included in the per-protocol population will require an assessment of the protocol non-compliance for a particular subject against pre-specified criteria. In certain situations criteria may be pre-specified to identify subjects who should be excluded from the population only for analysis of certain variables or even analysis of certain variables at particular times. Therefore, it is usual that exclusion from the per-protocol population will result from major non-compliances with the protocol that are usually pre-specified in the SAP, if not already included in the protocol. For example, if a visit for a given subject is outside a particular time window this may not be considered sufficient to exclude a subject; while use of a concomitant medication which could affect the primary end-point would result in exclusion from the per-protocol population. However, all protocol non-compliances should be identified and reported so that the statistician can decide whether these have introduced any imbalance between treatments, which could have an effect on the outcome of the trial.

In order for this to occur, the sponsor should ensure that all non-compliances from the protocol are fully documented and collated before the trial is unblinded. Non-compliance could be documented in monitoring visit reports, telephone calls, emails, file notes and comments in the CRF; therefore all these documents can be reviewed in this context. There should be a process for collating all non-compliances so that this is available for evaluation for per-protocol population decisions and for assessment of the impact of the analysis (see section 1.3.5). This could be achieved by ensuring that the database captures protocol non-compliances. It is often seen on inspection that the process for capturing and collating this information is poor, such that not all non-compliances are identified and/or access to this information is not provided to the statistician.

For analysis population decisions, the criteria for inclusion/exclusion from the per-protocol population is usually defined and documented in the SAP, if it is not already included in the protocol. The data can then be evaluated against these criteria, often by using a suitable data validation program applied to the data to identify or flag those subjects that fail to meet each criterion. This review and decision process should be documented so that it is clear when it occurred, as it should be undertaken prior to any efficacy analysis. For blinded trials, it is recommended that it can be demonstrated that this process was undertaken prior to unblinding of the data. For open-label studies it is extremely important that analysis datasets are predefined in the protocol before access to any data. The lack of a formal process to adequately document these decisions and when they are taken has been seen in several organisations during inspections.

As the CSR or publication reflects the conduct of the trial and provides the summary of the results, it is important that it contains a listing of all the significant non-compliances that occurred during the trial and how these contributed to the analysis. Section 4.7.6 provides further details on CSR production.

9.7.2   Availability of final data

As described in Chapter 8, provision of the 'final data for analysis' should follow a formal database lock process; this may just be a final checked spreadsheet for trials that only require simple analysis (for example, summary tabulations). It is advised that the formal provision of these data segregates data management from the analysis activities. In all situations it must[5] be apparent that the data are final and the files should be suitably protected from deletion or editing once transferred to statistics; for example, by not simply placing them on a shared drive where a number of people have the ability to edit the data, with no audit trail.

For many situations, there may be a requirement to write programs, or use those already written, to extract datasets from a database (for example, structured query language (SQL) or SAS programming to extract SAS datasets) or to enter data from a central laboratory (for example, use of the SAS program to read in data from an MS Excel file to form a SAS dataset). There may also be specialist web-based applications written to download data. All data from the various sources would usually be entered into the trial database at some stage. All such programming and applications should be tested and validated (see section 8.5.3). There should be a process in place to ensure that any data from test extractions undertaken (for example, the blinded data used to develop programs for analysis) are deleted prior to the final extraction following database lock.

9.7.3   Analysis datasets and statistical programming

The statistical analysis usually requires analysis datasets to be created by merging or transposing data and creating derived variables. This process and the statistical analysis itself may be undertaken by menu-driven options in the software, using previously created programs/macros/systems, or by writing new code in the statistical software. Where programming is undertaken, there is an ability to change variable values by 'hard coding'. Such programming, whereby a variable's value (data point) in the dataset is changed directly (for example, using an 'if–then' function), is not acceptable and formal controls should be in place to prevent or control this. It is recommended that programming be undertaken such that the process is controlled, with author version control applied to written routines; often organisations have 'good programming practice' guidelines. Where standard macros/programs have previously been developed, these should be validated and subject to change control and all bespoke programs should be tested for fitness for purpose (validation).

9.7.4   Interim analyses

Interim analysis may be planned in the protocol and is an essential requirement of some trial designs, for example sequential trials and dose escalation trials. The analyses form part of a formal review and may also be described in charters for trial data monitoring or trial steering committees. All unblinded interim reviews of the data should be pre-planned, specified in the trial protocol and, where it is a blinded trial, conducted by personnel who have no further involvement in the conduct of the trial or the final analysis. Ad hoc (unblinded) and unplanned reviews of any trial data, particularly where statistical testing of the data comparisons takes place, are not acceptable as they affect the statistical validity of the final analysis. This is because frequentist methodology would require an adjustment of the significance level of the test to account for previous analyses. However, in blinded trials, blinded reviews of trial data can be part of the data cleaning process and can be used for the development of the SAP. In addition, some changes to the trial may be possible based on blinded analysis (for example, the sample size may be adjusted based on a protocol pre-specified blinded calculation of variability based on data already collected).

Interim analyses must[4] be conducted at the intervals specified in the trial protocol. There have been examples seen on inspection where this has not occurred as required by the protocol, such that the analyses have been conducted at an incorrect time interval or with too few or too many subjects. One problem seen is where the interim analysis is planned on a time basis rather than a 'subjects recruited' basis and the trial recruitment is slower than anticipated, so a decision is made not to undertake the analysis due to insufficient subject numbers. The decision to cancel the interim analysis must[6] be documented as a protocol amendment. However, the importance of non-compliances from the protocol with regard to the timing and number of subjects depends on the reasons for the interim analysis and any stopping rules which have been described in the protocol. Therefore, the timing and the purpose of the interim analysis together with full details of stopping rules (for example, for futility, safety and efficacy) should be carefully described in the protocol to facilitate compliance. An interim analysis SAP may be prepared to expand the detail of the analysis (such as including templates).

9.7.5 Oversight by a qualified statistician

Programming activities may be undertaken by programmers rather than qualified statisticians. It is recommended that there is demonstrable oversight of the analysis by a statistician. The planned analysis may potentially need to be changed due to, among other factors, data distributions not being as expected (for example, non-parametric methods have to be used) or breaches of model assumptions. In this case, the statistician's oversight will ensure that the planned analyses remain statistically valid, otherwise the SAP will need to be adjusted before unblinding. There should be evidence of the statistician's checks of the analysis.

9.7.6 Detection of suspicious data

Both the data management and statistics functions are in a position to identify suspicious data that could be indicative of fraud. For example, they could identify that some subjects had been entered into a trial more than once, as although they were under different names, their dates of birth remained the same. This instance led to a serious breach report being submitted to the MHRA. There is a potential that, where central monitoring is being used, checks for unusual patterns of data are formally undertaken. It is recommended that there is a formal process of how such issues are escalated with a view to an investigation as to whether a serious breach of GCP or the trial protocol has occurred. In this respect, staff within data management and statistics functions must[3] be trained in any such procedures and be aware of this aspect of the legislation.

9.7.7 Audit trail

Within the statistical analysis process there must[5] be an audit trail to follow the data analysis, including the comparison of any created datasets and derived variables with the original data. There have been some inspections where this audit trail has been lacking and the computer system files for programs and outputs have been so poorly organised they were impossible to follow by anyone other than the person who undertook the work (and even they found it difficult).

The audit trail may be reviewed during inspections. For example, one marketing authorisation application contained two sets of data from clinical trials – one set with all clinical trial investigator sites included and another with one centre removed that had been found to be fraudulent. The assessor requested that the inspector confirm that the data removed were actually from that site and that the right data had been removed. By review of the audit trail and SAS programs and datasets, it was possible for the organisation to demonstrate this to the inspector. It was also possible to use the SAS output to verify the dataset against the in-text tables in the CSR.

An audit trail would mean that the output of the trial results contained in the CSR or publication was traceable to the statistical program output and datasets used. For example, a table of results including a t-test and 95% confidence interval should be able to be verified against information to show by whom, when and how this was undertaken. This should be available for review by an inspector, if requested. This is often achieved by printing on the CSR output the information pertaining to the computer program that generated the output, the dataset name and the run time and date of the program. The program and the output it created would then be on the system for an inspector to verify. Some organisations keep a spreadsheet or log of all the files and datasets and how these relate to the final output in the CSR. This is a useful document to have in place as it is often used by the inspected organisation to demonstrate the audit trail. Records and computer files must[2] be maintained to enable the inspector to verify the flow of data from the extracted datasets to any subsequent created variables or datasets used in the analysis.

It is recommended that where runs of the statistical analysis are undertaken and output generated this is retained such that it is not overwritten by subsequent runs; for example, vendors involved in statistical activity could keep archive folders containing all official output delivered to the sponsor which subsequent runs do not overwrite.

Where there are numerous individuals involved in programming or analysis, formal procedures should be in place to ensure consistency of organisation of the audit trail.

Documentation of processes should make it possible to reconstruct that the events occurred in appropriate sequential order: for example, for a blinded trial, that release of the randomisation code was done following the analysis populations' decisions, database lock, SAP finalisation and approval and that the running of the analysis programs was done following data extraction (Figure 9.1).

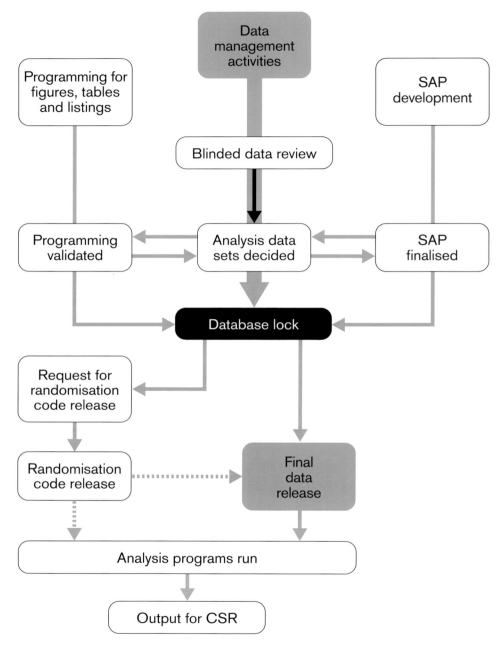

CSR, clinical study report; SAP, statistical analysis plan

Figure 9.1 Sequential flow of statistics activities around database lock for a blinded trial

9.7.8   Statistical output

The output of the statistical analyses can vary. For example, the statistician may provide documents to be used for a CSR or they may write directly into a CSR, or they may produce a formal statistical report as a separate document. The principle to follow is that all outputs of the statistical process are appropriately version-controlled. This would include documents containing just tables, figures and data listings for use in the CSR.

9.7.9   Quality control

It is essential to apply QC checks to the statistical analysis process to ensure that the output is accurate (the principles of QC are outlined in section 14.3). The sponsor is responsible for ensuring that this takes place and that it is applied at all stages of data handling.

It is acceptable for the QC checks to be undertaken on a risk-based approach, with the detail and level of checking varying depending on the item being checked. For example, output related to the primary objective of the trial, that is analysis of the primary end-point, should be subject to the highest-level checks for accuracy and these checks should be pre-specified. Inspections have found failure to document the QC and use of non-validated programs. The QC of the statistical analysis has been seen to be addressed using various methodologies including:

- independent analysis (dual programming and comparing output)
- detailed checks of output against raw data or data listings combined with review of code/programming (essentially computer system validation). It is expected that the programmers writing code will undertake checks to confirm that the program is functioning correctly
- use of previously validated code/macros
- checks and retention of any logs produced by the statistical software to ensure that code runs correctly
- checks on accuracy and quality of any new variables/datasets derived from final datasets provided at the end of the data management process
- review of any formulae in spreadsheets (where used for analysis)
- checks of any manual tabulations/in-text tables and values contained in the text of statistics reports or the CSR
- review to confirm that the SAP and/or protocol analysis has been followed.

It should be noted that spreadsheets and manual analyses are not acceptable to statistical assessors for trials to be submitted to support a marketing authorisation application; validated software with an ability to check the programming used to create the output is required.

'Any person who provides to the licensing authority or an ethics committee any relevant information which is false or misleading in a material particular shall be guilty of an offence' (Regulation 50 of SI 2004/1031). Therefore performing an appropriate level of QC checks is of particular importance when submitting the results of the trial. It is also important to note that, where statistical work has been undertaken by a vendor, the sponsor or applicant applying for marketing authorisation approval is responsible for the accuracy and quality of the output included in the CSR.

There should be a clear process and documentation of the QC process to demonstrate that it has been undertaken as planned.

9.8   Chapter legislative references

Throughout this chapter, specific terminology – 'must', 'required' or 'requirement' – has been used to interpret activities that are legislative requirements. These terms have been number-coded in the text where used, and the corresponding reference in the legislation can be found below.

1.   Schedule 1, Part 2 (4) of SI 2004/1031

2.   Regulation 31A (4) of SI 2004/1031

3.   Schedule 1, Part 2 (2) of SI 2004/1031

4.   Regulation 29 of SI 2004/1031

5.   Schedule 1, Part 2 (9) of SI 2004/1031

6.   Regulation 24 of SI 2004/1031

Trial master file and archiving

10

Editor's note

The conduct of a trial must be able to be reconstructed both during the trial and for some time after its completion from the documentation which is filed and retained within the trial master file (TMF). Maintenance of the correct and appropriate documentation in a manner suitable for managing the conduct of the trial and enabling evaluation by audit or inspection is essential for Good Clinical Practice (GCP) compliance.

This chapter covers the legislative requirements and gives recommendations on how effective TMF management can be implemented. The move to electronic records is also discussed as this provides new benefits and challenges.

10.1 Requirement for a trial master file

The planning, conduct and reporting of a clinical trial can generate extensive documentation, which includes internal documents generated by the organisation as a result of following its written procedures as well as documents produced to meet regulatory requirements. The documentation from a trial of an investigational medicinal product (IMP) must[1] be filed in the TMF. This requirement is set down in both Article 15 (5) of Directive 2001/20/EC and Regulation 31A of SI 2004/1031. A TMF is the collection of documentation that allows the conduct of the clinical trial, the integrity of the trial data and the compliance of the trial with GCP to be evaluated. Therefore, the documentation contained within it should be sufficient to adequately reconstruct the trial activities undertaken, along with key decisions made concerning the trial. Consideration must[1] be given to the TMF being a stand-alone set of documentation that does not require additional explanation from the associated sponsor or site staff. As such, the TMF forms the basis for an inspection to confirm compliance with regulatory requirements (Article 16 of Directive 2005/28/EC).

Guidance on the TMF can be found in ICH Topic E6 (R1) 'Guideline for Good Clinical Practice' (hereinafter 'ICH GCP') and EudraLex Volume 10 'Recommendation on the content of the trial master file and archiving' (hereinafter 'TMF guidance document'); however, the documentation referred to in the ICH guidance will form part of the TMF but will not necessarily form the entire TMF.

The documentation generated during the conduct of a trial can be quite extensive, and effective organisation within the TMF is essential, not only to facilitate inspection and audit by persons unfamiliar with the trial, but also for those involved in conducting the trial, as these persons will require regular access to the documentation to undertake their various tasks. The documentation in the TMF should be complete, legible, accurate, unambiguous and, where appropriate, signed and dated. Signatures on documents are recommended only where it adds value; many documents require wet-ink signatures as a result of internal written procedures, without clarity on what the signature is actually for. Some documents should be expected to be signed as part of GCP requirements (for example, the clinical trial protocol).

10.2 Trial master file organisation

10.2.1 Sponsor and investigator files

The TMF is normally composed of a sponsor file, held by the sponsor organisation, and an investigator site file, held by the investigator. These files together are regarded as comprising the entire TMF for the trial and should be established at the beginning of the trial. In organising the TMF, it is essential to segregate those documents that are generated or held by the sponsor of the trial from those of the investigator, as some documentation held by the investigator should not be provided to the sponsor. This requirement is firstly due to subject confidentiality issues (for example, the sponsor must[2, 3] not have documents such as consent forms and subject identification lists). Under certain circumstances subjects can specifically consent to this information being sent outside the investigator site, for example if required by the protocol or central monitoring procedures. Secondly, where the investigator site file contains source documents, the case report forms (CRFs) contain source data or the CRFs are the investigator's independent copy of the transcribed data, providing this to the sponsor would remove the investigator's control. This could lead to the sponsor making uncontrolled and unauthorised edits to the investigator's documentation.

The clear segregation referred to above would be expected in all situations apart from those where the sponsor and investigator are essentially the same. This can often occur for trials sponsored by NHS Trusts or universities, where the chief investigator is an employee of the sponsor. In these situations, the chief investigator is most likely to be acting as a clinical investigator in the trial and also, in many cases, has been formally delegated a number of sponsor functions from the NHS Trust R&D office. This means that documentation typically held by the sponsor will need to be accessed by the chief investigator. Examples have been seen on inspection where the R&D office of the sponsor maintained the sponsor file in the belief that this would be an expectation to comply with GCP. However, it resulted in extensive and needless copying. In such a scenario it is perfectly acceptable for the management of the TMF to be delegated to the chief investigator with the chief investigator maintaining all the necessary documentation. The sponsor must[4] still maintain an adequate level of oversight to ensure that the correct documentation is being maintained. (Chapter 1 provides details on how to maintain this oversight.) One example of such oversight would be the availability of guidance or written procedures within the organisation to assist the chief investigator in maintaining the files, together with monitoring and/or audit of the TMF and with the R&D office holding oversight documents such as risk assessments, governance or chief investigator questionnaire returns.

10.2.2 Sponsor trial master file levels

The organisation of a sponsor file can become quite complex, especially when the trial is multinational or multi-centre. Typically documentation is organised in the sponsor file at three levels, as illustrated in Figure 10.1. This approach is recommended as it allows particular sections of the TMF to be made available upon request, although amalgamation of the files may be a more suitable approach if, for example, a single-country trial is being performed (with combination of global and country-level files) or when running a single-site trial, where all three levels can be combined.

10.2.3 Identification of the location of trial master file documentation

The sponsor organisation should identify where all of the potential documentation that should be filed in the TMF is located, as the TMF must[5] at all times retain the

Global/trial-level files

These would contain documents that are relevant to the conduct of the trial at any site (for example, the investigator's brochure). (Note: The protocol would ideally be such a document, but may, due to country-specific requirements or requested changes, be a country-specific document)

Country-level files

These would contain the country-specific documentation that is relevant to the conduct of the trial at any site in that county – for example, the approval from the country's competent authority (MHRA in the UK).

Site-level files

These would contain documentation that is specific to the conduct of the trial at a particular investigator site – for example, the protocol signed by the principal investigator or the site staff delegation list.

Figure 10.1 A typical organisation of a sponsor file

essential documents relating to the trial. The documentation does not all necessarily need to be in the same location, but it must be clear where it is held from TMF procedures or indexes as it must[6] be readily available both during the trial and during the archiving retention period following the trial. For example, it may be appropriate for an organisation to determine that serious adverse event (SAE) cases will all be retained in the pharmacovigilance department, including the suspected unexpected serious adverse reaction (SUSAR) receipt confirmation, rather than printing it off the pharmacovigilance database and filing in the TMF. This detail may, dependent upon its complexity, necessitate formal documentation in a written procedure. In large commercial organisations, the TMF could include documents from a variety of different departments other than clinical operations; for example, data management, statistics, pharmacovigilance, clinical trial supplies, legal, regulatory affairs, as well as those provided or held by vendors (see section 10.2.6). This contrasts with a small, single-centre, non-commercial trial, where the documentation is likely to be much less and could be limited to just the investigator and pharmacy files. Some documentation may be non-trial-specific, for example the validation of a computer system that is used for numerous trials, but is still needed to demonstrate the quality of the trials. Figure 10.2 illustrates how different departments may, within a large organisation, hold documentation that is considered part of the TMF.

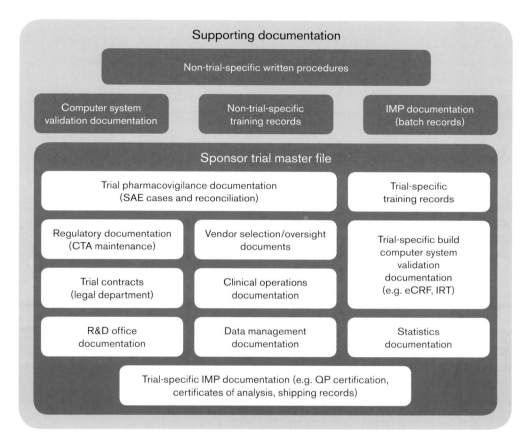

Figure 10.2 Potential documentation sources for the sponsor trial master file (not exhaustive)

CTA, clinical trial authorisation; eCRF, electronic case report form; IMP, investigational medicinal product; IRT, interactive response technologies; QP, Qualified Person; R&D, research and development; SAE, serious adverse event

10.2.4 Indexing

It is essential to have a suitable indexing system in place for the TMF. This ensures that the documentation is appropriately sorted and filed, which facilitates audit, inspection and trial management. It is recommended that the documentation is filed in date sequential order (usually with the most recent on top) to enable a clear audit trail of, for example, communications with sites, research ethics committees (REC) and competent authorities.

Investigator site files are typically indexed and organised by the trial sponsor and maintained with the assistance of the trial monitor. As a result, an investigator who is working with several sponsors may have several different files organised in slightly different ways. Some non-commercial trial sponsors may not provide investigator site files and in such circumstances the investigator will need to organise the filing themselves. In such cases, if the host organisation (for example, an investigator site's R&D office) has a standard indexing system available for use, this would prove useful to the investigator.

10.2.5 Written procedures for controlling the trial master file

The extent of the potential distribution of TMF documentation and the number of trials a sponsor conducts will inform the decision as to whether a formal procedure is necessary to document the locations of all records associated with the TMF as well as the content of the TMF (for example, standard indices) or whether the protocol providing an overview of the TMF arrangements, together with a trial-specific index in the TMF, is sufficient. The use of a formal procedure and a standard indexing system (rather than creating 'trial-specific' indices repeatedly) in organisations sponsoring several trials is recommended as it tends to facilitate compliance. If there is a change in written procedures or to the format of indices, organisations are recommended to perform a risk assessment regarding the necessity to 're-file' previously filed TMFs, as this resource-intensive exercise may be of little benefit.

10.2.6 Vendor involvement in the trial master file

The complexity of the TMF is increased by the use of vendors in assisting in the management and/or conduct of the trial. The role of the vendor in the trial would be expected to be formally documented in an agreement between the sponsor and the vendor, outlining the functions transferred to the vendor (see section 1.3). In conducting these allocated functions, the vendor will be generating documentation that must[1] reside in the TMF. In addition, the vendor may have been delegated the functions of managing the sponsor's TMF. It has become increasingly common that, in addition to a contract being in place that delegates specific functions from the sponsor to the vendor, formal 'plans' (similar to a technical agreement) may also be prepared and approved between the two parties. These are extremely useful as they can provide, at a sufficient level of detail, the written procedures to be used when performing the delegated functions as well as providing detail as to how the quality systems of the two organisations will interact. One such plan that may be considered is a TMF plan, particularly when the interactions between a vendor and sponsor are quite involved and complex and the agreement would not provide a sufficient level of detail of the practical working relationship. Such a plan would be extremely useful for those involved in managing, auditing and inspecting the trial documentation and this plan (where used) must[1] be filed in the TMF.

The content of such a plan could typically address:

- who holds the official TMF (or which parts each party holds when this is divided)
- the process for filing documentation in the TMF during the live phase of a trial
- the access arrangements for both parties to enable trial management and oversight
- the structure and indexing of the TMF
- where an electronic TMF (eTMF) is being used, the details of the system, processes to be followed, training requirements etc.
- documents that both parties must retain
- arrangements for managing correspondence, so that there is not a huge amount of duplication
- how the TMF would be made available if either party was inspected
- arrangements for when the trial is completed
- lists/attachments of applicable written procedures.

Where sponsors have delegated functions to the vendor, this may involve maintaining the TMF (or sections of it). The vendor will also be generating documentation if it is following its own written procedures; for example, internal quality control (QC) checklists for documents (for example, subject information sheets). Vendors may provide all the documentation back to the sponsor on completion of the trial, but if the vendor's internal records are supplied to the sponsor, the vendor would need some assurance that these will be retained by the sponsor, as GCP inspectors have seen situations where these records were not retained. These records are important in demonstrating that the vendor followed its own quality system. Alternatively, these internal vendor records could be retained and archived by the vendor and it is acceptable for the vendor to do so, but this would need to be clear in any agreement or TMF plan with the sponsor.

Vendors can be subject to a GCP inspection and this would require access to the records that were generated in undertaking the duties and functions delegated from the sponsor. If this documentation has been provided to the sponsor, the sponsor and vendor are both responsible for ensuring there is a documented arrangement to make the TMF readily available as required[7] for inspection both during and after completion of the trial. It is recommended that this is contained in the contractual arrangements between the two parties.

If the documentation is returned to the vendor from the sponsor for inspection, or indeed if the vendor's documentation is inspected at the sponsor site, it is recommended that the vendor is able to demonstrate that the documentation is the same as that which was sent to the sponsor. The lack of this ability could be a problem if the documentation revealed an offence had been committed, in particular on the part of the vendor, as the vendor would not know whether the documentation had been changed in some way. A recommended solution to this, in line with due diligence, would be for the vendor to maintain its own copy of key documentation, which could be on paper or electronic media (subject to appropriate QC and archive controls). This arrangement would need to be part of the contract or TMF plan to ensure sponsor agreement to the vendor retaining a copy of the TMF documents.

Where the sponsor has delegated the maintenance of the TMF to the vendor as well as many other trial conduct functions, there will still be a requirement[4] for the sponsor to hold or have access to some trial documentation in order to undertake oversight of the conduct of the clinical trial. In this situation, many of the documents will be copies of those held in the TMF of the vendor (for example, the protocol). However, there will be documentation that demonstrates the oversight of the sponsor (for example, internal correspondence that may not be in the TMF of the vendor), but this documentation must[1] eventually form part of the TMF. In GCP inspections of the sponsor where virtually all the trial conduct functions had been subcontracted, the sponsor would be expected to provide documentation to demonstrate oversight of the trial conduct. In such situations the quality system of the sponsor should reflect its oversight functions (see Chapter 14) and this would include written procedures for the handling of trial documentation that demonstrates this oversight is taking place. This may take the form of sponsor oversight files and defining what needs to be maintained. It is recommended that it is clear that sponsor oversight can still be demonstrated if the files of the sponsor are amalgamated with the vendor TMF at the end of the trial. One common problem occurs where the oversight is done extensively by email – for example, demonstrating review and approval of key trial documents – but these emails are not made available to the inspectors.

10.3   Content of the trial master file

10.3.1   Essential documents

Often encountered on inspection is the view that if a document is not listed in ICH GCP and EudraLex Volume 10 as being an 'essential document' then it need not be contained in the TMF. This is not the expectation of MHRA GCP inspectors. Firstly, Regulation 31A (4) of SI 2004/1031 defines essential documents as:

> *'The essential documents relating to a clinical trial are those which (a) enable both the conduct of the clinical trial and the quality of the data produced to be evaluated; and (b) show whether the trial is, or has been, conducted in accordance with the applicable requirements of Directive 2001/83/EC, the Directive, the GCP Directive and Commission Directive 2003/94/EC.'*

Secondly, two of the principles of GCP stipulated in Parts 2 (4) and (9) of Schedule 1 to SI 2004/1031 respectively state that: *'The necessary procedures to secure the quality of every aspect of the trial shall be complied with'* and *'All clinical information shall be recorded, handled and stored in such a way that it can be accurately reported, interpreted and verified, while the confidentiality of records of the trial subjects remains protected'.*

These principles and definitions together can be interpreted to mean that all records created from following trial procedures, as well as those listed in guidance relating to the conduct of the trial, should be retained to demonstrate compliance. The documentation listed in section 8 of ICH GCP and Chapter 3 of the TMF guidance document are useful guides for the minimum documents that are considered essential; however, this list is not recommended to be used as a definitive checklist for TMF content. Examples of documents that are essential to reconstruct the trial but that are not contained in the above include Qualified Person (QP) certification, the regulatory green-light document to release and ship investigational medicinal products (IMP), and the database lock documentation. Therefore, the 'essential documents' list is a subset of the potential documentation that could be regarded as essential for reconstruction of the trial conduct.

Where the risk-adapted approaches to trial management are being followed (see section 10.3.4), some documents listed in the guidance may not be in the TMF –

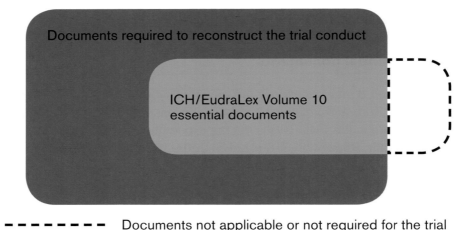

Documents not applicable or not required for the trial

Figure 10.3 Documentation to reconstruct the conduct of a trial

for example, IMP temperature storage records, IMP accountability, laboratory reference ranges – and the rationale for this would be in the trial risk assessment. This is illustrated in Figure 10.3.

Additionally, during inspections, verbal information provided during interview, particularly at investigator sites, reveals activities that occurred which were not transparent from the documentation in the file, such as the training that the principal investigator provided to team members. Therefore, it is recommended that an assessment of all activities is undertaken to determine whether they need to be documented to enable reconstruction of the trial conduct from the paperwork alone. This is an important point to consider, because if a trial needs to be reviewed by the competent authority some years after its completion, personnel involved may no longer be available. The TMF must[1] therefore be a robust record of all aspects of the clinical trial.

Superseded issued versions of documents (for example, the investigator's brochure), should be retained within the TMF (unless it is clear from a formal TMF procedure or index where they reside) as these are necessary to reconstruct activities in the earlier part of the trial, when that version of the investigator's brochure was being used as the reference document for expectedness assessment. Retention of draft versions of documents may be necessary if these are required to demonstrate compliance with the document production and review process, but if this is possible to demonstrate by other means (for example, use of summary or checklist documents), then these documents may not be required.

10.3.2   Correspondence

The conduct of a clinical trial can generate large of amounts of correspondence, such as emails, letters, meeting minutes and telephone call reports, which may be internal within an organisation (for example, within the sponsor, vendor or investigator site) or between organisations (for example, between sponsor and vendor, or sponsor and investigator). Correspondence is an important component in reconstructing the trial conduct, with some vendor organisations relying solely on email correspondence to confirm sponsor approval of processes, documents, and decisions. Only relevant correspondence that is necessary for reconstruction of key activities and decisions (for example, the medical advisor allows a subject to remain in the trial who has taken a banned concomitant medication, or confirmation that the IMP can continue to be used after a temperature excursion), or correspondence that contains other significant information, must[1] be retained. If some correspondence is not retained (particularly certain emails which may not add any value by being retained, such as email correspondence between investigator site staff and the trial monitor discussing holidays or suitable hotels to stay in near the site), then there should be a formal process to assist individuals in the evaluation of whether it contributes to the reconstruction of the trial or not. Electronic correspondence may be retained electronically, provided the requirements for eTMF are considered.

It is recommended that correspondence is effectively organised; this could be done by segregating correspondence into topic area (for example, protocol development) or into relevant sections (for example, correspondence with the MHRA and REC). It is also recommended that correspondence is always filed in chronological order and that duplication of documentation (for example, chain emails) is avoided. Electronically attached documents that are not present elsewhere within the TMF must[1] be included where necessary for reconstruction (for example, reports/data reviewed in dose escalation meetings).

Sections including correspondence must[1] be complete. On inspection, it is often seen that only copies of letters received rather than those sent out and received are filed (such as those sent from the sponsor to the REC or from the investigator to the REC), such that the TMF only contains half of the audit trail.

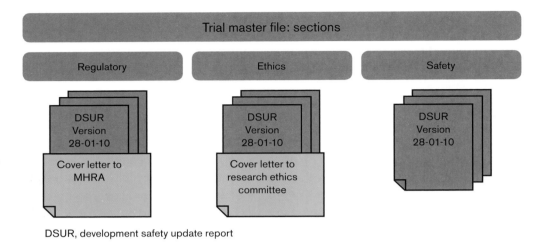

DSUR, development safety update report

Figure 10.4 An example of possible duplication of documentation

10.3.3   Document duplication

It is recommended that duplication of documents within the TMF is avoided, where possible, as this can hinder the effective use of the TMF. For example, a development safety update report (DSUR) submission to the MHRA and REC could result in three copies of the same document being filed in the TMF (see Figure 10.4). This is unnecessary, as the submission letters could contain the version of the DSUR, and the actual DSUR could then be located only once in the TMF within the safety section, provided the indexing covers this approach. This approach is recommended to be used for other documentation in the TMF, such as MHRA submission letters, as the aim is for the documentation to provide clarity on the document submitted and provide only one copy of each document in the TMF.

10.3.4   Impact of the risk-adapted approach on trial master file content

The risk-adapted approach to clinical trial approvals and trial management was implemented on 1 April 2011 (see section 2.4). Trials that have been categorised as Type C, involving unlicensed medicines, would be expected to have few, if any, modifications to the documentation contained in section 8 of ICH GCP and Chapter 3 of the TMF guidance document. Trials categorised as either Type A or B are, however, highly likely to have such modifications. This would be in relation to the sponsor's risk assessment of the trial, with a focus on those activities that are important to meeting the objectives of the trial. This assessment would be reflected in the documentation generated and retained for the trial.

This approach would easily result in differential documentation requirements, for example:

- Section 8.3.23 of ICH GCP and section 3.2.23 of the TMF guidance document state: *'Investigational products accountability at the site – to document that investigational product(s) have been used according to the protocol'.* In some cases this may require temperature records for the storage of the IMP to be retained: for example, an unlicensed product being used in a trial categorised as Type C may be unstable outside a particular temperature range and/or has limited stability data and/or a short shelf life. Conversely, such records may be irrelevant where the IMP is an authorised product, used in the same way as in normal clinical practice in a trial categorised as Type A, as the storage arrangements used as normal practice are deemed to be appropriate and no further requirements need to be imposed for the purposes of the trial.

- Section 8.2.12 of ICH GCP, section 3.1.12 of the TMF guidance document and MHRA guidance on the maintenance of regulatory compliance in laboratories that perform the analysis or evaluation of clinical trial samples, expect certification or accreditation, or established QC and/or external quality assessment or other validation of laboratories. For a trial categorised as Type C, a contract laboratory may be used to undertake drug or metabolite sample analysis, and in such cases this validation documentation would be appropriate. In a trial categorised as Type A, however, using the hospital laboratory for haematology and biochemistry analysis as per normal clinical activity, the addition of the Clinical Pathology Accreditation (CPA) certificates to the TMF adds no value in terms of either risk to subject safety or to the data quality. In addition, as the laboratories require evidence of standards for normal clinical practice, such documentation could be made available upon request, if required.

- Section 8.3.10 of ICH GCP and section 3.2.10 of the TMF guidance document list monitoring visit reports of on-site visits. For trials categorised as Type A and B, central monitoring may be used extensively in place of on-site monitoring visits. This may result in documentation being generated that is not included in the guidance, such as a monitoring plan, reports of remote contact with sites, questionnaires obtained from site and checked reports from

341

interrogation of the clinical database (as part of statistical central monitoring), that must[1] be filed in the TMF.

MHRA GCP inspectors will not rigidly apply the list of documentation in the guidance as a checklist and, particularly for Type A and B category trials, will take a pragmatic approach to the TMF content. The recommended approach for both sponsors and investigators to take when assessing the need for retention of documentation is:

- Is a document listed in the guidance actually going to be produced (if the process that normally produces it is not taking place based on the risk assessment)?
- Is the information available in a different format that is filed elsewhere in the TMF?
- Does this document add value in terms of establishing the quality of the conduct of the trial?
- Has this document been produced by following an organisation's written procedure?
- Does having this document in the TMF matter in terms of meeting the objectives of the trial and producing reliable results?

10.4   Control of the trial master file

The sponsor's TMF is the repository of all the information that is necessary to reconstruct the trial, therefore its security and maintenance are vital. The arrangements for who should access the TMF in order to add or remove documentation are important points to consider and must[8] be controlled. It is recommended that this is done using the risk-adapted approach. The two key factors that influence risk are:

- The number of trials the organisation is conducting (creation of a specific department to manage TMFs may be appropriate compared with an investigator maintaining their own TMF in their office.
- Use of the trial data (if the trial is to be used to support a marketing authorisation or will be important in determining treatment via its publication).

The investigator's TMF should be stored securely such that only trial staff (and monitors, auditors and inspectors) can gain access to the documentation.

Some organisations have controls in place for placing documentation in the TMF or removing it from the TMF while the trial is in progress. It can take the form of formal submission of TMF documents with some form of TMF tracking (for example, generation of a submission record or a simple signature and date on the index of the file). Some organisations may archive the documentation on an ongoing basis to prevent loss, particularly where eTMFs are in use. A lack of control would obviously entail the risk of missing documentation at the end of the trial. It is recommended that this risk and the implications of the loss should be evaluated before the implementation of additional paperwork or systems to track or manage the placing of documents in the TMF.

10

The TMF must[5] be kept up to date, with documents placed in the TMF in a timely manner, as Regulation 31A (3) of SI 2004/1031 states that *'The master file shall at all times contain the essential documents relating to that clinical trial'*. This can greatly assist in the successful management of a trial by the investigator, sponsor and monitor. The contemporaneous nature of the TMF may vary in trials and could be more anachronistic in trials that have more complex TMF arrangements with multiple parties involved. In this scenario it may be useful to define the timescales for submission and filing of documents to the TMF in written procedures or TMF plans. Documentation in the TMF that is relied upon for subsequent activities should therefore be in the TMF before these activities take place; for example, monitoring visits rely on the information in the previous report, so the previous report should be completed and filed in the TMF prior to the next visit. It may raise concerns on inspection if the TMF appeared so out of date that the organisation's ability to manage and oversee the trial conduct was questionable. It should be remembered that MHRA GCP inspections can be unannounced or performed at short notice and even routine inspections may not contain a notification of the trials to be inspected until shortly before the inspection, thus the TMF must[5,7] be maintained in an 'inspection-ready state'. This particularly applies to TMFs after the trial has completed, as these TMFs must[6] be 'complete and legible'.

There should be a process to ensure that any documents that have been, or are currently contained, in the TMF have traceability of any changes made to them to comply with Regulation 31A (6) of SI 2004/1031. Strict version control should be applied to key trial documents and failure to do so is frequently identified on inspections. (Section 4.4 provides details on how to maintain version control of key trial documents.)

10.5 Electronic trial master file

10.5.1 What is an electronic trial master file?

Many eTMFs are document management systems containing all the necessary controls listed in section 10.5.3 and these would make the system completely acceptable. Acceptability of a system of storage of documents within folders in the operating environment of a computer system would require the minimum security features in section 10.5.3. This is because these folders have typically been shared areas where everyone in the organisation has access and documents could easily be moved, deleted or replaced with a lack of version control, so there is ambiguity over which is the current version and which is a superseded version.

Table 10.1 Comparison of paper and electronic trial master files

Criteria	pTMF	eTMF
Accessibility to same documents from various locations and organisations with suitable equipment and connections	✗	✓
Potential environmental benefits	✗	✓
One controlled access to the official version of the documents (no circulation of copies, for example, from vendor to sponsor)	✗	✓
Searchable (including across trials)	✗	✓
Better control and audit trail	✗	✓
Interaction with electronic systems (for example, clinical trial management systems)	✗	✓
Back-up easy to create and available	✗	✓
Ease of compilation of common technical document	✗	✓
Extensive training needed	✗	✓
Scanning equipment required	✗	✓
Computers and internet not required (not susceptible to system/internet downtimes)	✓	✗
No computer system validation required	✓	✗
Simple and easy for small trials	✓	✗[a]
Inspection readiness	✓	✓

[a] Unless an eTMF system is already in place.

eTMF, electronic trial master file; pTMF, paper trial master file

10.5.2 Considerations for use of paper and electronic trial master files

There is an increasing use of eTMFs instead of paper-based TMFs in the pharmaceutical industry and MHRA GCP inspectors agree with the potential advantages of the use of such systems for some trial sponsors. However, the advantages for small organisations conducting one or two trials may not be as great and it is recommended that the organisation makes a suitable assessment prior to making the investment in an eTMF. Nevertheless, the same controls must[8,9] be in place for managing the eTMF as for managing a paper TMF – that is, controls in terms of security, control over unauthorised edits and access or ease of retrieval of documents. Table 10.1 illustrates some comparisons of the two systems.

10.5.3 Controls, security, training and validation

The minimum requirements for an eTMF system should enable appropriate security to be in place, which would include role-based permissions for activities being undertaken through the use of secure passwords. Accounts should be created and deleted within a formal approval process and in a timely manner. This is analogous to the paper system where the TMF is kept in a secure location, with restricted access.

Further controls for when more complex document management systems are being used are expected. For example, where the system is being used for approval of documents via a workflow system, password-enabled electronic signatures could be used. The system must[9] have an audit trail in place to identify date/time/user details for creation, uploading, approval and changes to a document. It is also recommended that a system for locking documents or the entire eTMF is considered to prevent changes to documents, such as when the eTMF is archived. Finally, all members of staff involved in the conduct of the trial must[10] receive training in using the system and this should be documented.

The eTMF could contain digital documents in their original format, potentially with digital signatures, or records that have been converted from another format (such as paper documents that have been converted to digital images, which may contain wet-ink signatures). Records that exist only in a digital format are often only printed onto paper at the time of an inspection as they are normally accessed in their digital form. This can result in loss of any version control applied in the computer system (for example, a dated filename). An example of this could be the 'edit checks' specification used by data management. Such documents, when uploaded into the eTMF, may also have the same potential issue, which reinforces the requirement that all documents should have clear version control that is maintained on transition from one type of media, or from one system, to another.

Unlike a paper TMF, documents loaded into the eTMF will need the addition of metadata to enable the document to be identified within the system. Metadata are data which are associated with the document (but not the document itself), so typically would be identifying codes for the trial, site, protocol and product. The type of metadata is recommended to be formally defined to ensure consistency across all documents.

The eTMF will require validation to demonstrate that the functionality is fit for purpose, with written procedures in place to manage this process and for change control. The validation of the system is recommended to follow previously published standards (see section 14.5 for further details). The documentation for this process must[1] be retained. Consideration may also be given to the provision of a helpdesk for system users, where appropriate.

There is also the potential for the investigator site file, held by the principal investigator, to become electronic, with the system provided either by the sponsor, a vendor or the host site organisation. The documentation in the investigator site file will contain source documents – for example, subject screening and identity logs, consent forms, drug accountability records – and the control of these must[2, 3] remain with the investigator unless specific consent has been obtained from trial subjects for their personal information to be released from the trial site. A situation where all the site records are sent to the external sponsor for uploading onto an eTMF system, which the investigator then accesses via a portal, would breach this requirement. The sponsor may wish to consider the EMA GCP Inspectors Working Group paper, 'Reflection paper on expectations for electronic source data and data transcribed to electronic data collection tools in clinical trials' (EMA/INS/GCP/454280/2010), as the considerations and recommendations will have applicability to source documents contained in eTMFs.

10.5.4   Scanning or transfers to other media

The use of eTMFs and electronic archiving generally require the scanning of some paper records to generate electronic copies of the documents. When original paper TMF documents are transferred to an electronic format (or other media) the system of transfer should be validated in order to ensure that the transfer of documents is without loss and to ensure that certifiable copies are made (such that there should be a demonstrable 1:1 mapping between the content of the original TMF and the eTMF, which essentially means a QC check of the original TMF against the eTMF). Some eTMF systems require a review of each scanned document before it is approved within the eTMF, but all transfers should be certified for accuracy and completeness by someone with appropriate authority (for example, the trial manager), as part of the quality system. This does not necessarily mean that the individual reviews every document, but that they have approved the validated system that is being used. The organisation should maintain records to demonstrate that the transfer system is effectively validated.

10

It is recommended that there is a formal process in place for regular checks of documents in the eTMF, usually on a sampling basis, including escalation procedures where issues arise. This process could assess, for each document reviewed, one or more of the following:

- accuracy of the metadata attributed to the document
- quality of the image (for example, readability)
- whether it was the correct document (as expected)
- that the document had the correct number of pages
- the eTMF audit trail associated with the document (with a link to any changes)
- chain of custody documentation and timeliness of uploading into the eTMF
- approval process (where applicable).

Scanned images must[6] be at appropriate resolution so that when viewed at actual size on the screen (same size as the original) the image is clear and legible. Post-scan adjustments to the image to increase legibility are acceptable, provided the limits of what may be undertaken are clearly specified in a formal procedure. It is not acceptable to use the scanning process to remove or add material to the image (for example, to remove the header a fax machine has added), or undertake physical 'cut and paste' or 'correction fluid' activities on the original paper record. Documents within an eTMF must[6] remain complete and legible in all aspects giving information about the way the document was prepared. This holds especially true for contracts and forms completed by hand. It would not be acceptable, therefore, to create a new electronic version of a form that had been completed by hand and then file that instead of the original (or the scanned, unaltered version of the original).

When a vendor is used for eTMF management, appropriate pre-qualification checks should be undertaken prior to placing the contract (see section 1.3.2). It is recommended that where TMF documents are moved from the sponsor to the vendor for scanning, a formal procedure is in place to ensure chain of custody records are maintained (for example, use of a TMF record transmittal form).

There is a move towards scanning of subjects' medical records within the NHS and the same principles of ensuring authentic copies also apply to this situation, prior to any destruction of original source documents.

10.5.5   Destruction of original paper records

The use of an eTMF would be considered as a prerequisite to the sponsor's being able to destroy paper records and reduce storage requirements. The Clinical Trials Regulations does not consider the transfer of documentation to other media, but does require the documents to be readily available, complete and legible, and contain traceability of any changes made. EudraLex Volume 10 guidance states that sponsors should ensure that essential documents are not destroyed before the end of the required retention periods; however, transfer of the document to an eTMF repository could enable earlier destruction of the paper original. The eTMF system would need to have all the characteristics as defined above, such that there is confidence on inspection that the eTMF is complete and the documents are authentic copies. Experience of eTMFs to date has not yet provided sufficient evidence that inspectors would not need to request some original paper records for inspection, and thus early complete destruction of such records is not currently recommended or should only be undertaken on a risk-adapted approach. A duplicate paper TMF need not be retained; the reasons for this include the following:

- A document may only have existed and been used in an electronic format (for example, a spreadsheet used for QC of edit check programs).
- A paper document may be a copy of an original located elsewhere (for example, investigator's signed CV).
- Documents do not have wet-ink signatures, thus the electronic version is an exact copy of the paper version that has been in the TMF (provided there are no additional annotations made, handwritten or otherwise – for example, receipt stamps, fax machine header).

This indicates that the eTMF would contain some documents that are more likely to have the original paper copy requested than others, such as agreements with wet-ink signatures and signed letters. The current recommendation is to undertake a risk assessment in order to decide which documents do not need to be retained on paper, particularly focusing on whether or not the paper version could be obtained upon request (for example, reprinted or obtained from another location).

10.6 MHRA GCP inspection of trial master files

10.6.1 General principles of trial master file inspection

The TMF is the basis of inspection for the MHRA conducting GCP inspections in the UK (and elsewhere). As indicated previously, GCP inspections in the UK require[6, 7] the TMF for the trial to be readily available and for the TMF to be produced at any reasonable time by the organisation during the trial conduct and for at least 5 years after the trial completion. The requirements and logistics of TMF provision will be discussed with the organisation prior to the inspection and this is where planning the arrangements for the TMF at the trial start can be beneficial, especially in complex trials with vendor involvement. Organisations should have considered how to make the TMF available to the inspectors should an inspection be announced. MHRA GCP inspectors will be clear about the levels of the TMF they wish to review, which is usually the whole of the country-level and the site-level documents. For the latter, specific sites may be requested during the inspection if there are many to choose from. There will also be a requirement to view some documentation from the trial-level TMF – for example, the investigator's brochure. The inspectors will not expect to have to request documentation individually for a trial as the whole TMF should be provided if asked for.

The inspectors will require[7] direct access to the TMF, which means reviewing the TMF as used by those conducting the trial. Inspectors have in the past been provided with an 'artificial TMF' or 'snapshot' which consisted of a copy of the official TMF being used and led to issues with documentation not being consistent with that of the official TMF. The organisation must[1] be aware of the locations of all the documentation that comprises the TMF, as there have been inspections where only the clinical operations files have been provided that contain the documentation listed in section 8.0 of ICH GCP.

The MHRA GCP inspectors will not wish to be supervised during the review of the TMF. Documents will not be removed from the site without the organisation being made aware, and inspectors make every effort to ensure that the documents remain as provided (for example, returning documents to their original position in the file). MHRA GCP inspectors have the right to seize documents under the Human Medicines Regulations 2012 (SI 2012/1916).

10.6.2 Inspection of the electronic trial master files

The legislation does not differentiate between paper and eTMFs, therefore all the requirements are the same; however, the use of an eTMF at an inspection presents additional challenges both to the inspector and to the organisation.

It is an expectation that the eTMF should adequately replicate the paper-based system that it is replacing. There have been issues reviewing eTMFs on inspection and this has resulted in organisations receiving major inspection findings and/or an increased number of inspector days on site. It is recommended that the organisation consider that the requirements for inspectors will also reflect the requirements of any auditors, and the system should be designed and developed or purchased with this requirement in mind.

While it is acknowledged that some training or familiarisation for an eTMF will be required, it is recommended that this is very brief (taking no more than an hour), otherwise additional inspection days may be required. This also implies that the system is user friendly. MHRA GCP inspectors will require[7] direct access to the eTMF system (not a copy), without reliance on an eTMF 'super-user', so the system should ideally facilitate a read-only 'inspector or auditor view' access.

The eTMF will require the use of suitable equipment for the inspector to view the documents. It is recommended that this equipment facilitates the presentation of the documents at actual size, which in most cases would be A4 paper, and that the size is not reduced due to other areas on the screen (for example, directory or index structures and toolbars). The organisation should not expect the inspectors themselves to provide suitable equipment to view the eTMF.

It is anticipated that the time taken to review documents in the eTMF system will be similar to the time it would take to review them on paper, otherwise additional days may be required to conduct the inspection (at a cost to the organisation) or reference made back to the original paper records. It is therefore recommended that the system should have a sufficient speed of access, and not require the use of a nomenclature document or time spent opening files that are not self-evidently named in order to determine their content. Using the system and equipment should ideally be akin to flipping the pages of a book, with a system tool available to mark documents for subsequent retrieval and examination as well as the ability to compare documents side by side.

Finally, the inspector may have to copy and retain documents from the eTMF, so it is recommended that the organisation have facilities to allow this.

10.7   Archiving

10.7.1   Document retention times

Retention of the documents within the TMF (including the investigator site file) and the medical records of trial subjects is a legal requirement.[11] The sponsor and the principal investigator must[6, 12] ensure that the documents contained, or that have been contained, in the TMF, as well as the medical files of trial subjects are retained for at least 5 years after the conclusion of the trial. Trials where the data are used to support a marketing authorisation have further requirements as per Directive 2003/63/EC. Here the documentation should be retained for at least 15 years after completion or discontinuation of the trial or for at least 2 years after the granting of the last marketing authorisation in the EC (when there are no pending or contemplated marketing applications in the EC) or for at least 2 years after formal discontinuation of clinical development of the investigational medicinal product. Additionally, the sponsor or other owner of the data must retain all other documentation pertaining to the trial as long as the product is authorised. This documentation shall include the trial protocol (which must include the rationale, objectives and statistical design and methodology of the trial, with conditions under which it is performed and managed, details of the investigational medicinal product, the reference medicinal product and/or the placebo used), any written procedures used for conducting the trial, all written opinions on the protocol and procedures, the investigator's brochure, case report forms on each trial subject, final clinical study report and audit certificate(s), if available, and staff training records. Additionally, the final clinical study report shall be retained by the sponsor or subsequent owner, for 5 years after the medicinal product is no longer authorised.

Trial subjects' medical files must[12] be retained for at least 5 years in their original format and in accordance with the maximum period of time permitted by the hospital, institution or private practice. Scanning or microfiching of subjects' medical records is acceptable provided the process is validated such that the institution can demonstrate that it is an authentic copy of the original and it is kept in a format that means that the data can be retrieved in the future. It is recommended that the notes of subjects who have been involved in clinical trials are clearly identified to prevent premature destruction. Many UK hospitals attach stickers to the notes with a 'do not destroy' or 'retain until' date clearly marked.

In addition to these retention times for the trial documentation, records relating to the full traceability of the IMP for advanced therapies have longer retention periods. These are 30 years after the expiry date of the product or longer if required by the clinical trial authorisation. This will include the relevant documentation contained in the sponsor and investigator files as well as the trial subjects' medical records. Further information can be found in Annex 3 and the EU detailed guidance on GCP for advanced therapy medicinal products (2009).

It is the responsibility of the sponsor to inform the hospital, institution or practice as to when these documents no longer need to be retained. As such, the expectation would be that the retention requirements of the sponsor for the documentation and medical records held by the investigator should be agreed either in the protocol or a separate agreement. The sponsor would be expected to have systems in place to alert the investigator when the records are no longer required to be retained. The sponsor should notify investigators in writing when their trial records can be destroyed and up until that point the investigator or institution should take measures to prevent accidental or premature destruction of these documents. The ultimate responsibility for the documents to be retained by the investigator or institution resides with the investigator or institution. If the investigator becomes unable to be responsible for their essential documents (for example, relocation, retirement) the sponsor should be notified in writing of this change and informed to whom the responsibility has been transferred.

The EU Regulation on Medicinal Products for Paediatric Use 1901/2006, which was adopted in December 2006 and came into force in January 2007, enables the use of data from published literature for the application of Paediatric Use Marketing Authorisations (PUMAs). To this end, the archiving requirements should meet the requirement of Directive 2003/63/EC. The data may not be used for a marketing authorisation application (MAA) when the TMF has only been maintained for 5 years.

It is important that where an organisation has centralised records that may be relevant to a number of trials – for example, written procedures, staff training records or maintenance and calibration records for equipment used in the trial –

that these are also considered in the arrangements for archiving and retention as they may be required to be produced in addition to the TMF to demonstrate compliance.

The protocol or the written procedures of the sponsor should contain details of the retention times for all the trial documentation as outlined above or the process used to determine how long particular documentation will be retained and how this should be documented.

The requirements for the retention of sponsors' records also apply to the records retained by vendors or other agents of the sponsor, unless arrangements have been made to transfer the documents to the sponsor. The details of the retention time of documents held by the vendor should be formalised in an agreement between the sponsor and the vendor or be clear within the vendor's written procedures that will have been reviewed by the sponsor.

Investigators can retire, hospitals can close and vendors (some of which are also investigator sites, such as commercial Phase I units) can go out of business or be acquired by other organisations. The sponsor should ensure that agreements cover such eventualities, to ensure that the documentation remains available for inspection for the specified retention time. Sponsors outside the UK must[1] ensure that provision is made to make the archived documents for trials conducted in the UK available to the MHRA throughout the retention period, in particular for documentation held by vendors. This issue has occurred on several occasions in the UK when Phase I units have closed and there has not been any contact with the trial sponsors to ensure the long-term availability of their investigators' files and data until the MHRA was informed.

10.7.2   Named individual responsible for archiving

It is a legal requirement[8] that the sponsor appoints a named individual within the organisation to be responsible for archiving the documents which are, or have been, contained in the TMF, and that access to these documents must be restricted to those appointed individuals and auditors or inspectors. This can be undertaken either by having a specific archivist role or by combining the archiving duties with another role, but in either case there must[10] be clear documentation to support the appointment and appropriate training provided. The named individual responsible for archiving must[13] have a clear legal link to the sponsor, in that they are the sponsor themselves or employed or contracted by the sponsor. Although an investigator site institution is not required to have a named individual responsible for archiving (unless they are a sponsor in their own right), it is recommended that, where an organisation has many trials, there is a person responsible for this activity.

10.7.3   Ownership of documentation

Where there is a change of ownership of data or documents connected with the clinical trial – for example, transfer of a marketing authorisation to another organisation – then the sponsor must[14] record the transfer and the new owner must[14] be responsible for data retention and archiving.

10.7.4   Review of trial master file prior to archiving

Before the TMF is archived, it is recommended that it is checked to ensure that it is complete and that all necessary documentation has been filed. This would often be done by the trial monitor (particularly at the close-out visit at the investigator site) but may also be undertaken by other appropriate individuals. It is recommended that this check is documented and that, for organisations which sponsor numerous trials, a written procedure is produced to cover this process. A documented check usually involves completing a checklist of the expected documentation, although it should be remembered that this needs to be comprehensive so as to record all of the documentation that has been filed to allow reconstruction of the trial conduct.

Before archiving, it is important to assess the contents of the TMF for any records that could be disposed of (for example, duplicates), and those that may be subject to rapid deterioration or need special requirements in order for them to be retained (such as needing to be transferred to other media). Examples include:

- thermochromic paper print-outs (which fade and become illegible over time)
- electronic media (CDs, USB flash drives, floppy disks)
- electromagnetic tapes
- photographs and films
- dummy IMP/medical device samples/packaging
- contaminated paper documents that may cause deterioration (from fungal or insect infestation, for example)
- plastic wallets that remove ink from documents.

The investigator may have delegated IMP activities to the site pharmacy, resulting in files being located within the pharmacy itself. These documents form part of the investigator site file and therefore may need to be combined with it. Alternatively, the archiving facilities or arrangements of the pharmacy should be assessed by the sponsor. Sponsors should be aware that some clinical trial documents are not kept in the site pharmacy file (for example, production worksheets for aseptic services either in-house or with service providers). The storage and retention requirements of these should also be assessed.

10.7.5 Tracking of archived documentation

It is important that the sponsor maintains records of the trials conducted and the archiving arrangements for the TMF for those trials, particularly if the organisation sponsors many trials and an external archive facility is being used. Removal of the records from the archive is anticipated to be a relatively rare occurrence and the records should track transfer of documentation to and from the archive facility (particularly important where contract archives are being used) and, where appropriate, such as for large organisations, location of the documentation on site when it is temporarily removed from the archive. The process should be controlled or overseen by the named individual responsible for archiving. For TMFs that are returned to the archive it is recommended that the contents are checked to ensure all the originally archived records are still present.

Where the sponsor and investigator are essentially the same, such tracking systems are probably unnecessary: for example, where one trial has been conducted and the documentation is stored in a suitably assessed location in the hospital, such as the investigator's office.

10.7.6 Sponsor archiving on behalf of the investigator

The investigator should retain control of the documentation contained in the investigator site file. The investigator site file should never be sent to the sponsor organisation except where the sponsor and investigator are essentially the same.

This does not mean that an external sponsor cannot arrange archiving on behalf of the investigator; this is acceptable, subject to the following being implemented:

- The archive arrangements are formally agreed and documented between the sponsor and investigator or host institution.

- A formal procedure is in place such that the documents are only released from the external archive with the approval of the investigator or host institution. It is recommended that this is tested for robustness. Permission from the investigator or host organisation should also be required to permit access to the contents of investigator site archived materials at the archive facility.

- The records go directly between the investigator site and an archive facility independent of the sponsor, thereby ensuring that the sponsor does not have uncontrolled access to the investigator files.

10.7.7   Contracting out archive facilities

The storage of the sponsor's or investigator's documentation may be transferred to a vendor (for example, a commercial archive), but the ultimate responsibility for the quality, integrity, confidentiality and retrieval of the documents resides with the sponsor and the investigator respectively. It is strongly recommended that the sponsor/investigator undertakes an assessment of the suitability of the facility prior to use – via an audit, for example – and that consideration is given to ongoing assessment. There should be a formal contract in place between the sponsor/investigator organisation and the archive company. Where the archive company has several document storage locations, it is recommended that the sponsor/investigator makes sure it is made aware of the storage location of its TMF, as some contracts allow the archive company to move documents between its facilities and the sponsor/investigator may be unaware of the exact location of its records.

10.7.8   Storage areas

The storage area for the TMF records must[6] be appropriate to maintain the documents such that they remain complete and legible throughout the required period of retention and can be made available to the competent authorities upon request. This may be assessed on a risk-adapted approach. Where a sponsor is conducting many trials in support of marketing authorisations, the requirement for long-term storage in appropriate conditions will be higher than for an investigator-initiated small Type A category trial where its publication is not likely to affect prescribing practice. Adequate and suitable space should be provided for the secure storage of all essential records from completed trials. Thus, for an investigator storing a TMF or investigator site file the sponsor may consider that the office filing cabinet may provide a suitably secure environment for a 5-year retention period, whereas a large sponsor that is required to retain documents in excess of 15 years may need more specialist facilities with sufficient level of controls. Some areas to be considered when performing such a risk assessment include:

- **Security** How accessible are the documents, are there locks in place on doors/cupboards, what is the risk of unauthorised access, are there windows on the ground floor?
- **Location** What risks are there from water (burst pipes, flood), fire (what activities take place in the room next door/above/below), what runs in the ceiling/floor void?
- **Size** Is the archive facility large enough and does it have appropriate off-floor shelving to accommodate the expected documentation?
- **Environmental** Are there risks from excessive temperature, humidity, sunlight, contamination (dust, fumes, smoke)?
- **Pests** Are there risks from rodents or insects?

British Standard BS 5454:2000 *Recommendations for the storage and exhibition of archival documents* is a standard for commercial archive facilities and sponsors may refer to this for consideration in maintaining purpose-built archive facilities as well as taking it into account when assessing potential contract archiving companies.

It is essential that sponsors make a documented assessment of the storage conditions at the investigator site for the investigator site file, and that the investigator provides this information. The importance of this is illustrated by an example where the archive facility of an investigator site was found on inspection to contain an automatic water pump to extract flood water. This risk to the documentation was highlighted to the organisation by the inspector, but it was not acted upon in a timely manner. Subsequently the pump failed to operate during a river flood and the investigator files sustained extensive water damage.

10.7.9 Electronic archiving

The use of electronic systems for such activities as data management, statistical analysis, reporting, trial management systems and eTMFs means that electronic documentation and data are likely to need to be retained. The data may be on a server or on transportable media (for example, USB drives, CDs, tapes). It is recommended that more than one copy of the data is retained: for example, where the data are archived in a specific server, this would be subject to back up, with the back-up media stored in a separate location. Consideration may be given to storing the data in differing formats on different types of media or even on the same media from different manufacturers.

Access to archived data must[8] be suitably restricted either by user access levels to the archive area of a server or by controls to access the storage area where the media are retained (as for paper). Additionally, the electronic documents or data that have been archived must be protected from unauthorised changes to maintain authenticity.

It is important that future access to records and data is maintained. This could include maintaining the system (hardware and software) to access the data in its original format, or the use of a new system to emulate the old software or migration of the data into a new format to ensure continual access with new software. This issue should be addressed by the organisation via written procedures.

Media used to store the data may potentially deteriorate or become obsolete. For example, it has been seen on inspection that a paper file contained a 3.5-inch floppy diskette containing the randomisation schedule. Computers with the ability to use such media are now rare and future potential access would not be guaranteed, thus transfer to an alternative would need to be considered. The media should be stored under appropriate conditions. The transfer of data to new media as technology advances would need to be considered by the organisation. It is also recommended that periodic test retrieval or restores are undertaken to confirm that ongoing availability of the data is being maintained.

Where data have to be migrated to new media or a new format, then the transfer should be validated and fully documented, so that it can be subject to audit, to ensure and demonstrate that there has been no loss, change or corruption to the data or metadata and that authenticity is maintained.

10.8   Chapter legislative references

Throughout this chapter, specific terminology – 'must', 'required' or 'requirement' – has been used to interpret activities that are legislative requirements. These terms have been number-coded in the text where used, and the corresponding reference in the legislation can be found below.

1.   Regulation 31A (4) of SI 2004/1031
2.   Schedule 1, Part 2 (9) of SI 2004/1031
3.   Schedule 1, Part 2 (13) of SI 2004/1031
4.   Regulation 3 (12) of SI 2004/1031
5.   Regulation 31A (3) of SI 2004/1031
6.   Regulation 31A (7) of SI 2004/1031
7.   Regulation 31A (2) of SI 2004/1031
8.   Regulation 31A (9) of SI 2004/1031
9.   Regulation 31A (6) of SI 2004/1031
10. Schedule 1, Part 2 (2) of SI 2004/1031
11. Regulation 31A (1) of SI 2004/1031
12. Regulation 31A (8) of SI 2004/1031
13. Regulation 31A (11) of SI 2004/1031
14. Regulation 31A (10) of SI 2004/1031

10

CHAPTER 11

Investigator sites

Editor's note

The development of any new compound will eventually require evaluation within the subject population who suffer with the condition that the new medicinal product is intended to treat. The conduct of clinical trials within the subject population usually follows trials that have taken place on healthy volunteers. In some disease areas (for example, oncology), due to the proposed action or potential side effects associated with the new treatment, Phase I trials may bypass the stage of healthy volunteers and be first tested in subjects who have that condition. A trial site is defined as a hospital, health centre, surgery or other establishment or facility at or from which a clinical trial, or any part of such a trial, is conducted (Regulation 2 of SI 2004/1031).

This chapter predominantly covers trial conduct at investigator sites within the NHS, but the principles outlined here may also apply to privately owned organisations such as Phase I units, research centres and hospitals. The development of alternative treatment strategies and alternative uses of established medication, generally the focus of research that is not commercially sponsored, also requires evidence of efficacy and safety and thus the guidance in this chapter is equally applicable to the generation of such data, particularly if the data will change prescribing practice.

Note that this chapter provides only an overview of the principles involved in conducting clinical trials from the perspective of an investigator site. Most of the concepts and activities are described elsewhere in the guide in more detail (for example, safety reporting) and reference should also be made to those chapters.

11.1 Research site

The source of subjects for a clinical trial is drawn from the various standard healthcare systems available to the population.

Examples of these organisations include:

- general practitioners and community clinics (primary care)
- secondary care (hospitals)
- tertiary care (specialist referral centres)
- private or charity-funded hospitals and clinics
- ambulance NHS Trusts.

Careful consideration will need to be given by the sponsor and the individual investigators to the operational aspects of running a clinical trial within each proposed type of organisation, prior to commencing recruitment of subjects. For example, insurance arrangements will differ between a private hospital and an NHS hospital covered by a blanket indemnity, out-of-hours cover for medical doctors involved in clinical trials may vary among organisations, and the informed consent process may depend on the setting of the trial (for example, paramedics could be taking consent). There will also be additional aspects to consider, such as the need for access to an intensive therapy unit or hospital emergency department if not available at a trial site. Specific considerations for units conducting Phase I trials are described in Chapter 12.

11.2 Investigator site research team

Before undertaking a clinical trial, it is essential to ensure that appropriate staffing and resources are available to conduct the trial. The principal investigator (PI) needs to ensure that sufficient staff are involved in the trial to ensure that all activities can be undertaken effectively. This includes both non-clinical activities, such as case report form (CRF) completion, data queries and management of the investigator site file, as well as subject-focused clinical care and medical cover. Insufficient resources can lead to issues such as missed tasks and data points, protocol non-compliance or inadequate supporting documentation that is essential to verify compliance with Good Clinical Practice (GCP) and the protocol.

It is not always possible to define set roles and responsibilities for some individual job functions (such as a research nurse or trial coordinator) as these can vary considerably from site to site and ultimately depend on what has been delegated to the individual by the PI based on resourcing, experience and the specifications of the protocol. For example, in some NHS Trusts a research nurse may solely be involved in clinical care aspects of the subject (such as blood draws and administration of the investigational medicinal product (IMP)). In other NHS Trusts, the role of the research nurse may also include trial coordination as a significant proportion of the role.

11.2.1 Investigator

In relation to a clinical trial, the term 'investigator' in Regulation 2 of SI 2004/1031 is defined as:

> 'the authorised health professional responsible for the conduct of that trial at a trial site, and if the trial is conducted by a team of authorised health professionals at a trial site, the investigator is the leader responsible for that team'.

In the UK, the term 'chief investigator' found in SI 2004/1031 is used for the healthcare professional who takes primary responsibility for the conduct of the trial, whether or not they are an investigator at any particular trial site. This definition is similar to the term 'coordinating investigator' found in ICH Topic E6 (R1) – 'Guideline for Good Clinical Practice' (hereinafter 'ICH GCP') to denote an investigator assigned the responsibility for the coordination of investigators at different centres participating in a multi-centre trial.

The role of the chief investigator may be undertaken by a sponsor's representative (for example, the sponsor's medical director or similar) or it may be contracted out to another investigator (who may or may not be involved in the recruitment and treatment of subjects at an investigator site). It is not uncommon for the sponsor to appoint a chief investigator per country or region to facilitate the oversight of a large number of investigator sites and to assist in the identification and management of local requirements.

The additional responsibilities of a chief investigator, according to the Clinical Trials Regulations, include:

- initial application and signatory for research ethics committee (REC) opinion
- appealing against an unfavourable REC opinion
- ensuring the trial master file (TMF) and the medical files are retained for at least 5 years (jointly with the sponsor).

Aside from the role of oversight and facilitation, the chief investigator may be delegated additional sponsor responsibilities. In the case of non-commercial sponsors, any of the sponsor responsibilities may be delegated to the chief investigator (see Chapter 1 for additional sponsor responsibilities). In addition, regardless of whether the sponsor is commercial or non-commercial, the process of applying for REC opinion is led by the chief investigator for the trial (as described by Regulation 14 of SI 2004/1031), with assistance from the sponsor or delegated external vendor to assist with the completion of the application form.

Article 2 (f) of Directive 2001/20/EC defines the term 'investigator' as:

> 'a doctor or a person following a profession agreed in the Member State for investigations because of the scientific background and the experience in subject care it requires. The investigator is responsible for the conduct of a clinical trial at a trial site. If a trial is conducted by a team of individuals at a trial site, the investigator is the leader responsible for the team and may be called the principal investigator'.

Although the definition of investigator is essentially the same in SI 2004/1031 and Directive 2001/20/EC, the UK regulations do not specifically define the term 'principal investigator', although the title is commonly used to describe the lead investigator at a trial site; therefore in the UK the terms chief investigator and PI can be interchangeable when a clinical trial is conducted at a single site and the chief investigator is the investigator for that site.

The PI is responsible for the conduct of the trial and for the leadership of the trial team at their site, although activities can be delegated to appropriate members of the trial team. As such, it is essential that there is clear, documented evidence of the PI's oversight and involvement in the trial and that the PI is kept appraised of any issues regarding the trial. The following examples are commonly used to provide suitable evidence of that oversight and active trial management:

- acting as the signatory on consent forms (it is not necessary for the PI to take consent for every subject)
- eligibility assessments
- participation in subject visits
- sign-off of completed serious adverse event (SAE) forms
- review of safety information (for example, line listings or suspected unexpected serious adverse reactions (SUSARs) from other sites)
- regular, minuted meetings with the trial team
- emails

- attendance or availability at monitoring visits
- documented review of incoming data (for example, laboratory, electrocardiography (ECG), imaging) in a timely manner
- review of completed CRFs and responses to medical queries
- provision of protocol or specialised training to the team.

A PI must[1] be an authorised healthcare professional; however, they do not have to be a medically qualified doctor, although it should be noted that there are a number of trial-related activities that are required[2] to be performed by a medically qualified doctor (such as eligibility, decision to dose and safety reviews). Therefore if the PI is not a medically qualified doctor, these activities must[2, 3] be formally delegated by the PI to a medically qualified doctor (see section 11.3.4).

The terms 'sub-investigator' or 'co-investigator' are used for authorised healthcare professionals working alongside the PI at a trial site. Examples include other consultants in the unit, nurses, GPs in the same surgery or training-grade doctors such as research fellows or registrars. A sub-investigator or co-investigator may undertake part or all of the PI's activities. The PI must[3] ensure that these individuals are adequately trained and familiar with the protocol, informed of any changes to the protocol and provided with safety information including the investigator's brochure (IB) and all safety updates. New team members who join the trial after the trial has started must[3] also receive training in GCP and the protocol, and be delegated appropriate responsibilities (usually via the delegation log), prior to undertaking these activities.

11.2.2   Other team members

The investigators are supported by a team of professionals responsible for carrying out various aspects of trial activities. Table 11.1 provides a list of job roles and functions that are typically found in a trial site setting. However, the list is not exhaustive and the various functions may be undertaken by the same individual.

11.3   Site set-up

The approach made to an investigator site to participate in a clinical trial is usually made to the health professional intended to become the PI. This approach can be a request from a sponsor based on previous experience of using that site, recommendations from other clinical colleagues, the investigator's or site's specialist expertise, the specific subject population served by the site; or an

Table 11.1 A typical investigator site research team

Role	Typical activities undertaken
Research nurse	Recruitment, consent, screening, subject assessments, investigational medicinal product administration, record keeping
	Case report form entry, facilitating handling of data queries, sample handling (taking and processing of samples, arranging sample storage and shipment)
Trial/study coordinator or data manager	Management of trial documents and data entry (a research nurse may additionally take on the role of trial/study coordinator and therefore the role of trial/study coordinator may perform a wide range of functions)
Pharmacists and/or pharmacy technicians	Investigational medicinal product management: supply ordering, handling, storage, dispensing, accountability and destruction
Technical specialists	Taking X-rays and scans, recording electrocardiograms, performing specialist activities
Laboratory technicians	Handling and processing of routine samples (biochemistry and haematology)
	Handling and processing of trial-specific samples (for example, blood biomarkers, throat swab, nasal lavage)
Specialist assessors	For example, in oncology trials, the radiologist may take on an important role in interpreting scans (such as RECIST score measurement)

RECIST, Response Evaluation Criteria in Solid Tumours

approach can be made after the clinician has expressed an interest in participating in clinical trials as an investigator's site (for example, via a trial-specific website or suggested by a site management organisation).

Once participation has been agreed in principle there is a significant amount of organisational and logistical work involved in order to open the site to recruitment. This may be facilitated to a greater or lesser extent by the sponsor, but all sponsors are reliant on the organisation to provide accurate and realistic information that reflects the subject population available for approach, the research infrastructure at the investigator site, and any site-specific requirements and arrangements that are necessary for running the clinical trial successfully at that site. This information may be assessed via questionnaires returned to the sponsor or by pre-trial selection visits where the information and facilities are reviewed to ensure that they meet the sponsor's requirements.

11.3.1 Required approvals

Before any clinical trial activities can be conducted at a trial site (this includes trial-specific consent and screening; administering an IMP to the subject; trial-specific medical or nursing procedures, or trial-specific tests or analysis), the PI at that site must ensure that all the required approvals are in place.

The sponsor of an IMP clinical trial is required[4, 5] to obtain initial authorisation from the competent authority in the form of a clinical trial authorisation (CTA) and a favourable REC opinion prior to starting the trial. The task of obtaining and maintaining the competent authority approval may be performed by the sponsor themselves or delegated to an individual or organisation, while applying for REC opinion is led by the chief investigator for the trial. These activities are described in detail in Chapters 2 and 3 respectively. The PI will need to ensure that there are processes in place for them to be informed of the trial approval and any subsequent updates to the authorisation as well as the initial and subsequent (as relevant) favourable REC opinion status of the clinical trial.

In addition, it will be necessary to apply for site-specific assessment (SSA) or NHS management permission, depending on the type of site. This is commonly obtained from the organisation's R&D office (NHS hospitals); the Primary Care NHS Trust (GPs); the organisation's management in the case of private facilities; or a REC in the case of private Phase I clinics (see section 3.2.4).

The conduct of the trial can only take place at sites included in the SSA. It is not acceptable to send subjects outside the NHS Trust to have trial-specific samples taken or undergo trial-specific procedures without an SSA applicable to those sites, or an exemption (see section 3.2.4).

PIs should also be aware of any conditions stipulated in the local approval (for example, submission of SAEs and SUSARs within a particular timeframe to the R&D office or the provision of annual update reports). Depending on the wording of the approval letter, non-compliance with these local requirements can affect the approval for the conduct of the trial at that site: that is, the MHRA approval is conditional to obtaining a favourable REC opinion which in itself may be conditional on a local approval. Careful consideration should therefore be given by the departments giving local approval as to any local conditions they impose and by the trial team to ensure that these conditions are met.

Other applications may also be needed – for example, Administration of Radioactive Substances Advisory Committee (ARSAC) certification. Further guidance on the approvals required for a particular trial is available within the Integrated Research Application System (IRAS) which is described in Chapter 3.

Copies of the approval documentation should be obtained by the PI to confirm that all the necessary approvals are in place and retained in the investigator site file (ISF). However, ultimately the check that all these approvals are in place and that the site is authorised to start the trial should be given by the sponsor in writing. See section 1.5.2 for further details on this process.

11

11.3.2 Investigator agreements and contracts

For host investigator sites activities should be formally delegated to the PI by the sponsor and this may be in the form of an investigator agreement or another appropriate document. These usually encompass the clinical activities undertaken by the site for the trial plus any trial-specific responsibilities (see section 1.3.7.2).

A model clinical investigation agreement or clinical trial agreement (mCTA) was developed between the industry and the NHS. NHS Trusts will sign the mCTA if it remains unmodified. If changes are made the NHS Trust may need to obtain an external legal review before signing the contract, which may significantly delay trial start-up. This standard agreement or tripartite agreement (which includes the contract research organisation who may be managing the trial on the sponsor's behalf) is intended to simplify the review and approval process. For further detail please refer to the National Institute for Health Research (NIHR) and Association of the British Pharmaceutical Industry (ABPI) websites.

Bespoke contracts may also be used but generally require extensive review and often lead to identification of deficiencies during inspection due to the contracts not being followed as they contain non-standard requirements which, unless the R&D office or investigator are aware of them, may not be fulfilled. Examples of these deficiencies include failure to notify the sponsor of requested information in the required timeframe (such as status or recruitment updates) and inappropriate sponsor control of the data generated at the investigator site.

If the investigator site subcontracts any part of the work it has agreed to undertake to another organisation then this should be first agreed with the sponsor (and the necessary site-specific approval obtained where necessary – see section 3.2.4) and a contract or service-level agreement put in place prior to the subcontracted work being undertaken. Examples of subcontracted services include imaging conducted by a private facility specifically for the trial or laboratory services provided by another organisation.

In non-commercially sponsored clinical trials, the chief investigator may take on some of the sponsor's responsibilities. Typically these will include pharmacovigilance (assessment and expedited reporting of SUSARs, production and submission of development safety update reports (DSURs)), reporting serious breaches, end-of-trial notification and the production of the clinical study report (CSR) or publication. In all cases, there should be adequate delegation of these tasks to the chief investigator by the sponsor. The delegated responsibilities may be in the form of an investigator agreement or a list of standard responsibilities as a condition of R&D approval usually appended to the approval letters (see Chapter 1 for the sponsor's responsibilities).

11.3.3 Training requirements

Appropriate training must[3] be provided to staff involved in the conduct of clinical trials. The extent of this training will depend on the activities undertaken by that member (or group) of staff. For example, it may be appropriate that some staff only receive an overview of the clinical trial, which could be in the form of a written summary; or they could simply be made aware of the local trial team contacts and have an awareness of, rather than a detailed knowledge of, GCP requirements. Examples of investigator site staff for whom reduced GCP and trial-specific training requirements could be considered include:

- chemotherapy unit nurses involved with the administration of the IMP, but with no additional roles in the trial
- pharmacy staff involved in general dispensing of clinical trial medication under the oversight of a clinical trial pharmacist
- laboratory staff processing routine samples for clinical trial subjects.

It is expected that a named contact within each relevant department is given the opportunity to input into the conduct of the trial at the site; they can then identify potential issues (such as differences between the standard of care and the trial-related procedure) and gain more detailed knowledge of the trial, GCP requirements and links with the trial team. They will then be able to pass on the relevant knowledge to other members of their department as required. Examples of such key staff may include the pharmacy clinical trial lead, or the laboratory or radiology clinical trial contact person. Requirements for training are described further in Chapter 14.

11.3.4   Delegation of tasks

The PI may delegate activities to appropriate members of the research team but must[3] ensure that the member of staff holds the appropriate qualification for the role they are to undertake (that is, medical degree or nursing qualification) and has been provided with appropriate GCP and protocol-specific training as well as any training necessary for the role/activity to be undertaken (that is, informed consent training or use of a particular piece of equipment).

In order to demonstrate that the PI has authorised appropriately trained and qualified individuals to undertake certain trial-related tasks, a delegation of authority log is used at the site. This document may be combined with the site staff signature log, but should clearly state the name of the person, their role and the activities they are delegated by the PI as well as being signed and dated by the PI prior to the activity being undertaken by the individual. It is not acceptable for the PI to simply sign off the delegation log at the end of the trial.

The delegation is not just a paper exercise; it is documented evidence of the appropriate delegation of the investigator's responsibilities. Issues with these logs are commonly seen on inspection. For example:

- The delegation log was reconstructed retrospectively; the dates of entries were not in chronological order. Therefore there was no evidence to demonstrate appropriate delegation prior to tasks being undertaken.

- Key personnel were not listed on the delegation log, including sub-investigators involved in the clinical trial.

- The investigator site file contained logs pre-signed by the PI; therefore anyone could add their name and assign tasks, without appropriate review and delegation.

Large departments (for example, pharmacy, clinical laboratories or chemotherapy units) may have activities delegated by the PI to a named person (for example, clinical trials pharmacist or ward sister) who would then take responsibility for the conduct of that activity by the department. Investigators and these delegates should perform a risk assessment to determine the training requirements for the trial and GCP in relation to the tasks to be performed. For example, a dialysis unit may be involved in a number of trials, where almost all staff are involved in the care of the subjects while on the trial. For most members of staff this will not be any different from their normal duties when subjects come in for dialysis. It may not be practicable to provide large numbers of staff with detailed training in the protocol, or to restrict care to a small number of staff who have received this level of training, as this may be unfeasible for the subjects and the effective running of the department. In these cases it may be appropriate to include GCP training as part of the standard induction training for that role/department, thereby ensuring that all staff have a level of GCP training. This general GCP training must[6] be documented and retained; this could be in a departmental training log or in individuals' training records.

The need for further trial-specific training can be assessed by taking into consideration the tasks performed by the staff and assessing whether these tasks are the same as those performed for standard clinical care (for example, administering chemotherapy). If this is the case, trial-specific training and delegation of responsibilities may not always be required. However, all staff involved in clinical trials must[3, 7] understand the minimum requirements for GCP in relation to record keeping and reporting of deviations and adverse events to the trial team.

When documentation at a department level is required, this is commonly achieved by a departmental authorisation log, signed by the individual authorised by the PI. Evidence must[6] be retained of departmental trial-specific training conducted by the named person to the staff involved in these delegated activities. The retention location can be referred to in the investigator site file.

11.3.5 Team communication

It is essential that effective communication links exist for the dissemination of information to the trial team, but consideration needs to be given to protecting the blinding where necessary. Procedures to manage blinded trials should be put in place in advance of the trial initiation and will define which members of the team have access to unblinded information (for example, pharmacy staff if a randomisation list is used, or a nurse who has to prepare an infusion in theatres from labelled medication) and how records will be segregated to protect the blinding while maintaining appropriate documentation (see section 6.13.4).

It is recommended that consideration is given to how provision of information can be documented. For example, it should be possible to demonstrate that the safety information regularly provided to the PI from the sponsor has been disseminated to the other physicians so they are made aware of the updated information. This could be addressed by the receiving member of staff countersigning CIOMS I forms or other trial-related correspondence; documenting the provision of information within meeting minutes; or sending email confirmation of the reading to the PI or trial coordinator.

Communication with ancillary sites (for example, laboratories or imaging departments) is key to avoid any issues. These sites need to be notified of a subject's participation in a trial so that scans or laboratory results can be appropriately labelled to ensure subject confidentiality (for example, provision of images to a central reader ensuring the subject identifiers have been removed) or the blinding maintained (for example, reporting of trial-related blood results such as platelet values). These sites must[3] also be informed of information relevant to their role within the trial such as protocol amendments or changes to site processes.

11.4 During the study

11.4.1 Patient recruitment

Depending on the type of trial, there are a number of ways in which subjects may be identified for potential entry into the clinical trial. These include:

- identification through knowledge of a subject's pre-existing condition: that is, subjects are identified from a database or from a review of hospital records and then usually followed up by an invitation to attend a clinic to discuss the trial
- discussion during multi-disciplinary team meetings where treatment options are reviewed
- attendance at the clinic, surgery or hospital emergency department undertaking the trial
- subjects responding to advertisements
- support groups for the subjects' condition
- identification and contact of individuals under section 251 of the NHS Act 2006.

There may be an element of pre-screening to ensure that the trial(s) being offered to the subject as potential treatment options are appropriate. This pre-screening may take the form of reviewing the subject's hospital notes and associated imaging and laboratory results. No additional trial-specific screening activities (such as imaging tests or laboratory tests that do not form part of standard of care) must[8] take place until informed consent to participate in the trial is obtained from the subject.

In certain circumstances, potential patients for a clinical trial may be preliminarily identified using data that are anonymised but have a controlled way back to identify the person for recruitment. Many NHS datasets are available in an anonymised format for research, and linkage of these datasets creates a methodology to find subjects who meet certain inclusion and exclusion criteria. Such linkage of data only takes place when justified (and when no other methodology is available) and with the approval of the Ethics and Confidentiality Committee (ECC). The Clinical Practice Research Datalink (CPRD, www.cprd.com) has been set up to allow anonymised NHS clinical data to be linked to enable many types of research, with all required approvals. This work is in conjunction with the research networks of the National Institute for Health Research (NIHR) that has thousands of researchers and clinical trial sites. All identification work with patients is actually done by doctors and other healthcare professionals in the NHS.

After a subject has been identified as suitable for approach regarding a clinical trial, a general discussion about the nature and significance of the trial as well as the risks and implications of participation will take place. This is usually done face to face with the subject within the clinical environment, but examples have been seen where the initial approach is a telephone conversation (following an ethically approved script), followed up by the subject information sheet being posted to the subject. This is appropriate, if transparent in the REC application and granted a favourable opinion.

The level of detail provided in the initial approach may vary, as in some instances detailed discussions may not be considered appropriate: for example, if the introduction to the trial forms part of the consultation where the subject's diagnosis of the condition is presented. However, the intended outcome of the initial approach is always the verbal presentation of trial-related information and the provision of the correct version of the ethically approved subject information sheet to the subject for their further consideration. It should be possible to reconstruct when this provision of information has taken place in order to demonstrate that the subject was given time to consider the trial before informed consent was obtained. This can be in the form of a comment in the subject notes or recorded in a separate log.

11.4.2   Informed consent

Informed consent may be taken by a member of the trial team (for example, investigator, research nurse or non-medical investigator). The individual taking consent must[3] have been delegated this activity, and have undertaken appropriate training both in the specific clinical trial and in obtaining informed consent. The consenting procedures and personnel (that is, those members of the investigator's team who will be performing consent) should be clearly described in the REC application, and a favourable opinion given. It is the responsibility of the investigator to ensure that the approved consenting process is followed at the site. Any substantial changes to the consenting procedure following a favourable opinion must[9] be notified to the REC and a favourable opinion given. Where taking informed consent is the role of someone who is not a medically qualified doctor, it is expected that a medically qualified doctor who is part of the trial team is readily available during or following the consent process if the subject requires or requests further discussion relating to the medical care to be provided as part of the trial.

After the subject has been provided with the subject information sheet and has been given adequate time for consideration and discussion (including further discussions with the medically qualified doctor and research nurse if required) then written informed consent is sought. There are no statutory requirements specifying how long potential subjects should be allowed to consider the trial. This will depend on the need for treatment – for example, the decision to enter into a clinical trial in an emergency setting may need to be made in a very short timeframe – but it should be clearly defined in the REC application.

Informed consent is obtained by revisiting the information provided earlier to ensure that the subject understands the trial, its risks and what participation in the trial will entail. This may be assessed by asking the subject to explain what they understand about aspects of the trial (such as their understanding of the procedures, frequency of visits, dosing requirements, restrictions and possible side effects of the IMP) and by answering any additional questions which may have arisen during the time for consideration. If the person taking consent is satisfied that the subject understands, the subject is then asked to sign and personally date the current version of the approved informed consent form, and to indicate their approval of various statements by initialling against them, assuming that they agree with each statement and that they are freely giving their consent to enter the trial. There should be a process to ensure the appropriate management of any statements that are not consented to, as this may affect the subject's participation in the trial (or part of the trial).

Where mail-based trials are run, identified potential subjects may not necessarily have face-to-face contact with a member of the trial team to perform the consent process and therefore may be mailed the consent forms to sign and send back to the trials centre.

It is not uncommon to include a sub-study in a clinical trial: for example, pharmacokinetic or genetic studies. Subjects are not obliged to participate in these sub-studies and therefore separate informed consent forms may be utilised for the main trial and the sub-study. If the main trial and the sub-study informed consent forms are similar in design, this can lead to errors (such as subjects signing two sub-study informed consent forms but failing to sign consent for the main trial). Making sure the different consent forms can be readily distinguished from each other (for example, using different colours of paper) can avoid such confusion.

It is recommended that investigators also track which subjects have given consent to the sub-studies. This will help ensure that sub-study samples are taken from subjects as required, and that those samples are not taken from subjects and sent for analysis without their consent. Other useful aspects of consent to track are those subjects who have consented to their GP being informed of their participation in the clinical trial and those who have consented to an HIV test being performed.

A positive HIV test may preclude the subject from the trial, but investigators have a duty of care to ensure that clinical care to subjects is provided for. This may include offering counselling to the subjects if the test is found to be positive; informing the GP (if subjects have agreed); or referring subjects to specialist centres.

Occasionally, the investigator's section of the consent form is countersigned by the PI after the date of the consent previously completed by the subject and person obtaining consent. This can demonstrate PI awareness of the consent obtained for this subject. However, if this (or a similar practice) is used for this purpose, it should be stated within the investigator site file or the organisation's quality system for clarity.

There are occasions where trial subjects will be unable to give informed consent (that is, minors, or those with physical or mental incapacity); this requires the conditions and principles described in Parts 1, 3, 4 and 5 of Schedule 1 to SI 2004/1031 to be followed. Further details are given in Chapter 3.

In order to demonstrate that subjects were provided with the most up-to-date information (including safety information) for the trial, it should be clear which version of the subject information sheet subjects had given consent to. Issues can arise if, for example, the informed consent form did not make reference to the version of the subject information sheet and the site did not retain a copy of the subject information sheet given to subjects. It is therefore recommended that a copy of the subject information sheet and informed consent form are kept together in the medical notes, with the originals in the investigator site file. A copy of both these documents should be given to the subject.

Informed consent is an ongoing process for trial subjects. If there are changes to the trial design, the medication used or the risks associated with participation, then subjects may be asked to reconsent if the information constitutes a substantial amendment to the trial. It is common that significant emphasis is placed on obtaining the initial consent, but the process of reconsent may be less well managed. Investigators are advised to take a measured approach to determine which subjects need to be reconsented and which subjects only need to be informed of new developments. For example, subjects near to the end of a trial or those who have completed the end-of-trial visit may not need to consent to any new or revised procedures because they have already gone past certain milestones in the trial. However, they would still need to be informed about any new safety information that may have long-term consequences.

Investigators should reconsent subjects in a timely manner. Examples have been seen where subjects have not been approached for reconsent for more than 12 months following the update of a subject information sheet, even though they had attended site visits on many occasions in that period. It is generally expected that subjects are reconsented at the next visit defined in the protocol, following the update (and favourable opinion) of the subject information sheet. Careful consideration should be given when the durations between visits are long, as once a visit is missed investigators may not see the subject for many months. Investigators may also consider contacting subjects to arrange an unscheduled visit when new safety information has come to light that may affect the subjects' willingness to remain in the clinical trial.

It is recommended that the investigator site track the consent status of each subject when a new version of the subject information sheet/informed consent form is implemented, to ensure all those required are reconsented in a timely manner.

Where the sponsor or an investigator instigates an urgent safety measure to protect the subjects of a trial against any immediate hazard to their health or safety (see section 2.3.7), subjects must[10] be given the option to reconsent to continue in the trial with the modified trial procedures or withdraw from the trial. The rationale for the urgent safety measure should be made available to the subjects; reasons may include new safety information, the steps taken or new procedures required to minimise the risks to the subjects. This information may be initially presented in an unapproved subject information sheet or as a letter to the subjects. Investigators should provide this written information to the subjects and document the discussion in the medical notes. In addition, subjects may be asked to sign an unapproved consent form to document their consent to continue to participate in the trial in light of the new information.

Consideration should also be given to what actions would need to be taken in the event that a subject withdraws consent for their data to be used or for their samples to be analysed (see section 3.3.5).

11.4.3 Screening and eligibility

Once the subject has consented to the trial, then trial-specific screening activities may commence. A full medical history, a full medical examination and additional laboratory tests and imaging may be undertaken to determine whether the subject is eligible for entry into the clinical trial. The results must[11] be compared to the inclusion and exclusion criteria and any other requirements or restrictions (for example, wash-out periods and prohibited medications) as defined in the approved protocol and this review should be documented prior to confirming the subject is eligible. It is sometimes seen on inspection that subjects have been entered into the trial before the laboratory/ECG results required to confirm their eligibility were available (and subsequently found to be ineligible after trial enrolment and dosing) or without there being evidence of a medical review of these results beforehand.

The decision whether a subject is eligible for entry into the clinical trial is considered to be a medical decision and therefore must[2] be made by a medically qualified doctor. Part 2 (11) of Schedule 1 to SI 2004/1031 states that:

'The medical care given to, and medical decisions made on behalf of, subjects shall always be the responsibility of an appropriately qualified doctor or, when appropriate, of a qualified dentist.'

This decision should be clearly documented in the medical notes or CRF and signed by the medically qualified doctor making the decision, prior to dosing of the subject. At a minimum, the notes or CRF should contain a statement similar to 'This subject meets the inclusion criteria and none of the exclusion criteria and is therefore eligible for entry into the XXX trial'. If the medical decision for entry is within the CRF, it should also be reflected in the medical notes. The statement in the notes could be made by any healthcare professional (for example, the research nurse) if it is clear that the decision has been made by a medically qualified doctor. For example, the medically qualified doctor may sign off the eligibility assessment page in the CRF. The information used to make this decision must[12] be present in the medical notes or other available medical records. Where necessary, there should be documentation to support results which either require interpretation (for example, laboratory tests if the protocol does not state defined acceptance criteria) or a response by the investigator's team in relation to statements of clinical significance.

Protocol waivers are not acceptable as no person must[11] conduct a clinical trial otherwise than in accordance with the protocol, and sponsors should ensure that these requests are rejected (see section 1.3.5.1). A protocol waiver occurs when the sponsor (or delegate) gives approval for a subject to enter into the trial although the subject does not meet the eligibility criteria as defined in the approved protocol. Waivers seen on inspection include the age of subjects being outside the inclusion criteria or laboratory values being outside the stated acceptance criteria (but considered to be not clinically significant). If there are problems with recruiting subjects into the trial due to restrictive inclusion and exclusion criteria, then consideration should be given to amending the protocol.

Re-screening may be justified when investigators believe the elevation of some laboratory parameters to be an anomaly or if the cause of the elevation has been identified (for example, an infection) and the abnormality was only temporary. However, it is unacceptable to screen the subject repeatedly in order to meet the eligibility parameters. It is recommended that guidance be provided by the sponsor regarding the acceptable extent and conditions for re-screening.

Once the subject is deemed eligible for entry into the trial then a statement of participation should be entered into the subject notes stating that the subject is taking part in a clinical trial and providing appropriate trial identifiers. This permits other researchers to identify previous participation in clinical trials as this may be prohibited by future trials. It should also allow other treating healthcare professionals to be informed that their subject is on a clinical trial, and where to obtain additional information. Commonly, hospital records are marked in some way to permit easy identification by other hospital staff and to assist in appropriate long-term retention.

11.4.4   Ongoing medical oversight

Investigators should be closely involved in ongoing subject management throughout the course of the trial. This may include physical examinations, handling of adverse events and trial-specific assessments at key time points as defined in the protocol. The medical review of any subject assessments (for example, laboratory reports or ECGs) should be clearly documented. Abnormal laboratory parameters should be reviewed and clinically significant events should be recorded and reported when necessary. Abnormal values considered to be not clinically significant should also be documented to demonstrate the investigator's oversight. This may take the form of signing and dating print-outs of laboratory reports and ECGs, records in paper or electronic medical notes, and CRF pages.

In addition to routine safety monitoring, the protocol may prescribe certain courses of action when certain safety parameters have been breached. For example, reduction in the glomerular filtration rate (GFR) or neutrophil count will usually require a delay in treatment, stopping treatment or dose reduction in some oncology studies. A number of serious findings were observed on inspection because investigators either ignored, neglected or were unaware of the stopping rules; subjects had suffered serious adverse events as a consequence.

Sometimes the REC or competent authority may stipulate additional safety monitoring requirements and it is important researchers are aware of these requirements. For example, in a trial reviewed on inspection, the REC required researchers to remain at the subjects' home for an hour post-dosing, but on a number of occasions researchers left five minutes after subjects had been dosed.

The subject's GP should be notified of their participation at the outset of a clinical trial, if the subject has consented to this. This is particularly important when subjects are recruited through advertisements, rather than referred via another healthcare professional. Investigators may want to confirm eligibility with the GP in writing in relation to subjects' past medical history, prohibited medication and any previous (or ongoing) participation in clinical trials. In addition, it is invaluable for GPs to be aware of their patients' participation, as they may need to be aware of known contraindications or potential side effects. There may also be prohibited medication that the GP may need to avoid prescribing for concurrent or unexpected illnesses (for example, infections).

11.4.5 Equipment and facilities

It is important that the facilities used for the recruitment and treatment of subjects are appropriate for the work to be undertaken. For example, some optometry tests require control of the light level under which the test is conducted and the six-minute walk test has some very specific requirements.

In addition to the facilities, the equipment to be used should be fit for purpose and as such there must[6, 7, 12] be records to demonstrate the calibration and maintenance of equipment used to measure trial parameters (for example, scales, spirometer, DEXA scanner), equipment essential in crash trolleys (for example, a defibrillator), and equipment used for the processing of samples (for example, centrifuges, refrigerators and freezers). It is recommended that, when the software associated with equipment is updated by suppliers, checks are performed to ensure that the results obtained on that piece of equipment after the update would be equivalent to the results obtained before the update.

The outputs from this equipment may be important in several respects; for example, for determining eligibility (ECG, scales, CT scanner), for ongoing safety (ECG), for efficacy end-points (CT scanner), and for protection of IMP or sample integrity (temperature data loggers, refrigerators and freezers). Therefore care must[12] be taken to protect the safety of the subjects and the integrity of the trial data. Issues that have been observed on inspection with regard to equipment include:

* Expired collection tubes and consumables were used in the trial and therefore the validity of the samples could not be assured.
* Monitoring and testing equipment was not recalibrated or retested according to the manufacturers' recommendations (for example, thermometer, centrifuges, ECG equipment).
* Apparatus for ascertaining efficacy end-points was not calibrated or serviced (for example, treadmill for walk test); therefore the validity of the results could not be assured.

- There was an absence of monitoring records for freezer temperature for pharmacokinetic (PK) samples, therefore it was not possible to demonstrate the integrity of the samples.

11.4.6   Prescribing of study medication

Prescribing of trial medication is conducted by medically qualified doctors, although prescribing by consultant nurses and supplementary prescribers is permitted subject to the delegation of this activity by the PI and it being permitted by the host organisation. There are many ways that IMP can be prescribed for use. Usual methods include paper prescriptions, electronic prescribing systems (such as those used to prescribe chemotherapy, for example) and interactive response technologies (IRT)-led prescribing. However, a record in the subject's medical notes, clinical trial worksheet or CRF by the investigator (or appropriate delegated prescriber) is also acceptable. Prescribing of trial medication is further described in Chapter 6.

It is essential that the records supporting the provision of IMP permit the reconstruction of the IMP accountability as issues may arise if it is not possible to demonstrate that the subject received the correct IMP, at the correct dose, at the correct time point. The documentation generated in relation to IMP can be considered as part of the risk assessment and may be suitable for adapting on the basis of risk. However, the decision to dose a subject should be clearly documented and consideration should be given to including this in the hospital notes in addition to the prescription.

Counselling on the medication to be taken is especially important for subjects taking part in clinical trials. The level of counselling will depend on the medication and the complexity of the trial, but consideration should be given to ensuring the subject is aware of directions for taking the medication, the differences between strengths of medication (if multiple strengths are given to permit dose titration) and the importance of returning unused medication at each visit. In addition, provision of compliance worksheets or treatment schedules may be considered if the treatment regimen is complicated or multiple tablets are to be taken.

Where unused IMP is returned to the site by the subject, a process should be implemented for the timely review of the returns (if necessary, by the pharmacy department in order to maintain trial blinding) to ensure, where multiple strengths or multiple IMPs have been supplied, that the correct medication at the correct strength has been taken and to check the subject's compliance with the treatment regimen. The unused IMP should be segregated from undispensed medication until permission for its return or destruction is received from the sponsor. If issues are discovered with the medication returned, then these should be notified to the PI immediately so that action can be taken as necessary.

11.4.7   Adverse events

Adverse events should be recorded in the medical notes either by the investigators or by the research nurse. This information is then transcribed onto a CRF adverse event form (if required by the protocol) which will require the assessment of seriousness and causality for each adverse event. If a signature of the investigator is not required on this form, investigators should endorse the relevant CRF page (if transcription has been performed by the nurse) or record the seriousness and causality assessments in the medical notes. Care must be taken when the adverse event form is amended after it has been signed off by the investigator; any changes are expected to be endorsed by the medically qualified doctor to document their agreement with the change.

Serious adverse event (SAE) reporting should follow a robust process to ensure that reporting of SAEs to the sponsor is timely (that is, within 24 hours of the trial team's awareness of the event) and complete, and that decisions regarding causality can be clearly attributed to a medically qualified doctor. It is common for the paperwork associated with reporting an SAE to be completed by a trial coordinator or research nurse; investigators are, however, expected to document their approval by signing the SAE form. It is also recommended that the site clearly documents when it was made aware of the SAE.

For a single subject, there may be multiple sets of notes for different departments or different hospitals, depending on the various treatments at different locations. The investigator needs to consider all of these sources in terms of available information recorded and develop a process to ensure they are checked during the subject's participation in the trial so that the investigator is informed of any adverse events in a timely manner. For example:

- In GP practices, the subjects may report adverse events to a locum or their own GP (when the investigators are not the subjects' GPs) or the subjects may be admitted to a hospital and the discharge letter is received by the GP surgery and uploaded by an administrator. Under these circumstances, it is expected that the investigators will be informed immediately. This could be achieved by flagging up in the electronic health record to alert the investigators of any events occurring to a trial subject.

- A clinical trial may take place in a large NHS Trust with a number of hospital sites. Subjects may be managed by other specialities within the NHS Trust for concurrent illnesses (for example, an oncology subject may be referred to a cardiologist located at a different hospital within the same NHS Trust). In addition, some intensive therapy units may have their own set of drug charts and medical notes. The investigators should establish a process to ensure that they are informed of any unplanned hospital admissions (for example, admission to the hospital emergency department; the instructions in the medical record can alert the emergency department staff to inform the investigator).

When subjects are recruited by a site management organisation (SMO) or a hospital through advertisements, subjects' GPs should be informed of their patients' participation in a clinical trial (if consent is given for this) to allow them to alert the investigators to any adverse events.

For further information on adverse events refer to Chapter 5.

11.4.8 Contact details and out-of-hours arrangements

There are a number of methods by which trial subjects are provided with the contact details of the research team, including wallet-sized subject cards and information contained on the site-specific sections of the subject information sheet. This information permits the subject to contact site staff in the event of questions arising or to notify them of adverse events or issues that have arisen. This information may also be used if the subject is seen at another hospital (for example, in an emergency situation), to access additional information about the trial or to access code-breaking processes. It is therefore imperative that systems are in place to facilitate this contact. The three most commonly used methods of contact are described below:

- **Investigator's office number** This number is suitable during hours when the office is manned, but arrangements should be in place to forward the call to an alternative number or to provide additional contact details on the voicemail.
- **Ward or switchboard landline number** This arrangement has the benefit of the number being permanently manned. However, arrangements need to be made to ensure that staff taking the call are aware of the trial and the out-of-hours arrangements, and either have access to trial information so that the call

can be handled appropriately (this may be suitable if there is a large trial team providing 24-hour coverage), or hold trial team personal contact information. There should be alternative back-up contacts if the nominated person(s) are unavailable.

- **Trial-specific or personal mobile phones and pagers** These are commonly used, but care should be taken that an appropriate voicemail message is left, as described above. If callers are asked to leave a message rather than being referred onwards to an alternative contact (for example, how long to await a call-back before trying an alternative contact) then frequent checks for received calls should be made by the mobile phone holder.

Whichever system is used for cover, it should be assessed and tested accordingly to ensure that the chain of contact functions as intended.

Out-of-hours arrangements for trials that are hospital based, such as in an oncology unit, tend to be routinely challenged on a daily basis and subjects are usually well trained to contact their trial team out of hours if they become unwell after they have received a course of chemotherapy. Higher-risk areas are when the out-of-hours arrangements are not routinely used and the medically qualified doctors responsible for the out-of-hours service are not familiar with the trial (for example, where out-of-hours cover for a GP surgery is contracted out to a third-party provider). Investigators and sponsors need to assess the suitability of these out-of-hours service providers prior to use. Another additional factor for determining frequency and extent of out-of-hours arrangements is whether the trial is blinded or open. The process for unblinding should be clearly defined and tested when non-trial personnel are involved in providing out-of-hours medical cover.

Appropriate arrangements should also be in place to ensure that there is cover for those staff who are travelling (and therefore may not have access to the information and systems required), and for staff who are on holiday or on sick leave, to ensure that access to the trial team and code-breaking arrangements are maintained at all times.

11.4.9 Emergency code breaking

There are various methods available for the unblinding of trial subjects should this become necessary in an emergency: for example, to manage the treatment of a subject following an SAE. Most of these methods are dependent on the investigator site to manage the process, although back-up arrangements may exist through the sponsor. Prior to initiating the blinded clinical trial at their site, the PI should therefore ensure that a robust unblinding process has been implemented; that either the code breaks are on site in a designated place or working access codes for the IRT have been provided; and that all staff involved in the trial and process are aware of the arrangements. Consideration should be given to testing the code-break process if it involves a number of steps or staff (this testing is sometimes combined with the testing of the out-of-hours process). Any testing must[6] be documented and retained as evidence that it took place, and either that it is satisfactory, or if not, that corrective action has taken place.

Examples of code breaks include a master list held by the pharmacy; code-break envelopes; scratch-off panels on medication containers; or electronic availability via the IRT system. Some sponsors prefer to be contacted prior to performing the code break; however, the sponsor should not be able to delay or refuse the investigator's request to break the blinding if the investigator (or treating medically qualified doctor) deems it necessary for the management of a subject. On inspection, examples of this practice have been seen that had the potential to jeopardise the safety of the subject. Where IRT is used to perform the code break, the PI and other staff delegated with the code-break activity should ensure that they have accessed the IRT system prior to receipt of the IMP to determine that they hold the correct access level. These staff are advised to have the number of the IRT helpdesk readily available as this may be needed if the automated process does not work.

If a code break is needed to permit the appropriate medical management of a subject, the reason for the code break and the circumstances should be clearly documented (for example, in the hospital notes, in code-break envelopes, in the IRT system or on a specific form) and communicated to the PI and sponsor at the earliest opportunity. Care should be taken to limit the knowledge of the randomisation arm the subject was assigned to, in case this could affect the blinding of other subjects or future trial assessment of the subject (for example, analysis of samples or scoring of questionnaires, categorising of adverse events).

11.4.10 Handling of laboratory samples

Investigator sites routinely take blood and tissue samples from trial subjects, process, store and then pack and ship the samples to local and central laboratories. Sample processing and handling may be defined in the protocol or in a laboratory manual.

Testing of routine safety samples such as biochemistry and haematology is often done at the local laboratory. However, in some trials sponsors may prefer to send these samples to a central laboratory, for example to preserve the blinding of a trial, or to ensure consistency in reporting results. Care should be taken to prevent sending these samples to the local laboratory by mistake. In some cases, this may unblind the treatment of the subject when the unblinded results are made available to the investigator. When a local laboratory is used it is important to indicate clearly that the samples come from a trial subject. This enables the local laboratory to report the results or adverse events promptly.

Samples must[11] be taken according to protocol requirements. For example, for pharmacokinetic (PK) trials it is important that samples are taken at specific time points such as pre-dose and at specified times post-dose, in line with predicted PK parameters such as C_{max}. Sampling kits are often provided by the sponsors and should be stored in an appropriate environment and reviewed to ensure kits remain in date. Care should be taken to ensure the correct collection method is used and the handling process is followed: for example, standing time, centrifuge time and speed, and storage of the sample. For PK or safety samples it is important to record the stages in the processing, so that if there are anomalies in the results, the processing of the samples can be reviewed to rule out any potential processing issues. Sample tubes must[13] be labelled with trial subject identity rather than subjects' names and hospital numbers, to prevent any breaches of subject confidentiality.

Samples are usually stored in clinics or a local laboratory temporarily before shipment to the central laboratory. Storage temperatures should be according to trial-specific requirements and it is expected that the storage temperature will be monitored.

Complex manipulations may be required for certain studies and records should be maintained for calibration of equipment, preparation of the reagents and processes used. For example, the preparation of peripheral blood mononuclear cells (PBMC) for immunological assays involves isolation, cryopreservation and thawing of the specimens, which requires the preparation of a number of reagents, the use of specialist equipment and a number of key processes. The site staff must[3] be trained to perform the task, prepare the reagents and document key steps of each process.

11.5   Study documentation

Appropriate documentation is an essential part of any clinical trial as it supports the work undertaken and permits the reconstruction of the trial. Essential documentation is covered throughout this guide. This section covers documentation generated at the investigator site (that is, source documentation and its transcription) rather than that provided by the sponsor.

ICH GCP defines source documentation as *'Original documents, data, and records (for example, hospital records, clinical and office charts, laboratory notes, memoranda, subjects' diaries or evaluation checklists, pharmacy dispensing records, recorded data from automated instruments, copies or transcriptions certified after verification as being accurate copies, microfiches, photographic negatives, microfilm or magnetic media, X-rays, subject files, and records kept at the pharmacy, at the laboratories and at medico-technical departments involved in the clinical trial).'*

These documents contain source data which are defined in ICH GCP as *'All information in original records and certified copies of original records of clinical findings, observations, or other activities in a clinical trial necessary for the reconstruction and evaluation of the trial. Source data are contained in source documents (original records or certified copies).'*

Clinical information is required by Part 2 (9) to Schedule 1 of SI 2004/1031 to *'be recorded, handled and stored in such a way that it can be accurately reported, interpreted and verified, while the confidentiality of records of the trial subjects remains protected'.*

Clinical trial data originate from a variety of sources. Past medical history is readily available for subjects recruited at GP sites from their medical records. Where subjects are recruited via general advertisements and the investigator is not the primary care provider, past medical history will need to be obtained from the subject and the record of this may be the only source document available for the eligibility assessment. However, this could be subsequently verified by other means; for example, by the subject's GP.

Laboratory data, CT scans and reports are kept centrally within hospital computer systems and are therefore retrievable when necessary, while keeping in mind that the investigators need to demonstrate their assessment of these reports during the course of the trial. Similarly, records of drug administration could be accessed from different sources: for example, a drug chart, an infusion chart, a pharmacy worksheet, electronic prescribing and dispensing records. If these records are adequately maintained and archived as well as being readily retrievable, a separate manual record may not be additionally required.

It is the responsibility of the PI and trial team to maintain the ISF with all appropriate documents. See Chapter 10 for details on what should be included in the ISF. Investigators should consider documents, records and notes that are relevant for assessing eligibility and adverse event/SAE, ongoing subject management and efficacy data, and supporting documents to demonstrate integrity of the IMP and samples. These documents may be maintained by different departments and at different locations within the hospital. Care should be taken to avoid duplication and accidental destruction that might prevent the reconstruction of the trial data.

11.5.1   Source data

Subject notes and hospital records may exist in paper or electronic format or be a combination of both (in accordance with the hospital or health centre policy). Any format used should permit the reconstruction of the clinical care given to the subject and describe subject-specific significant events that have occurred during the conduct of the trial.

It is recommended that:

- All entries are completed contemporaneously or are the transcription of audio recordings made during/immediately after the consultation with the subject.
- All entries are signed and dated by the person making the entry. This could be a wet-ink signature or an appropriately controlled electronic signature. If retrospective entries or annotations are made then this should be obvious, and they should be signed and dated with the date the entries were added (electronic entries should have clear audit trails).
- All entries include details of staff involved in the consultation and are countersigned where decisions have been made by staff other than the person making the entry. For example, if a nurse is making the entry and it is decided that the dose should be amended then this should be countersigned by the physician making that decision.

Examples of key events to be recorded in the subject notes include:

- provision of the subject information sheet/invitation to consider trial

- obtaining informed consent
- eligibility decision and any required supporting information not available elsewhere within the notes
- randomisation or trial entry
- trial visits or follow-up phone calls required by the protocol
- treatment and dosing decisions, including changes to concomitant medication
- any trial-related decisions relating to the clinical care of the subject
- adverse events (recommended to include seriousness, causality, severity)
- withdrawal, termination or end-of-trial involvement including any protocol-defined follow-up.

In rare situations, the source document may come from a source outside the investigator site. For example, in trials of emergency situations, where the onset of head injury or aneurysm may be vital for eligibility assessment, the limit for the commencement of treatment from the start of injury is defined in the protocol. Under these circumstances, the ambulance records (which include pick-up time and time of onset of disease) are vital to the trial.

Sometimes investigator sites are provided with trial-specific source worksheets or labels to facilitate the recording of trial-specific information in the subject's notes and therefore these should be retained within the notes. If an organisation does not allow the retention of these within the subject notes, the use of any additional tools should be reconsidered in order to minimise potential duplication. The notes should still clearly document the subject's clinical care. Investigators should be aware that there should only be one set of source data for a clinical trial. The definition of the source data should be agreed with the sponsor and documented at the site initiation or in the form of a source data agreement unless it is clearly defined in the protocol.

Care should be taken to minimise duplicate sets of notes and these should be combined as soon as possible. The trial team should be aware whether hospital notes are split within the organisation (for example, department-specific subject notes such as haematology/oncology, nurse-specific notes) and ensure that these are available for periodic review (including during the eligibility decision) to identify any adverse events or events that may need to be recorded or reported. Previous volumes of notes should be reviewed before the eligibility decision is taken.

11.5.2   Electronic health records

Electronic health records (EHR) are commonly used in GP practices as well as some hospitals. Hospitals and GP sites should therefore implement procedures that allow for read-only access for research purposes by monitors, auditors and inspectors, with access restricted to trial subject data. Some investigator site organisations have already started to develop systems that allow these authorised personnel to access data on subjects enrolled in clinical trials.

However, it is acknowledged that on occasions when EHRs are used as source data, it is possible that monitors may not have direct access to the system for reasons of confidentiality. In these circumstances, monitors and inspectors may only have direct access with the supervision of site personnel. However, this can be time-consuming for both parties. An option may be for the site to print out a paper copy of the subjects' case notes for the monitor to review. Where these records are printed out it is recommended that site personnel sign and date the print-outs to verify that they are a certified copy of the electronic records and also that they represent the complete, chronological set of notes. It has been observed on inspection that a paper print-out omitted information that was contained in the EHR.

The electronic record may be updated retrospectively to include omitted information or input from an external source (for example, hospital discharge letters). As a result, the monitor may not be aware that what they have reviewed has been modified. Therefore, there should be a process for retaining the previous print-outs, as these will serve as an audit trail (by comparing older versions against the latest print-outs).

Any new information that is added retrospectively for a particular visit or date to the subjects' medical notes (whether these are paper or electronic) must show when the entry was made and by whom, so that the documentation provides an audit trail of the events.

The disadvantage of an EHR system is that the investigator and the research nurse may be in the same consulting room, with only one person able to log onto the subject record at any one time, making contemporaneous notes while the subject is there. It is therefore not always possible for investigators to demonstrate their involvement and input into clinical decisions and assessment of adverse events when the record shows that entries are made by the research nurse. The site should design a process to address this shortcoming. For example, investigators may endorse the decision by logging into the system using their own password at the end of each consultation.

Electronic images of radiographs, CT scans or other forms of electronic data that are relevant to a clinical trial are treated as source data. Care must[12] be taken when data are stored in a workstation (or other stand-alone computer) to ensure that the data are not subject to change or adulteration, or corrupted or deleted accidentally. In one example seen on inspection, the output from an R-R interval measuring device was in a Word document format and the data were stored in a workstation and backed up on the investigator's USB memory stick. There was therefore potential for the data to be edited in an uncontrolled manner. On another occasion, scan images were kept on a workstation for weeks and subject identifiers, dates and types of scan were editable. Consideration must[12] be given to the control of these data files to protect unauthorised changes and back-up of these stand-alone systems to prevent accidental corruptions or deletion.

Many advanced workstations allow images to be imported from external sources, such as when subjects are seen and scans taken at a referral hospital, or when photographs are used to assess wound healing, where assessment may be visual and subjective. These images are imported and editable, therefore some control must[12] be in place to ensure they are not modified. In some trials, the source data may be an image or diagram that is then evaluated, usually subjectively, in some way to generate a numeric value that is related to the end-point of the trial and thus analysed. Examples include radioactive scans of the digestive system showing dispersal of an IMP and tracings/photographs of skin lesions. These images are the source data and must[6] be retained, with the ability to view as the original image: for example, an image should not be saved at such a low resolution that reconstruction of the evaluation is impossible. If the evaluation involves annotation of the image, for example, then this documentation should also be retained to form part of the audit trail from source data to the end-point numerical value.

In addition, images taken on a particular date may or may not be transferred to the picture archiving and communication (PAC) system immediately, which could lead to an issue with back-up as well as the possibility that the data are corruptible.

The editing function also enables site operators to edit the image by removing the subject identifiers and inserting subject numbers before the image files are transferred to a sponsor. Quality control processes should be implemented to ensure the correct re-labelling of these images.

Further guidance on the use of electronic health records is available in the EMA GCP Inspectors Working Group paper, 'Reflection paper on expectations for electronic source data and data transcribed to electronic data collection tools in clinical trials' (EMA/INS/GCP/454280/2010).

11.5.3   Worksheets and case report forms

Worksheets, paper CRFs and electronic CRFs (eCRFs) should be completed in a timely manner (this may be during the consultation with the subject if they are used as source documentation). The records should:

- be legible
- be complete (following the CRF guideline)
- reflect data present on the source documentation
- clearly indicate if changes have been made (these changes should be initialled, dated and explained where necessary)
- be approved by the PI or delegated member of staff upon completion (this may be per page or per CRF dependent on the CRF template used).

There are situations where trial-specific observations or tests are not performed routinely on site and therefore, to facilitate data collection, a worksheet for each visit might be warranted to avoid missing data. This may be particularly important for studies with high throughput and time-dependent data requirements such as hourly PK blood sampling or vital signs in an intensive therapy unit setting. A worksheet may be provided by the sponsor or prepared by the site team. In all instances, consideration should be given to version control to ensure that any worksheets used are updated in line with amendments to the protocol (eligibility criteria, additional efficacy data points). When worksheets are used as source data, they must[6] be retained; and they can be held in the subject file, if hospital policy allows.

With the increased use of electronic data capture (EDC) processes, data entry is often performed by the site staff. Refer to Chapter 8 for principles to consider when performing data entry and when using eCRFs.

11.5.4   Documentation of decisions

Key decisions and discussions relating to the clinical care of subjects as well as management of the trial must[6] be adequately documented throughout the course of the trial, and retained. Ideally, the documentation will include the rationale behind the decision and allow reconstruction of the decision-making process (for example, by attaching correspondence and meeting minutes). Key decisions and discussions may include:

- treatment decisions, that is, dose escalation or reduction; treatment breaks due to toxicity
- implementation of an urgent safety measure
- disagreements with a sponsor regarding substantiality of an amendment or whether an issue constitutes a serious breach or not
- rationale to support why a course of action was taken, especially if the action is not defined in the protocol
- implementation and training of amendments to the trial team
- communication with support departments
- training of new members of the team.

11.5.5   Supporting documentation

The PI should ensure that processes are in place for the collection and retention of supporting documentation to ensure that the trial files when archived are 'stand-alone'. This does not mean that duplicate copies of centralised documentation needs to be retained (for example, IMP temperature records or staff training records), but it should be clear within the ISF that these records are held centrally and can be requested.

Care should be taken to ensure that meeting minutes are recorded and retained where trial specifics are discussed. These meeting minutes may cover discussions for a number of clinical trials sponsored by different organisations and clinical management of non-trial subjects. A local procedure may be needed to determine how these discussions are recorded and filed, and how monitors could review these documents.

Examples of supporting documentation may include:

- relevant emails and other correspondence
- equipment records (including maintenance and calibration)
- temperature records
- staff training records
- non-trial-specific meeting minutes where aspects of the trial were discussed.

Refer to Chapter 10 for further details on the retention and management of essential documents for a trial.

11.6   Chapter legislative references

Throughout this chapter, specific terminology – 'must', 'required' or 'requirement' – has been used to interpret activities that are legislative requirements. These terms have been number-coded in the text where used, and the corresponding reference in the legislation can be found below.

11

1. Regulation 2 of SI 2004/1031
2. Schedule 1, Part 2 (11) of SI 2004/1031
3. Schedule 1, Part 2 (2) of SI 2004/1031
4. Regulation 12 of SI 2004/1031
5. Regulation 13 of SI 2004/1031
6. Regulation 31A (4) of SI 2004/1031
7. Schedule 1, Part 2 (4) of SI 2004/1031
8. Article 3 of Directive 2001/20/EC
9. Regulation 24 of SI 2004/1031
10. Schedule 1, Part 2 (1) of SI 2004/1031
11. Regulation 29 of SI 2004/1031
12. Schedule 1, Part 2 (9) of SI 2004/1031
13. Schedule 1, Part 2 (13) of SI 2004/1031

Phase I clinical trials

12

Editor's note

Phase I clinical trials represent the first stage of the clinical programme. In the UK, Phase I clinical trials are usually conducted in dedicated Phase I units; however, they may also be conducted at site management organisations, non-commercial clinical research facilities or hospitals (NHS and privately owned). Since 2007 UK Phase I units have had the option of being accredited by the Voluntary MHRA Phase I Accreditation Scheme (hereinafter the 'Scheme',) which aims to give assurance that units within the Scheme meet satisfactory standards for avoiding harm to clinical trial subjects and for handling medical emergencies should they arise. This chapter will primarily focus on the requirements of the Scheme but will also cover expectations of those units not currently in the Scheme.

This chapter should be read in conjunction with Chapter 11 which provides an overview of the principles involved in conducting clinical trials from the perspective of an investigator site. Reference should also be made to available European Medicines Agency (EMA) guidance on first in human (FIH) clinical trials and readers may also find the Association of the British Pharmaceutical Industry (ABPI) guidelines on the subject helpful.

12.1   Introduction to Phase I clinical trials

Phase I clinical trials tend to be performed in a small number of healthy volunteers. However, there may be situations where the investigational medicinal product (IMP) is first tested in patients with the disease for which the IMP is being developed – for example, IMPs for the treatment of cancers – where administering an IMP to healthy volunteers would be considered unethical due to the anticipated risk–benefit profile of the product.

The majority of Phase I trials have different risk factors from later-phase trials, as the sponsor and investigator will have little or no experience of the IMP in humans. The healthy volunteers or subjects participating in these clinical trials are not expected to receive any therapeutic benefit from the IMP and therefore these trials are also referred to as 'non-therapeutic' trials. However, some clinical trials may be referred to as Phase I clinical trials because the trial subjects are healthy volunteers even though the IMP is already authorised. These trials may also be conducted when the sponsor wishes to explore different formulations or routes of administration in an authorised product, or conduct a bioequivalence/bioavailability trial.

The purpose of a Phase I clinical trial is usually to establish:

- if the IMP is safe in humans (within the anticipated therapeutic dose range)
- what the body does to the IMP (pharmacokinetics)
- early indicators of effectiveness (preliminary assessment of pharmacodynamics or biomarkers).

There are various types of Phase I clinical trials, but the clinical development process begins with the IMP being given for the first time to healthy volunteers (or patients, where appropriate); these are known as 'first in human' (FIH) clinical trials. The IMP is usually administered in single doses of increasing amounts and the subjects are not expected to derive any therapeutic benefit from the IMP.

The FIH clinical trial is likely to be followed by several additional Phase I clinical trials: for example, multiple ascending dose trials, food effect trials, and trials related to specific genders or age. Sometimes, these various types of trials are combined into one protocol. However, this has its own risks and consideration should be given to clear stopping criteria and interim analysis of the data before progressing to the next phase of the trial.

Other types of Phase I trials include bioequivalence and bioavailability trials. These are generally associated with the authorisation of generic compounds and are used to test the comparability of the new 'test' product against the licensed innovator or 'reference product'.

Some FIH trials may be administering a novel compound, which requires a review by the Clinical Trials Expert Advisory Group (CTEAG) (see section 2.5), as these compounds are thought to carry a 'higher risk' as the outcome of administering the IMP cannot be entirely predicted through animal models.

12.2   Voluntary MHRA Phase I Accreditation Scheme

12.2.1   Background

The profile of Phase I clinical trials, and in particular FIH clinical trials, was raised following the TGN1412 incident in March 2006, where six clinical trial subjects became seriously ill and were admitted to an intensive therapy unit. Following the incident, an expert scientific group (ESG) was set up to review Phase I clinical trials. The ESG made a number of recommendations, one of them being that a national voluntary accreditation scheme be established for units conducting Phase I clinical trials in the UK, in order to maximise subject safety and to create additional public confidence in the regulatory oversight of Phase I clinical trials.

In response the MHRA developed the 'Voluntary MHRA Phase I Accreditation Scheme', which has resulted in formalised routine inspections with an increased scope and depth, exceeding the legislative requirements and providing the public, researchers, the MHRA and research ethics committees (RECs) with more information about the units wanting to conduct these types of trials.

12.2.2   Operation of the Scheme

The Scheme operates on a voluntary basis. Applicants are required to complete and submit a detailed application form to the MHRA GCP Inspectorate. After reviewing this form, the MHRA GCP Inspectorate will perform an inspection of the unit. Once any necessary corrective and preventative actions have been implemented and reviewed (including supporting evidence) the unit is issued with an accreditation certificate, which contains an expiry date. A re-inspection is performed before a renewal of the certificate is granted. Units are required to submit any significant changes to the MHRA GCP Inspectorate for continued assessment. Significant changes are those that affect the basis upon which the accreditation was granted. For example:

- relocation, refurbishment or addition of facilities (for example, extension of the existing unit, permanent use of facilities at another location)
- changes in key personnel (usually those listed on the accreditation certificate, but there may be others who are key to attaining and maintaining the Scheme's requirements such as medically qualified doctors, investigators authorised for FIH trials, senior nurses, clinic managers or pharmacists)
- significant contractual changes in agreements with local hospitals.

If changes result in the criteria for the Scheme no longer being met, the Scheme requires that the MHRA GCP Inspectorate be informed immediately. If substantial changes occur during the conduct of a clinical trial, then the sponsor, MHRA Clinical Trials Unit (CTU) and relevant REC should be informed where appropriate, and must[1, 2, 3] be informed in accordance with the legislation, for example, if these changes also result in a serious breach, urgent safety measure or early termination of the trial. If the criteria for the Scheme are no longer being met, the accreditation for the unit may be suspended. In addition, if serious concerns are raised with regard to compliance at the unit, the accreditation may also be suspended.

The GCP Inspectorate circulates relevant documentation concerning a unit's accreditation status to the local REC responsible for the unit's site-specific assessments. This includes the application form, inspection report, responses to the report and final certificate, and is exchanged under the terms of the MHRA's memorandum of understanding with the Health Research Authority (HRA).

Since the Scheme was launched in 2007, the majority of commercial units conducting Phase I clinical trials in the UK have been accredited as part of the Scheme. A summary of the activities assessed for units conducting Phase I trials is given in Table 12.1. This also defines what is considered good practice and what is required for accreditation into the Scheme. Detailed information on the Voluntary MHRA Phase I Accreditation Scheme and a list of accredited units are available on the MHRA website.

12.3 Authorisation and ethical opinion for a Phase I clinical trial

As with any clinical trial, the sponsor is required[4] to obtain and maintain authorisation and a favourable REC opinion for the trial as per Chapters 2 and 3. However, for FIH clinical trials with certain novel compounds, the trial must be reviewed by the CTEAG before approval for the clinical trial can be given. Further guidance on this process can be found in Chapter 2 of this guide.

Units that are in the Scheme must assess each clinical trial independently of the opinion of the sponsor to confirm whether it requires review by the CTEAG, and document this assessment (some units have integrated this into their risk assessment).

Table 12.1 Summary activities assessed for units conducting Phase I trials

Required for all units conducting Phase I trials
Contracts and agreements
Contract/agreement with the sponsor (including any in-house agreements) must ensure that investigators are notified immediately if/when new safety/toxicology data come to light (unless this requirement is clearly documented in the protocol).
Planning and resource
The unit must have appropriate numbers of staff with adequate training to handle medical emergencies.
Subject recruitment
There must be a procedure in place to address 'over-volunteering'.
Subjects must be provided with 24-hour emergency contact numbers (that are tested) for when they are outside the unit. The unit must also hold the contact numbers for volunteers to ensure that they are contactable outside the unit should the need arise.
There must be a robust procedure in place to identify subjects accurately to ensure that the person screened is the person dosed (for example, utilising photographic identification, which is a requirement for the Scheme).
Required for units in the Voluntary MHRA Phase I Accreditation Scheme and for all other units depending on risk *(some level will be required based on the risks associated with the types of trials being undertaken)*
Emergency procedures
The unit must have robust (and tested) arrangements for immediate maintenance of life support (resuscitation and stabilisation) and onward transfer of subjects to hospital, where necessary. Periodic all-staff testing of emergency scenarios should occur within the unit and be documented.
Facilities and equipment
An emergency trolley/bag should be available that is easily and rapidly accessible. This should be in each main dosing area and can be moved quickly to where it is needed. It should be stocked as per the current UK Resuscitation Council Guidelines or, for those items not present on the trolley or in the bag as per the Resuscitation Council list, there should be documented justification.
The contents (including expiry dates) of the trolley/bag should be checked weekly, and the checks documented. If a tamper-proof seal is used then the seal should be checked weekly.
There must be alarm points in areas where the subjects will be (for example, showers, toilets, in the ward and recreational area) or at a minimum a personal alarm held by the volunteers. Staff must also be able to open bathroom doors from the outside in an emergency.

Quality system

There must be written procedures for every aspect of the trial process, plus:

- medical emergencies, including stabilising subjects in an acute emergency and transfer to hospital (with provision of relevant medical and trial information)

- procedures for handling common medical emergencies (for example, syncope, hypotension, anaphylaxis, cardiac arrest)

- out-of-hours medical cover and contact with sponsor or investigational medicinal product responsible person(s)

- training and refresher training in emergency resuscitation procedures

- unblinding in an emergency (if blinded trials are undertaken)

- dose escalation (if not all aspects are part of the protocol).

Subject recruitment

Verification of the past medical history for the subject via the subject's general practitioner (GP), or other medic, such as hospital consultant for patient trials, to provide assurance that inclusion and exclusion criteria are being met, as required by the risk assessment. (This is a requirement for subjects participating in first in human (FIH) trials for units in the scheme.)

Training

Clinical staff must be appropriately and currently trained to initiate resuscitation (for example, basic airway management and ventilation, intravenous administration, cannulation and fluid therapy, giving adrenaline, cardiopulmonary resuscitation and use of an automated external defibrillator). Annual updates are required (as a minimum clinical staff should receive immediate life support training and annual updates for those units in the scheme).

Required for units in the Voluntary MHRA Phase I Accreditation Scheme and recommended for all other units conducting Phase I trials

Emergency procedures

Either an existing agreement with the hospital for supporting emergencies arising from their clinical trials or ability to demonstrate communication and notification of trial information (for example, dosing times) with the hospital's emergency teams. The hospital emergency response team and the intensive therapy unit must be aware of the research unit, the nature of the research (for example, first in human, biologicals), and that subjects from the unit could be referred at any time.

Facilities and equipment

Continuous monitoring equipment must be available; to include electrocardiography (ECG), pulse oximetry and vital signs (such as blood pressure, heart rate and temperature).

Beds (where used for dosing days) must be able to be tilted and adjusted for height.

Table continues

Table 12.1 *continued*

Planning and resource
The unit must be able to demonstrate that there are sufficient numbers of trained staff employed by or contracted to the unit that are available during dosing and overnight stays. The unit must have in place a policy or procedure that stipulates the minimum staffing levels during clinical conduct of the trial.
Risk assessment and contingency planning
There must be a formal procedure in place for contingency planning (this must include consideration of availability of specific antidotes/emergency treatments and predictable reactions based on the pharmacology of the investigational medicinal product).
Training
There must be documentation to demonstrate that medical doctors are authorised to act as principal investigators in first in human trials, as described by their job description, and this should be supported by a curriculum vitae and training record. It is expected that principal investigators should have relevant clinical experience, plus a postgraduate qualification, such as a Diploma in Pharmaceutical Medicine, Diploma in Human Pharmacology, MSc in Clinical Pharmacology, or equivalent.
For FIH trials requiring the Clinical Trials Expert Advisory Group (CTEAG) review, there must be staff present during and after dosing who are trained in advanced life support (ALS) with recent experience in handling medical emergencies.

12.4   Contracts, agreements and insurance

12.4.1   Contracts and agreements

Contracts or agreements should be finalised and signed prior to the commencement of any activities in the unit, and these should be reviewed to ensure they are kept current, as covered in section 1.3.7.

If the unit uses a vendor, the sponsor should be made aware of this arrangement and these contracts should also be finalised before using the vendors.

In addition, the Scheme requires that processes be in place to ensure that the sponsor provides any ongoing safety and toxicology data updates to the unit (or in-house unit) immediately, to ensure the safety of the subjects in these early phase trials. This is often ensured by including a relevant clause in the contract between the sponsor and unit (or in the internal agreement for in-house units). The sponsor's responsibilities regarding this should be clearly stated in the protocol.

12.4.2   Clinical trials insurance

The sponsor and relevant parties must[5] ensure that appropriate insurance provisions are in place to cover the trial: for example, that the insurance policies do not contain any policy exclusions that could impact on cover for clinical trial subjects. It is expected that Phase I units will have a mechanism in place for ensuring the sponsor's insurance is adequate. This may be documented in a number of ways, for example:

- A copy of the sponsor's insurance policy is supplied with the insurance certificate.
- The insurance certificate clearly lists the policy exclusions.
- Formal sign-off to verify that appropriate sponsor personnel have checked and confirmed the policy exclusions to the Phase I unit.
- A clause in the contract between the unit and the sponsor specifically details the sponsor's responsibilities for checking the insurance policy.

Insurance for clinical trials is covered in more detail in section 1.3.8. Guidance on Phase I insurance has been developed by industry groups in consultation with the Department of Health and the HRA. This guidance is available on the ABPI website.

12.5   Risk assessment and contingency planning

Performing a risk assessment for a trial has already been discussed in Chapter 4 (section 4.7.1); however, contingency planning in relation to specific Phase I aspects also needs to be considered before the trial begins. It is recommended that all Phase I units perform a risk assessment, but a defined process is required for those units in the Scheme.

This risk assessment allows the unit to assess the clinical trial in detail and make an informed decision as to whether their organisation should conduct the clinical trial. It also allows the unit to identify and mitigate any potential risks that may arise while conducting the trial. When performing the risk assessment, units should refer to the EMA 'Guideline on strategies to identify and mitigate risks for first in human clinical trials with investigational medicinal products' (EMEA/CHMP/SWP/28367/07). In order to perform the risk assessment, the unit should ensure

Table 12.2 Considerations for risk assessments

Considerations for risk assessments
Clinical aspects
Choice of subjects
Route and rate of administration
Dose escalation scheme: number of subjects per cohort; precautions between doses within a cohort; precautions to apply between cohorts; stopping rules and decision-making (allocation of responsibilities for decisions with respect to subject dosing and dose escalation)
Monitoring and communication of adverse events
Predictable risk of certain adverse reactions
Availability of specific antidotes
Availability of supportive emergency facilities and medical staff
Appropriate unit facilities: which wards are to be used for which clinical trials and availability of appropriately trained site staff and extra staff (if required)
Non-clinical aspects
Mode of action of the IMP
Nature of target of the IMP
Relevance of the IMP to animal species and models
Novel compound status (whether the trial needs review by the Clinical Trials Expert Advisory Group (CTEAG))
Determination of strength and potency of the IMP
Pharmacokinetics of the IMP
Pharmacodynamics of the IMP
Safety pharmacology of the IMP
Toxicology of the IMP
Experience in humans (for example, FIH) of the IMP
Estimation of starting dose of the IMP in humans for FIH trials (this should be re-calculated by the unit to verify that it is the correct starting dose)
Quality aspects
Quality of the IMPs and nIMPs used
Reliability of very small doses

FIH, first in human; IMP, investigational medicinal product; nIMP, non-investigational medicinal product

that the sponsor has provided them with all necessary reference information and documents – for example, the protocol and the investigator's brochure (including all necessary non-clinical data) – and assess whether the quality of the data provided to them by the sponsor is acceptable (that is, if any of the non-clinical data contained in the investigator's brochure are in draft form, the extent of Good Laboratory Practice (GLP) compliance will not be known, and this could impact on the quality of the data).

The risk assessment will vary for each trial; however, Table 12.2 covers some examples of the risks posed and some practical considerations.

The defined procedure for the risk assessment and subsequent contingency plan should cover the following aspects:

* who is responsible for performing the risk assessment
* how it is documented (including the documents, and any updates, used to perform the assessment)
* who should review and approve it
* circulation to relevant staff to ensure any requirements are implemented
* continued review, updates and communication
* who is responsible for ensuring it is complied with during the trial (for example, a medically qualified member of staff may be required to be available in the unit until 8 hours post-dosing and there must be documentation to illustrate compliance with this requirement).

Some units also have a template risk assessment form or plan, which can be used as a starting point for each study.

Common findings related to the risk assessment and contingency planning on accreditation inspections have included failure to implement a risk assessment/contingency planning process, lack of documentation to demonstrate the review and update of a plan in response to relevant changes (for example protocol amendments) and lack of documentation to demonstrate that the plan was complied with.

It is also a requirement for Phase I units in the Scheme to perform an independent re-calculation of the starting dose of the IMP for FIH trials, and often this is done as part of the risk assessment. The reason for the requirement for principal investigators (PIs) in FIH studies to have a relevant postgraduate qualification in a pharmacology-related discipline is to ensure that the PI is able to review and understand all the non-clinical information, raising questions and requesting further documentation where appropriate. The PI should be confident that the starting dose is correct (as the safety of the subjects is the responsibility of the PI), and therefore should be able to re-calculate it. This assessment and re-calculation should be documented.

12.6 Dose escalation in clinical trials

12.6.1 Dose escalation process

Dose escalation clinical trials involve increasing the dose at regular intervals following the review of available data from the previous dose level(s) (see Figure 12.1). The risk associated with this type of design is one of safety, should a decision to escalate be made with a set of inappropriate data. For example, it has been observed that due to an unvalidated set of data (that is, the complete set of required data was not available) the decision to escalate the dose resulted in a cohort of subjects being dosed at a higher level after the trial-stopping criteria related to C_{max} had been exceeded in the previous cohort.

The Scheme requires that dose escalation is a formally documented process, which defines the following:

- The minimum set of data required for 'active' subjects on which the dose escalation decision is to be based; that is, if not all the assessments at all the time points for all the subjects in a cohort are required, this needs to be clearly identified, taking into consideration the ratio of active treatment to placebo; otherwise, it is assumed a complete set of data will be reviewed before escalating the dose.
- The stopping rules (both for an individual and for the trial).
- How the data will be captured.
- How the data will be quality controlled to ensure it is accurate.
- The minimum quorum of study and sponsor personnel required to make the dose escalation decision.
- Who is able to authorise dose escalation decisions (if this can be delegated, it should be done formally by the principal investigator).
- How the dose escalation decision is to be documented, communicated to the team and retained (including retention of the dataset).
- The system for preventing dose escalation if the parameters required are not met (for example, there is an incomplete set of data because a full cohort of

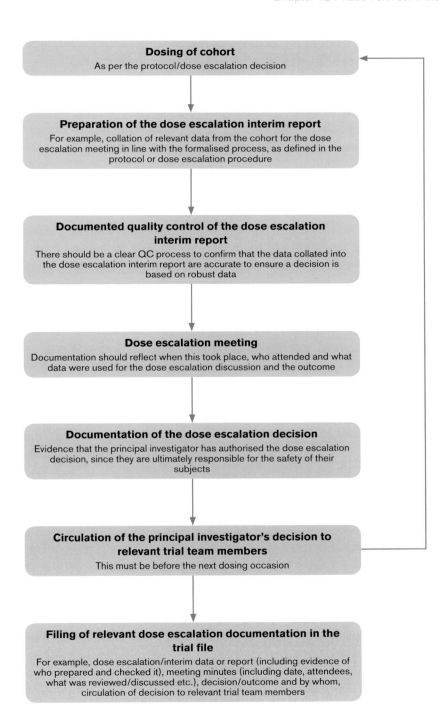

Figure 12.1 Dose escalation tree

subjects has not been recruited or a substantial amendment requires authorisation and/or favourable REC opinion to progress).

- Consideration for amalgamation and circulation of all data from each cohort to all principal investigators for multi-centre dose escalation trials.

Some units include the dose escalation processes in the protocol. However, the unit should have formal documentation of the minimum requirements for dose escalations and if any of the above aspects are not included in the protocol, then a separate document should ensure these are specified and agreed.

The sponsor may request that its own dose escalation procedures are used. However, it is expected that a unit which is part of the Scheme assesses these to be of the same standard as their own (as the unit's processes have been assessed for inclusion in the Scheme). Where this standard is not met, it is expected that the sponsor will implement any recommendations provided by the unit.

For safety purposes, many FIH clinical trials are designed to incorporate dose leaders (for example, the dosing of two subjects 24 hours before the remainder of the cohort, with usually one subject receiving placebo and the other subject receiving active treatment). Where this is the case, there should be a procedure in place to ensure the randomisation is designed to correctly assign the first two subjects accordingly. If there are designated unblinded staff within the unit, then it is recommended that they check the assignment of dose leaders prior to dosing.

12.6.2   Dose escalation data

It is very important that the data used to make the dose escalation decision are accurate and robust. Therefore, all data to be used for the dose escalation decision should undergo a documented quality control (QC) process. The sponsor and those units that are in the Scheme should also document their expectations for the review and QC of data received from the sponsor and other investigator sites in multi-centre dose escalation clinical trials.

12.6.3   Dose escalation decision

The trial master file must[6] contain and clearly reflect:

- the data reviewed (if this was blinded or unblinded – unblinded data must not be available to the unit, therefore its location should be identified)

- the personnel that reviewed the data and when they did so
- the decisions taken by the sponsor and the PI or an authorised delegate.

12.7   IMP management

Guidance on the receipt, storage and accountability of investigational medicinal product (IMP) is given in Chapter 6 and Chapter 11 of this guide. This section focuses on specific considerations for Phase I units.

12.7.1   Requirements for the authorisation to manufacture and import IMP

Any Phase I unit may perform dispensing activities; however, they will require a manufacturer's authorisation for investigational medicinal products (MIA(IMP)) where they are performing:

- manufacturing activities, unless they can apply the Regulation 37 exemption (private Phase I units are not classed as hospitals or health centres)
- receipt of IMP directly from outside the European Economic Area (EEA) (that is, importing).

See Chapter 6 for details on the manufacture and/or importation of IMPs and the associated requirements.

There have been several examples where manufacturing processes have been incorrectly deemed as dispensing at Phase I units. For example, at a commercial unit, bulk supplies of various strengths of active IMP and the corresponding placebo were present in the nursing office. Each subject's dose was prepared by 'dispensing' the allocated number of the required tablet strengths (active and placebo) into an unlabelled pot to make up that cohort's dose. This was then administered to the subject and the next dose 'dispensed'. However, there was insufficient evidence to fully reconstruct what subjects had actually been dosed and when in relation to the preparation activity. For example:

- No times were documented in relation to 'dispensing' activity concerning each subject (only dosing) to verify that doses were prepared and dosed sequentially per subject to ensure no potential for cross-contamination.
- Only a total number of tablets 'dispensed' was recorded in each subject's accountability records; therefore it was only possible to verify that they got the correct number of tablets, but not the correct strength.

- Only a total amount of bulk used for each cohort, not each subject, was recorded, therefore it could only be established that the correct total number of tablets had been 'dispensed'.

This type of activity is not deemed to be dispensing and should have been performed as an assembly and labelling activity and certified by a Qualified Person (QP) under an MIA(IMP).

12.7.2 Authorisation to start a clinical trial

Authorisation to start a clinical trial is described in section 1.5.2. However, it is common for an IMP to be shipped under quarantine to the Phase I unit, especially where the unit holds an MIA(IMP) and will be performing the final packaging, labelling and QP certification. Therefore the unit should have procedures in place to cover the quarantine of the IMP and its release.

12.7.3 Blinding considerations

Most Phase I trials are double-blind. However, as previously mentioned, bulk supplies of IMP may be provided to the units. In these circumstances the units should have a robust mechanism to ensure the blinding in the trial is maintained. Therefore, where unblinded IMP or documentation, such as randomisation lists or PK data, are received by the unit, it is expected that unblinded activities are delegated to designated unblinded staff, to avoid the potential for other unit staff to be unblinded. Inadequate maintenance of blinding has been seen on inspection a number of times. For example:

- A trial was using a type of diabetic injection gun where the label of the active and placebo vials could be viewed at the point of administration. There was no mechanism or supporting documentation to ensure the dosing staff remained blinded to the IMP administered.
- IMP pack labels specified that medication 'A' was active and medication 'B' was placebo; therefore if one subject needed to be unblinded this would essentially unblind the entire study.
- IMP patches labelled 'A' and 'B' were applied to the location according to the randomisation schedule held in the IMP file. However, there were insufficient controls to ensure that investigator site staff performing blinded irritancy assessments (primary outcome) and assessing adverse events did not have access to the randomisation schedule and were not present during the application of the patches.

12.7.4   Emergency unblinding (identifying a blinded IMP in an emergency)

As many of the trials performed at Phase I units are double-blind, it is expected that units have a defined process for emergency unblinding that is formally tested at regular intervals to ensure it is robust. Any testing of the systems should be documented and retained as evidence. All units should implement emergency unblinding procedures; however, it is a requirement for units in the Scheme, many of whom have integrated this testing into their emergency scenarios. Further guidance on emergency unblinding is available in sections 6.6.2 and 11.4.9.

12.8   Facilities and equipment

In accordance with Regulation 15 of SI 2004/1031 the REC is required to consider the suitability of each clinical trial site and investigator when giving its opinion on a trial. This is performed as part of the site-specific assessment (SSA) which, for commercial Phase I units, is usually managed by the REC. Further information on this process is detailed in Chapter 3 and on the Health Research Authority (HRA) website. Due to the nature of these trials it is expected that units have suitable procedures and facilities to deal with medical emergencies that may occur (as assessed in the risk assessment). These may vary slightly depending on the types of trial a unit conducts: for example, for 'consumer' units that run lower-risk trials these may cover the more common emergencies, unlike those units that are in the Scheme which require full resuscitation equipment and medication.

12.8.1   Emergency resuscitation trolley

The Scheme requires units to have an emergency resuscitation trolley that is easily and rapidly accessible, just as would be the case in a hospital. There should be an emergency resuscitation trolley (or bag) in each main clinical area that can be moved quickly to where it is needed. The emergency resuscitation trolley should be stocked in accordance with the current UK Resuscitation Council Guidelines (available at www.resus.org.uk). However, it is appreciated that there may be a decision not to stock certain items as there is no one in the unit qualified and experienced to use them; for example, a central venous catheter kit. This is acceptable, provided any deviations are clearly documented and justified. However, the minimum requirements for the resuscitation trolley for units in the Scheme are listed in the detailed information on the Scheme available on the MHRA website. A lack of documented justified deviations from the UK Resuscitation Council Guidelines has been a common finding when inspecting units for the Scheme.

There should be a documented weekly check of the contents of the emergency resuscitation trolley. This should include checks that the equipment is functioning properly, for example:

- Checking that there is adequate suction at the end of the nozzle, rather than simply checking that the suction equipment switches on when the power supply is activated.
- Checking that the defibrillator is functioning and the battery is fully charged.
- Checking that the expiry dates for medication and equipment are in date, and will remain in date until the next check.

The checks can be conducted in a number of ways: for example, documented weekly checks of tamper-proof seals for the drawers of the emergency trolley and/or the emergency drug box to ensure there has been no access to the trolley contents. However, it is important that there is a mechanism to ensure that any expiring items (for example, syringes, needles, drugs and oxygen cylinders) are replaced, as it has been frequently identified during inspection that trolleys contained expired items.

It is also recommended that units have sufficient processes in place to be notified of any drug or medical device recalls. This can be achieved via any contracts with the emergency drug supplier or by subscribing to the MHRA drug and medical device recall alerts.

12.8.2 Continuous monitoring equipment

Units should ideally have available continuous monitoring equipment which includes capability for ECG, pulse oximetry and vital signs measurements (for example, blood pressure, heart rate and temperature). For units that are part of the Scheme this is a requirement.

12.8.3 Equipment calibration and maintenance

It is expected that any equipment is maintained and calibrated (in accordance with the manufacturers' instructions) and the supporting records should be retained as evidence that the equipment is fit for purpose. This applies to all equipment including any continuous monitoring equipment, centrifuges, refrigerators and freezers, as well as study-specific equipment. For example, some trials require intravenous infusion of the IMP via infusion pumps/syringe drivers, which may be available at the unit or may be supplied by the sponsor. In either case it is expected that there is documented evidence of calibration to ensure that the infusion pumps/syringe drivers are working correctly (that is, they are delivering the correct volume per minute) and there are no occlusions. These checks should be carried out before the infusion pumps/syringe drivers are used in a trial, as these can be very sensitive pieces of equipment and can easily be out of specification as a result of transit/transport. These checks could be in the form of a manufacturer's calibration certificate or a documented 'fit-for-purpose' test run of the equipment in the unit before it is used in the trial.

12.8.4 General facilities

12.8.4.1 Emergency call buttons/alarms

There should be a mechanism for subjects to alert staff in the event of an emergency in any location that they have access to: for example, the ward, showers, toilets and recreational areas. If these areas are not constantly staffed then they should contain emergency call buttons. These should be easily accessible to subjects and should all be checked regularly to ensure they are working. This should be formalised and is a requirement for those units in the Scheme.

The mechanism used can range from a system similar to those in hospitals (call buttons and/or pull cords) to personal alarms carried by the subjects (which may be acceptable in certain situations, such as those units conducting 'lower-risk' trials). It is common to see pull cords in toilets or showers, but it must be ensured that these are easily reached by the subjects and they are not too far away or outside the shower cubicle.

Units must also ensure that staff are able to unlock and open bathroom and toilet doors from the outside in an emergency, so that the subject can be attended to promptly. Therefore, consideration should be given to:

- the type of lock installed
- easy accessibility of a device to unlock the door from the outside, such as a suitable coin or plastic card that is carried by staff or kept near the door
- the direction in which the door opens.

All these have been identified as problematic when tested during inspection.

12.8.4.2 Beds

The unit should have beds that tilt and are height adjustable. The Scheme requires this in areas used for dosing. Some units have bedrooms with bunk beds, which may be acceptable for subjects on an overnight stay on the day before dosing, but not suitable for dosing days, as in case of an emergency it would be very hard to reach the subject and attend to them. Where units use different configurations of beds in different wards, then the area to be used for dosing should be considered and documented as part of the risk assessment and appropriate contingency planning should be put in place. This may also apply to facilities that have sleep laboratories, cardiovascular/respiratory monitoring equipment, or other clinical areas set up for specialist activities that may not be appropriate for dosing activities.

Consideration should also be given to the ability of staff to observe the subjects while in the unit. This includes the location of the nurses' supervision station in relation to the location of the beds, staff presence on the ward for a period of time after dosing, and the use of mirrors and CCTV.

12.8.4.3 Restricted access

Units should ensure that subjects cannot access areas that are restricted to them, such as areas of IMP storage and sample processing. If the protocol has specific restrictions (for example, caffeine or food) access to areas where subjects can obtain these items should also be restricted. Access to toilets should be restricted if urine or faeces is to be collected, to prevent the loss or mix-up of samples. This is of particular importance for radiolabelled trials.

12.9   Planning and resources

Phase I trials tend to have many assessments being undertaken in multiple subjects and as a result can be quite resource-intensive. Therefore, planning the logistics and thus resources needed is an important factor for any Phase I unit, so should be considered as part of the risk assessment and contingency planning. Consideration should be given to having adequate appropriately trained staff available and how any unexpected absences are managed to ensure that activities and supervision can still be maintained. This process should be formalised for any unit undertaking Phase I trials and is mandatory for those units that are part of the Scheme.

The following must therefore be formalised for those units in the Scheme or considering applying:

- A process for allocating resource and ensuring the resource planner is made aware of any changes to the risk assessment, planned and unplanned absences and staff training/competencies for allocation of activities, plus any lapses in required training. The resource assignment should be clearly documented and communicated to the unit staff.
- A procedure stipulating the minimum staffing levels during the in-house phase of the study (including dosing and overnight stays). This should include the number of staff required to manage a medical emergency (should it arise) and their level of life support training. Consideration needs to be given to the number of subjects in the unit, the types of trials being undertaken and the number of wards that are occupied.
- The use of, training and oversight of contract/agency/bank staff.
- Documentation to provide evidence that the minimum staffing levels stipulated in the unit procedures or trial-specific documents (for example, the risk assessment or protocol) have been complied with.

The MHRA does not stipulate a specific acceptable number of staff, as this will vary depending on the type of trial, number of subjects and layout of the unit. However, the minimum requirements for level of life support and experience in medical emergencies for those units in the Scheme are listed in the detailed information on the Scheme available on the MHRA website.

12.10 Training

All units must[7] ensure that staff are appropriately trained and qualified (as discussed in Chapters 11 and 14) for their role in the clinical trial, the activities they are delegated by the PI, and their ability to manage medical emergencies.

Training requirements and oversight of that training are scrutinised on inspection in more detail for units in the Scheme, as detailed in Table 12.1. Training requirements should be considered as part of the risk assessment process and should include reviewing the availability of supportive emergency facilities and appropriately trained site staff (and additional staff if required) in accordance with the risk assessment.

All units should have formalised procedures for identifying and tracking staff training needs (for example, via training courses, written procedures and competency assessments) to ensure these are kept up to date. Many units use training matrices and tracking spreadsheets which are available to relevant personnel for scheduling training (such as life support training that needs to be regularly updated) and resource planning.

Therefore, in addition to the requirement[7] that all staff are qualified by education, training and experience to perform their tasks, clinical and medical staff of units in the Scheme are required to have specific life support training and 'hands-on' experience of medical emergencies, and those medically qualified doctors who act as PIs on FIH trials are required to have specific qualifications. These requirements are further described in sections 12.10.1 and 12.10.2.

12.10.1 Clinical staff

For units in the Scheme, all clinical staff working in the unit (including any bank staff) require immediate life support (ILS) training with annual updates, as a minimum, to ensure they are appropriately and currently trained to initiate resuscitation, for example:

- basic airway management and ventilation
- intravenous (IV) cannulation and fluid therapy
- administering adrenaline
- cardiopulmonary resuscitation (CPR)
- use of an automated external defibrillator (AED).

The unit should therefore clearly identify those staff they consider 'clinical' staff, so it is clear who is expected to have up-to-date ILS training.

12.10.2 Physicians/principal investigators

For medically qualified doctors working in units in the Scheme, there are specific criteria in relation to their activities that need to be demonstrated, for example in relation to medical emergencies and acting as a PI.

The regulations do not include any specific qualification or experience requirements. Therefore, units are encouraged to refer to the ABPI guidelines on Phase I clinical trials and the detailed information on the Scheme available on the MHRA website to develop their own in-house requirements.

12.10.2.1 Principal investigators

The Scheme requires that physicians are authorised to act as PIs and/or PIs for FIH clinical trials. This requirement should also be stated in a job description and supported by a *curriculum vitae* and training record.

Physicians acting as PIs for FIH clinical trials are expected to be able to calculate the proposed starting dose for FIH studies, review non-clinical data and question the sponsor to ensure that they have all the relevant information, and are able to interpret this information, before dosing subjects. Therefore, they need to have relevant clinical experience and a relevant postgraduate qualification in pharmaceutical medicine and/or pharmacology (for example, diploma in pharmaceutical medicine, diploma in human pharmacology, completion of speciality training in clinical pharmacology and higher degrees in pharmacology or equivalent. Qualifications such as membership of the Royal College of Physicians (MRCP) and equivalent are also highly desirable but are not considered to be a sufficient postgraduate qualification in pharmaceutical medicine and/or pharmacology).

It is recognised that there are a number of PIs who have no formal postgraduate qualification, but they do have a significant amount of experience in this field and therefore may be exempt from this requirement. There is a formal mechanism for these investigators to submit their justification for an independent peer review by the Faculty of Pharmaceutical Medicine. Further guidance on this process can be found in the MHRA 'Procedure for provision of advice via the Faculty of Pharmaceutical Medicine to MHRA on suitability of applicants to serve as principal investigators for FIH studies', available from the MHRA website.

Where units have PIs with varying authorisations (that is, FIH/non-FIH), it is expected that all the necessary certificates and experience are documented in their training records, and that there is a clear differentiation in their job descriptions. This is commonly found to be insufficiently apparent during inspection.

12.10.2.2 Advanced life support in relation to CTEAG-reviewed trials

The Scheme requires that units are able to demonstrate that appropriately trained and experienced medically qualified staff are available on dosing days for FIH clinical trials with higher risk factors requiring CTEAG review, to ensure that acute emergencies are appropriately managed, should they occur. These physicians must be trained to advanced life support (ALS) standards and have adequate 'hands-on' experience in handling medical emergencies.

These physicians do not have to be the PI or a permanent employee of the unit. Therefore, there are a number of different ways in which this requirement can be met. For example:

- Physicians may participate on an ongoing basis in periodic clinical attachments, for example, participation in a hospital resuscitation team rota or acute hospital department to ensure continued exposure to identifying and handling medical emergencies. Documented evidence must be maintained to list their experiences within the clinical setting, with sufficient detail, to demonstrate that their experience remains relevant and recent. Honorary contracts with the hospital should also be in place as required. If the unit employs physicians who have recently worked in relevant areas of clinical practice, processes and evidence must in place to ensure that the physicians' experience remains current.

- The unit may use contract physicians with up-to-date emergency medicine experience. Where this is done, there must be adequate:
  - » documentation of the assessment of the physicians' qualifications and experience
  - » contracts in place (including indemnity arrangements)
  - » evidence of training in ALS, Good Clinical Practice (GCP), appropriate unit standard operating procedures (SOPs) and the protocol
  - » supervision while in the unit.

- The unit is located within a hospital with critical care facilities. The unit will have 24-hour access to the hospital emergency response team, who can arrive at the unit within minutes of an emergency.

There should be a continued assessment that these requirements are met, whichever route is taken, to ensure it remains adequate. Therefore, a procedure must be in place to address and document the assessment of continuing competency (for example, by peer review, audit or other relevant means). There should also be supporting documentation for any requirements regarding specialist medical expertise that were identified by the risk assessment.

There is no requirement for a formal agreement with the local hospital for emergency care (and some NHS Trusts will not enter into one). However, the hospital should be aware of the unit and the types of trials that are undertaken. The Phase I unit should be able to demonstrate this communication with the NHS Trust, by email, letter, meetings or a formal contract if possible. It is also recommended that the Phase I unit (particularly if not located in a hospital) invite the local ambulance service and NHS Trust intensive therapy unit representatives to review emergency procedures and transfer to hospital. Those units that have done this have found it extremely valuable and have made improvements to their processes based on input from these groups.

12.11 Emergency procedures

Any unit undertaking Phase I trials should ensure they have formalised procedures to cover any anticipated medical emergencies they are potentially likely to encounter and that staff are appropriately trained (for example, classroom and/or scenario training). The following are required for those units in the Scheme; however, it is recommended those not in the Scheme also consider these aspects.

12.11.1 Access to emergency support

Units in the Scheme are not required to be based on a hospital site. However, whether based in a hospital or not, they are expected to be able to demonstrate communication and notification of clinical trial information (for example, dosing times) with the hospital's emergency team. The hospital emergency team and/or the intensive therapy unit should be aware of the unit, the nature of the research (for example, FIH clinical trials) and that they could be referred subjects from the unit at any time.

Although it is not a specific requirement of the Scheme, units are encouraged to practise transfers to hospital. However, it is expected that the unit has investigated and documented realistic transfer times to the nearest emergency care facility (either by testing it themselves, or being provided with average times by the ambulance service).

12.11.2 Emergency scenario requirements and training

The Scheme requires that units have robust formalised and tested arrangements for immediate maintenance of life support (resuscitation and stabilisation) and onward transfer of subjects to hospital, where necessary. This should be in the form of written procedures, combined with classroom and practical scenario training to cover the following activities:

417

- transfer of subjects to hospital (including provision of all relevant medical information for the trial and the subject(s) in question to the hospital)
- procedures for handling various medical emergencies (for example, syncope, hypotension, anaphylaxis, cardiac arrest) including stabilising subjects in an acute emergency
- out-of-hours medical cover and contact with sponsor or IMP responsible person(s)
- unblinding in an emergency.

It is important for unit staff to be trained and well prepared to deal with medical emergencies, should they arise. Therefore, periodic testing of these emergency scenarios, by creating various anticipated scenarios that allow staff to simulate what they would do in that emergency, should occur within the unit. This testing should cover a variety of situations (for example, cardiac arrest and anaphylaxis) and also include emergency unblinding activities. Consideration should be given to when scenarios are rehearsed in order to cover all staff working in the unit, including night/agency/bank staff and busier times when volunteers are in the unit. It is also recommended that, where possible, unannounced emergency scenario testing also takes place.

These scenarios should be seen as learning opportunities and therefore they should form part of the formal quality system. They should be documented to enable reconstruction of what was simulated, the assessment and the outcome. It is useful to distribute the summary of the training to all staff, so that any learning points can be shared with the whole team (whether they attended those scenarios or not). Following the training it should be ensured that any corrective and preventative actions following the scenario have been implemented.

In addition, the risk assessment for the trial may identify particular training needs, for example identification and management of an anticipated adverse event, and this could be incorporated into training scenarios for staff prior to the start of the study.

Attendance at this training must be documented and tracked to ensure that all staff are regularly involved. The number of training sessions a unit carries out will vary according to the size of the unit and the number of personnel it employs (permanent and temporary).

During an Accreditation Scheme inspection, the MHRA GCP inspectors will usually ask for a demonstration of an emergency scenario, along with testing of a transfer to hospital (via ambulance service or acceptable alternative method).

12.11.3 Out-of-hours medical cover

Subjects must be provided with 24-hour emergency contact numbers while they are outside the unit. There may be a number of ways in which a subject can contact the unit. It is expected that all methods of contact (including any sponsor emergency contact numbers) are formally tested to ensure an appropriate person is reached. Testing of the emergency contacts should be documented and retained and should clearly identify any issues and corrective actions.

In addition, the unit must also hold the contact numbers for subjects to ensure that they can be contacted outside the unit should the need arise, for example if new safety data come to light that would require further monitoring of the subject, or in the event of recall of an IMP that the subjects are taking between visits to the unit.

12.12 Subject identification and recruitment

It is important that any organisation conducting trials with volunteers has robust mechanisms in place for recruiting and identifying these subjects. This is extremely important, as volunteers will not have medical records associated with them (in the same way that hospital patients will have) and therefore there needs to be a mechanism for verifying that they exist, that the person screened is the same person dosed and that they do not take part in too many clinical trials (Table 12.1). For those units in the Scheme there are additional requirements to consider when recruiting volunteers in relation to FIH CTEAG studies.

12.12.1 Subject recruitment

Units use a variety of methods to recruit potential clinical trial subjects. For example, units may advertise in newspapers, websites or on local radio (advertisements should have been approved by the REC if trial-specific; see section 3.2.3.1), or seek referrals from medical professionals. A significant number of units also use an in-house volunteer database, which contains a list of people willing to be contacted about taking part in a clinical trial. Units will use this information to identify potential subjects and then contact them to discuss the clinical trial. Where units use a volunteer database, it is expected that:

* It is validated (where appropriate) and fit for purpose.

12

- Volunteers have consented to be included on the database (including a process for their removal if consent is withdrawn).
- It is possible to search and identify only subjects who are potentially suitable in line with the trial criteria.
- There is a mechanism for capturing significant safety information relating to a subject's participation in a clinical trial, to prevent them from being invited and recruited inappropriately to a similar trial in the future.
- There are adequate data protection procedures for the confidential information held, such as names, contact details or photographs.

It is expected that a search of the database should identify only those that fit the criteria for the trial: for example, if the clinical trial inclusion criteria required that subjects are aged 18–60 years, subjects outside this age group should not be identified and contacted. Also, if a subject experiences a severe adverse reaction to the application of a steroid cream in a clinical trial, they should not be invited to participate in a similar trial in the future. The unit should also have a policy for a washout period between trials: if a subject has recently completed a trial they should not be identified and invited to participate in another trial too soon.

12.12.2 Subject records

In settings where the investigator is not the primary care provider (that is, the GP or hospital consultant) for the subjects, for example a Phase I unit, a consumer unit or a site management organisation (SMO) which has its own facilities, it is important for them to maintain an independent record of the subject (apart from the CRF). These independent records ensure that any relevant information from prior trials (for example adverse events, abnormal laboratory tests) is recorded and maintained separately from the trial documentation. This should be made available to the investigators and monitors when the subjects are assessed for subsequent trials, in order to assess that there is no relevant prior history that could exclude them. These records can be paper or electronic (for example, part of the database described in section 12.12.1).

12.12.3 Subject identification

For units in the Scheme, there must be a robust procedure in place to accurately identify subjects. The most effective way of doing this is by using suitable photographic identification, thereby ensuring that the person screened is the person dosed (each time if there are multiple dosing occasions, and at any follow-up visits) and preventing the unit dosing a person who may have medical conditions of which the unit is unaware.

In addition, some units take and keep a digital photograph of the subject in the database. Ideally a copy of the photographic identification should be retained, as proof of the subject's existence. However, if it is decided that this will not be kept, the unit needs to consider how they will provide evidence in the trial documentation to prove the subject existed (for example, is there a GP letter or a medical referral letter?)

12.12.4 Generic screening and consent

It is acknowledged that that there are significant time pressures associated with conducting Phase I clinical trials. As a result, some units have a mechanism to perform what they call generic consent and screening. Where this is undertaken it is expected that there are defined procedures for this activity in relation to what assessments will be conducted (and ensuring no study-specific activities are undertaken). Expectations in relation to REC requirements surrounding generic screening documents (that is, subject information and consent form) can be found in section 3.2.3.7.

12.12.5 Confirmation of subject's medical history

Ideally, for any clinical trials involving volunteers, the unit should make every effort to verify their medical history to help assure themselves that the volunteer has not (either deliberately or accidentally) omitted anything that may affect their eligibility to be included in the trial, as this could impact on their safety. This could include, for example, questioning the subject about their own and relevant family medical history and contacting the GP for any relevant medical history. In addition, information can be gathered by conducting a physical examination and other relevant tests such as electrocardiography (ECG), safety bloods and urinalysis.

For FIH trials, those units that are part of the Scheme must have a robust and formalised procedure to seek confirmation of a subject's past medical history from the subject's GP or other medical professional (for example, a hospital consultant for patient studies) to provide assurance that subject is eligible for the clinical trial. This procedure should cover:

- How often the unit needs to contact the GP; for example, if the subject participates in more than one trial at the unit, is an updated GP letter required, or does the GP letter remain valid for a certain period of time?
- If the subject needs to be registered for a specified amount of time with their GP, and therefore has records that cover a certain length of time.
- Who is responsible for reviewing the GP report for its acceptability and impact on the subject's eligibility for the clinical trial, and how this is documented.
- What happens when the GP report is not received.

Although confirmation of medical history from the GP is required for those units that are part of the Scheme (for FIH studies), it is recommended that all units review what medical history is required. This can be done on a risk-based approach. The documentation of this decision may form part of the risk assessment process.

Once a subject has been recruited, the GP should also be notified of their inclusion in the trial, and of any significant adverse events that they may have experienced once the trial is finished.

12.12.6 Preventing subject over-volunteering

It is good practice for any organisation recruiting volunteers to identify mechanisms that prevent over-volunteering. It is a requirement for units in the Scheme to implement processes to address the over-volunteering of subjects. Preventing over-volunteering ensures that volunteers do not participate in too many trials at the same time and jeopardise their safety. Mechanisms that units can use to identify over-volunteering may include:

- registering with a national volunteer registration database (for example, The Overvolunteering Prevention Service (TOPS))
- contacting the subject's GP
- assessing bloods and urine results (for example, haematology and clinical chemistry) for key markers
- a physical examination to identify any signs of having participated in another clinical trial (for example, needle marks or residue from ECG patches).

12.13 Chapter legislative references

Throughout this chapter, specific terminology – 'must', 'required' or 'requirement' – has been used to interpret activities that are legislative requirements. These terms have been number-coded in the text where used, and the corresponding reference in the legislation can be found below. Note that where 'must', 'required' and 'requirement' have been used in relation to activities that are mandatory as part of the Voluntary MHRA Phase I Accreditation Scheme, there are no corresponding number codes.

1. Regulation 29A of SI 2004/1031
2. Regulation 30 of SI 2004/1031
3. Regulation 27 of SI 2004/1031
4. Regulation 12 of SI 2004/1031
5. Schedule 1, Part 2 (14) of SI 2004/1031
6. Regulation 31A (4) of SI 2004/1031
7. Schedule 1, Part 2 (2) of SI 2004/1031

CHAPTER 13

Clinical trial samples – analysis and evaluation

13

Editor's note

The nature and purpose of laboratory work performed as part of a clinical trial is very broad, encompassing a wide range of activities; the analysis can cover safety laboratory samples, pharmacokinetic (PK), pharmacodynamic (PD) and biomarker samples, and can include chemical and biological assays. In all cases laboratories generate data that are used directly or indirectly to make decisions on the safety and efficacy of medicinal products; consequently, it is of paramount importance that the data are reliable.

Local laboratories (that is, those laboratories that are attached to a hospital or investigator site) are often used for analysis of safety samples; however, laboratory work can also be contracted to specialist companies that are geographically remote from the investigator site. This can lead to a lack of awareness among laboratory staff of specific requirements that must be taken into consideration when processing samples from clinical trials. This chapter provides an overview of issues all laboratories should consider before embarking on the analysis or evaluation of clinical trial samples.

13.1 Organisation of laboratory work

The nature of laboratory work performed in support of clinical trials is very diverse and consequently the way laboratory work is organised will also be variable. The primary consideration for all types of laboratory work is that it must[1, 2, 3] be performed in accordance with the clinical protocol, Good Clinical Practice (GCP) and the laboratory's internal quality system.

There are various guidance documents available for organisations conducting laboratory work to refer to. These include the European Medicines Agency (EMA) reflection paper for laboratories that perform the analysis or evaluation of clinical trial samples (EMA/INS/GCP/532137/2010), the EMA guideline on the investigation of bioequivalence (CPMP/EWP/QWP/1401/98 Rev. 1) and ICH Topic Q (R1) – 'Validation of analytical procedures' (CPMP/ICH/381/95).

13.1.1　The quality system

Laboratory activities must[3] be performed in accordance with written procedures that are controlled and subject to periodic review. These written procedures or other policy documents should cover all key activities, such as sample receipt, storage, analysis and reporting, plus other activities, such as quality assurance functions and computer system validation (Chapter 14). The need for written procedures to cover specific laboratory activities should be assessed on a case-by-case basis. The number and nature of these procedures will depend on the complexity of the operation that the laboratory undertakes; however, it should be possible for an independent party to establish a reasonable understanding of how the laboratory operates by reading these procedures.

13.1.2　Laboratory personnel

Roles and responsibilities within the laboratory should be established prior to the initiation of validation and analytical work. Key roles will include personnel responsible for the management of the laboratory, scientific analysis and quality assurance.

Laboratory management is responsible for ensuring that all the key aspects required to perform the analysis or evaluation of clinical trials samples are in place prior to the start of work. Key aspects include the provision of adequate facilities and equipment, and an appropriate number of trained and experienced laboratory personnel. In addition to appropriate technical competence, it is important that personnel who work in laboratories that perform the analysis of samples collected as part of a clinical trial must[4] have an adequate understanding of specific GCP requirements. These include issues relating to trial subject safety, consent and confidentiality (see section 13.7 for further information).

13.1.3   Contracts, agreements and work instructions

A clear undertaking that the laboratory has agreed to perform the analysis or evaluation of clinical trial samples should be agreed prior to the initiation of any laboratory work. This will usually take the form of a legally binding contract between the trial sponsor or their representative(s) and the laboratory. If a laboratory performs the analysis of samples from several different trials for the same sponsor, it may be appropriate to perform all the work under a single master service agreement, although it is recommended that the content of the agreement is reviewed to ensure that it is applicable to all the work. It may also be necessary to issue a trial-specific work order which will detail information, such as the number of samples that will be received by the laboratory and any trial-specific assay requirements. It is appropriate to review long-standing contracts or master service agreements periodically to ensure that the terms and conditions remain relevant. Section 1.3.7 provides further details on preparation and oversight of contracts and agreements.

On inspection, examples have been seen where the agreements or processes surrounding the agreements were inadequate. For example, a written procedure did not identify what information should be included in a contract or agreement (when arranging contract clinical analysis with an external sponsor) and therefore did not ensure compliance with the clinical protocol and with the Clinical Trials Regulations. Contracts have also lacked clauses stating that the laboratory would routinely be supplied with the clinical protocol (or relevant part thereof) or protocol amendments. In addition, contracts have often been seen that only require that work be conducted to the principles of Good Laboratory Practice (GLP) and do not refer to SI 2004/1031.

If analysis is performed by a laboratory that is part of the organisation which is sponsoring the trial or undertaking the clinical phase of the trial, but is located in a department under an independent management line, it is recommended that a service level agreement is implemented between the two departments. For example, if two academic departments within the same university collaborate to perform different parts of a clinical trial, a formal arrangement (for example, a written procedure, memorandum of understanding or detail in the protocol) between the two departments is recommended.

All analysis or evaluation of clinical trial samples should be performed in accordance with a predefined plan. This may take the form of a work instruction/ plan or a series of laboratory written procedures, depending on the nature of the work. For example, work performed to determine the pharmacokinetic parameters of an investigational medicinal product (IMP) is often conducted in accordance with a formal laboratory protocol. In contrast, work performed by either a local hospital laboratory or a central laboratory that is generating routine clinical safety data will generally be performed in accordance with the facility's written procedures or standardised work instructions.

13.1.4 Communication

Data generated in the laboratory influence key decisions made during the conduct of a clinical trial. For example, interim analyses or dose-escalation trials will rely on analytical data to determine systemic exposure or specific safety tests required in relation to a drug, while routine clinical chemistry may flag safety concerns needing the investigator's immediate attention. In order to ensure that data are communicated to the relevant people in a timely manner, lines of communication between the laboratory and the sponsor or trial site should be established prior to the initiation of any work.

Many clinical trials are blinded to eliminate the possibility of bias. Laboratories that receive blinded samples should have a process to ensure that staff are aware that, if data are communicated to an inappropriate person, there is a possibility that the blind may be inadvertently compromised. The data may indicate what the subjects have received (for example, which subjects were given the drug and which were given a placebo). This situation could be avoided if it is agreed with the sponsor or the clinical investigator prior to the start of the work to whom data should be sent.

13.1.5 Subcontracting laboratory work

From time to time laboratories may need to subcontract work to other organisations. Prior to placing work with another laboratory, the sponsor or its representative should give permission for this work to be subcontracted and appropriate contractual arrangements put in place. See section 1.3.7 for considerations when contracting and selecting vendors.

13.2 Sample transportation, receipt and storage

13.2.1 Transportation and receipt of clinical samples

Issues associated with the transportation of samples are often overlooked because laboratories assume their responsibility for the samples starts when they are received. Although the clinical site that collects and packages the samples should ensure that every effort is made to ensure they remain fit for purpose, the laboratory should also exercise due diligence. For example, if laboratory staff receive samples shipped under ambient conditions they should check to determine how long they have been in transit and what temperatures they are likely to have been exposed to. This may be particularly important during periods of hot weather. Equally, when there is a requirement for samples to be transported chilled or frozen the laboratory should positively confirm that each consignment of samples arrived in an appropriate condition as the results may be affected if there was a temperature excursion. This is usually achieved by producing a signed receipt.

13.2.2 Sample identification

Laboratory staff should ensure that they receive the expected number of samples and that each sample is labelled appropriately. If samples are poorly labelled or missing, the sponsor or clinical investigator should be notified. If unexpected samples are received, laboratory staff will need to contact the trial site to confirm their identity. If there is any doubt about the source or identity of a sample, it should not be analysed until it has been identified. The exception to this rule is where any delay in the processing of the sample may lead to its degradation and/or loss. In such cases, it would be appropriate to analyse the sample and quarantine the results until its identity has been established. If the identity is not determined without any doubt, the results must[2] not be released.

13.2.3 Sample storage

Samples can often be stored for significant periods of time prior to analysis. The storage conditions in which samples should be maintained should be identified, for example, in the protocol, work instruction or associated trial documentation. It is also important that records are maintained which detail where samples are stored prior to analysis. Ongoing monitoring of refrigerators and freezers used to store samples should be conducted to identify any temperature excursions. There should be a process in place covering monitoring of refrigerator and freezer temperatures, and the actions to be taken in the event of a temperature excursion. Particular attention should be paid to the temperature of refrigerators, which quite often are subject to significant fluctuation. Storage conditions should be monitored using suitable calibrated equipment. Proof of calibration (for example, a certificate of calibration) should be retained with the monitoring data.

Inspections have highlighted issues in relation to monitoring of refrigerators and freezers. For example, at one laboratory, refrigerators attached to the electronic environmental monitoring system were set to register an alarm if the temperature fell below 1°C and or went above 10°C. However, the samples were required to be maintained at 2–8°C; it was not clear that excursions from these narrower limits would be detected or addressed.

The laboratory should make appropriate provision for the storage of samples in the event of a refrigerator or freezer failing.

13.3   Processing samples from clinical trials

13.3.1   Method validation

In the vast majority of cases the analysis of samples should be performed in accordance with a validated method. The nature of the necessary validation will be dictated by the complexity and type of technique(s) being employed and will need to be assessed on a case-by-case basis. In all cases, the aim will be to show that the method can be used to generate reproducible and reliable data.

Validation can be as simple as verifying that a technique already published in the literature is reproducible (for example, with established medicinal products or safety/biological markers) to full validation of, say, a new analyte for which there are no available data.

There are exceptional circumstances when samples taken during a clinical trial may be used to validate methods. This may be the case when new biomarkers are developed. This approach is acceptable provided the work has received the appropriate regulatory and ethical approval (for example, where the validation of a method is one of the trial objectives).

Therefore, based on a risk assessment of available published data and/or clear documentation of any justification to use the clinical trial samples for analysis, a finalised validated method should be in place and approved prior to undertaking any sample analysis on clinical trial samples. In inspections, there have been instances noted where clinical trial samples have been analysed in parallel with the validation study; had the validation not been reproducible, the sample data would have been rendered invalid and there may not have been adequate sample to repeat the analysis using a validated method.

13.3.2 Sample, standards and reagent preparation

In order to be able to fully reconstruct laboratory work, appropriate records must[5, 6] be maintained. One area that is often overlooked is the records associated with the preparation of buffers and reagents required by the analytical method. Laboratory analysts should ensure that it is possible retrospectively to verify how reagents were prepared – for example, this may take the form of notes in a laboratory book or proforma preparation worksheets that are cross-referenced to a written procedure. Additionally, there should be a process in place to ensure that the quality of reagents used in the assay is traceable to ensure they were fit for purpose. This may be done by the retention of a certificate of analysis in the study file or, if this level of information is not available, the source of the material should be recorded along with any relevant information (such as the batch number).

It may also be important to keep records of the use of some reagents (for example, the bulk reference product used to make calibration and quality control samples for batch analysis), so its use can be reconstructed if necessary.

13.3.3 Data recording

Data may be analysed, acquired and transferred by an analytical instrument and the values passed on to the sponsor or the clinical investigator without the need for any further intervention (for example, for routine clinical chemistry results or coagulation parameters). However, in more complex situations, such as the evaluation of biopsy samples or the determination of drug concentrations in body fluids, data are often presented in formal reports that are submitted to the sponsor or investigators. When this occurs, data must[5, 6, 7] be recorded accurately and legibly and should also be recorded promptly, where there are safety concerns (see section 13.7.1). In all situations, laboratory staff should ensure that they perform an appropriate level of quality control (QC) checks to confirm the accuracy of the data that have been generated and subsequently transcribed into the report. Any QC checks must[6] be documented and retained.

Any changes to data must be made so as not to obscure the previous entry. Where data are generated and recorded electronically, an electronic audit trail must[5] be maintained to make it possible to track any subsequent changes.

13.3.4 Repeat analysis

There may often be a valid reason for repeating the analysis of specific samples or batches of samples. For example, internal controls may fail or analytical equipment may malfunction. In clear-cut cases such as these, the decision-making process is relatively straightforward. However, there are also instances when the need to repeat the analysis of samples is less obvious (for example, if a sample from a low-dose group gives a result which is significantly higher than expected or if a sample from a control group shows the presence of drug). In order to prevent the selective reporting of results, acceptance criteria for data generated by each method of analysis and the circumstances where repeat analysis is permissible must[6] be clearly documented and retained.

Repeat analysis should only be undertaken in accordance with a written procedure. It is recommended this procedure includes the acceptable reasons for repeat analysis, any authorisation/approval for the decision to repeat, how it will be conducted (for example, repeat analysis is performed in duplicate to verify the repeat result) and documented. Appropriate documentation, including the rationale for performing the repeat, the original and repeat results, along with the reason why one result is accepted over another must[6] be maintained and retained in the trial master file (TMF) for full reconstruction of the data. It should also be clearly reflected in the clinical study report.

13.3.5 Unblinding and blinding

Clinical trials are often blinded. Maintaining the integrity of the blind is a key consideration for all those involved with the trial, as compromising the blinding may have a significant impact on the interpretation of the results. The sponsor is responsible for ensuring that measures are taken to protect the integrity of the blind. This will include ensuring that any laboratory data are only communicated to the appropriate people involved in the conduct of the trial. Laboratories that generate clinical trial data should be aware of whether the trial is blinded or not and exercise due diligence when communicating data to ensure the blind is not compromised.

Analytical laboratories may be asked to unblind trial samples so that analysis is not performed unnecessarily on samples collected from trial subjects that have been given placebo treatment. When this is the case, it is of the utmost importance that the laboratory has a written procedure to detail how results will be communicated in a blinded manner to the sponsor or its representative, especially if data are to be provided during the trial for preparation of an interim report or to inform dose-escalation decisions. The procedure may cover issues such as how to ensure that the final version of the randomisation code is obtained, the re-blinding of samples, storage of the information that allows samples to be unblinded and the way in which data are communicated to ensure that the blind is not compromised.

13.4   Laboratory facilities and equipment

The design and size of laboratories that analyse or evaluate samples from clinical trials will vary considerably depending on the nature of the work they undertake. However, in all cases they should be of a suitable size and design to allow an adequate degree of separation of different activities. The maintenance of samples' integrity as they pass through the laboratory is critical, so consideration should be given to the design of sample receipt and storage areas. For example, if a laboratory is likely to receive large numbers of chilled samples, provision should be made to ensure they remain at an appropriate temperature while they are being 'booked in'. Laboratories should be designed to ensure that ambient temperatures remain stable regardless of weather conditions or the heat generated by analytical equipment and refrigeration units.

13.4.1   Equipment maintenance

Laboratory techniques are often automated or use complex analytical instrumentation that requires periodic maintenance and calibration. In many cases it will be necessary to put in place service contracts with the equipment manufacturer or a maintenance company to ensure that instruments remain fit for purpose. If maintenance is performed by laboratory staff it is important that they have received an appropriate level of technical training. In all cases comprehensive records of maintenance, servicing and calibration must[6] be maintained and retained.

A procedure should be put in place to address system suitability tests; this procedure may stipulate that these tests are performed at appropriate intervals to demonstrate that the equipment remains fit for purpose between routine maintenance cycles. It is considered good practice to assess the functionality of analytical systems prior to the start of an analytical run.

In addition to analytical instruments, general laboratory equipment (such as centrifuges, balances, pipettes, refrigerators and incubators) should be subject to periodic calibration by appropriately qualified technicians. Additionally, checks should be performed on a regular basis to ensure equipment remains fit for purpose between calibration cycles. Documentation to demonstrate these checks have been performed must[6] be maintained and retained.

Calibration also needs to be appropriate, and on inspection examples have been seen where this has not been the case. For example, a laboratory balance was periodically checked with a 0.5 g check weight; however, the acceptance criterion for this two-place balance was $\pm$ 8 μg, which would have been impossible to determine with this check weight. In another example, a calibration certificate for the probe monitoring the −20°C freezer did not provide assurance that the probe could accurately function at the operating temperature of the freezer, which was routinely −27°C.

13.4.2 Computerised systems

The vast majority of today's analytical equipment is associated with computer software that is used to drive the instrument and to process the data. Many of these systems are commercial 'off-the-shelf' packages used by many organisations. Although full validation of these 'off-the-shelf' packages is not required by those purchasing them, organisations should subject all computerised systems used within the laboratory to an appropriate level of validation within their systems. However, a distinction can be made between bespoke systems developed exclusively for a particular laboratory and systems that are commercially available and widely used.

Examples of computerised systems that have been specifically designed for laboratory use may include laboratory information management systems (LIMS) or software that is required for specialised data processing. In these cases, the systems should be subject to a detailed validation process that is designed to test all expected functionality. In contrast, if a computerised system is commercially available, the level of validation needed prior to use may be more limited and used to confirm that the system is operating in accordance with the manufacturer's specification. In all cases, it will be appropriate to assess the functionality that will be used and implement a validation programme that demonstrates the systems are fit for their intended purpose.

Computer software is often updated to add functionality or to correct programming errors. Following changes to computer software, such as system upgrades or the installation of 'patches', it is likely that some level of revalidation will be required. The need for revalidation will need to be assessed on a case-by-case basis taking into account the complexity of the changes that have been made to the computerised system and their likely impact on functionality.

Prior to the validation of a computerised system, a validation plan should be produced detailing the nature of the tests that will be performed and their expected outcome. Records of each test should be maintained; this may include relevant screen shots and data files. On completion of the validation process it is often appropriate to generate a report that details the results of each of the tests that have been performed. Any limitations of the system highlighted during the validation process should be clearly described in laboratory procedures. See section 14.5 for the general principles of computer system validation.

The output from computerised systems can take many forms, from chromatograms to a digital image. Consequently, laboratory policies should clearly define what constitutes source data. However source data are defined, it must always be possible to use them to reconstruct the analysis and any subsequent changes made to data during or after analysis.

Inadequate validation of laboratory systems has been observed on inspection. For example, in one laboratory, the LIMS included functionality to use a barcode reader during sample receipt. While the LIMS had been subject to a level of validation, the barcode reader functionality had not been subject to an adequate level of validation to demonstrate that it operated effectively or reliably.

13.5 Reporting and archiving of data

13.5.1 Reporting

The way in which trial data are reported will vary considerably, depending on the nature of the analysis that the laboratory is contracted to undertake. In many cases, datasets may be reported without any additional interpretation, while in other instances the laboratory may produce a report that includes the results and associated interpretation.

If results are presented in the form of a report, it is not uncommon for the data to be summarised in tables. In such cases, original data (for example, chromatograms) will not always be reviewed by the study sponsor or regulatory authorities. Over the last several years, national monitoring authorities have identified a number of cases where data have been manipulated to ensure that results pass the stated acceptance criteria. For example, the inappropriate integration of chromatography peaks in order to ensure quality control samples or standards are accepted has been identified on a number of separate occasions. Consequently, every effort should be made to ensure that data are subject to an appropriate level of quality control checks prior to their finalisation and incorporation into a clinical study report.

In general, any change to the data must[5] be made so as not to obscure the previous entry. If data are generated, recorded, modified, corrected and stored or archived electronically, there should be an electronic audit trail maintained. Justifications for any changes to the data must[6] be documented, so it is possible to determine who made the change, when the change was made and for what reason.

It is always important to agree with the sponsor how data will be reported prior to the initiation of laboratory work. Regardless of how the data are reported, they must[7] always be accurate and complete.

13.5.2 Archiving

If a laboratory is contracted by the sponsor to retain source data, they must[5] be stored in a way that ensures their integrity and security. The length of time that the laboratory will retain data should be agreed with the sponsor prior to the initiation of the work and will usually form part of the agreement between the laboratory and the sponsor (see Chapter 10 for further information on document retention requirements).

It is important that all personnel are aware of the requirement to retain documentation. For example, it has been seen on inspection that it was not possible to verify that the laboratory method used was the one that had been validated, as the scientist who had performed the research had left the laboratory, taking the method development and validation records with him.

13.6 Maintaining quality within the laboratory

The quality of laboratory work is of utmost importance. A particular emphasis should be placed on ensuring that robust systems and procedures are in place that will be used to assess data quality and provide the oversight needed to ensure laboratory procedures are being adhered to. Quality requirements in the laboratory can be split in to two functions: quality control (QC) activities and quality assurance (QA) activities. Both are equally important but have a different focus and purpose.

13.6.1 Quality control

The accuracy of all laboratory processes should be subject to some level of QC checks. For example, if calculations are performed to produce a reported value, a representative sample of the calculations should be checked. The only caveat to this requirement is if a validated computerised system is used to generate the final result. Spreadsheets are commonly used to perform calculations and unless such spreadsheets are validated, locked and version-controlled, QC checks should be performed. QC checks will extend to a number of laboratory processes over and above the calculation of data points. Other activities that will require QC checks will include, but not be limited to, the assessment of manual integration of chromatograms, the recording of samples received by the facility and the production of sample collection kits.

Effective QC should be a central part of a laboratory's quality system and if implemented effectively will have a significant impact on the quality of the information that the laboratory generates. Section 14.3 provides further details on the principles of QC.

13.6.2 Quality assurance

The purpose of QA within a laboratory is very different from that of QC; however, they should not work in isolation from each other. The QA function will assess whether the laboratory's quality systems are operating effectively. Repeated issues associated with a laboratory activity that are identified by QC will often provide QA personnel with evidence that a given system is not working. The frequency and nature of QA checks will vary depending on the nature of the work conducted by the laboratory. However, in all cases the QA programme should be designed to assure that the laboratory works in accordance with the relevant national regulations.

Depending on the size of the laboratory operation, it may not be practical to employ dedicated staff to perform the QA function. In such cases, laboratory management may draw on resource from other areas of their operation. However, care should be taken to ensure that there is no conflict of interest. For example, it is unlikely to be appropriate to appoint an analyst who is involved in the generation of data to audit processes and policies that govern the analysis or evaluation of samples. Anyone who is appointed to perform QA functions must[4] be appropriately trained and be familiar with the processes and policies they are asked to audit. The audit process is further described in section 14.4.

Processes should be clearly defined to manage the handling and reporting of serious breaches that may originate within the laboratory. Examples of these may include the identification of fraudulent activity such as inappropriate data manipulation, or serious deviations from the clinical protocol or work plan that are likely to affect the integrity or interpretation of data. Further information on the identification of and reporting requirements of serious breaches can be found in section 1.3.5.3.

13.7   The trial subject

Many laboratories are geographically remote from any clinical activities and consequently it is easy for staff to overlook the fact that the samples they are analysing are collected from individuals whose rights and safety is of paramount concern. In addition to ensuring that the data they produce are of the highest standards, laboratory staff will also need to consider how the communication of those data affect the individuals participating in the trial.

13.7.1   Safety considerations

The well-being of trial subjects is of primary concern during the conduct of any clinical trial. The laboratory quite often has an important role to play in ensuring that any adverse reactions to IMPs are identified and reported as quickly as possible.

Prior to the initiation of laboratory analysis it is always appropriate for laboratory personnel to discuss with the sponsor or the investigator whether there is likely to be a need to expedite the reporting of the data they are responsible for generating. Examples of when expedited reporting will be necessary may be where the laboratory is responsible for assessing safety end-points that may indicate organ damage, or the data are needed to determine if a subject is eligible for dose adjustment.

In most instances, normal ranges should be established for safety tests prior to the start of analysis and if these ranges are exceeded a mechanism should be available for rapidly disseminating results to the relevant personnel. For example, the laboratory may define high and low values for certain parameters, but also define 'alert' values, to highlight very high or very low values. If these alert values are seen, then the laboratory should be able to quickly communicate this to the investigator to ensure appropriate care of the subject.

In one inspection it was identified that some central laboratory results were required for the investigator to assess whether the subject was eligible for enrolment into the trial. However, these results were not routinely reported by the laboratory until after the enrolment visit; therefore the investigator was forced to take additional samples for analysis by the local laboratory (which was not permitted as part of the protocol).

13.7.2   Consent

Laboratories must[2] only perform work that is detailed in the clinical protocol, a work instruction or the contract. The scope of the laboratory work should always be agreed with the sponsor or its representative before the work starts. It is important that there is a clear understanding between the sponsor and the laboratory on the nature of the work that will be performed, as it will allow the sponsor or investigator to ensure that the planned procedures are covered by the informed consent obtained from the trial subjects or their legal representatives. Procedures should also be implemented to ensure that the laboratory is informed in a timely manner if consent is withdrawn, to ensure that no further data are collected or generated from the sample. It is the site's responsibility to ensure that only appropriate samples are taken and sent to the laboratory (see section 11.3.2).

On inspection there have been numerous issues identified in relation to this issue. For example:

* As a result of the set-up of the analytical kits, laboratories have analysed and reported parameters in addition to those identified in the protocol and consented to by subjects. No consideration was given to ensuring that these unauthorised results were not captured, retained and reported.

- A laboratory received and reported results for samples that had not been consented to by the subject, as these samples had been taken and sent to the laboratory by the site in error.

13.7.3   Confidentiality

The trial subjects' right to confidentiality must[8] always be considered by the laboratory. If samples or associated documentation contain information that identifies a trial subject, measures must[8] be taken to ensure the information is masked and not disseminated further. The most common issue that laboratories are likely to encounter is the receipt of samples that detail the trial subject's name. All laboratories should have documented procedures for dealing with the receipt of such samples, including procedures for masking the information and informing the investigator site from which the samples originated.

13.8   Chapter legislative references

Throughout this chapter, specific terminology – 'must', 'required' or 'requirement' – has been used to interpret activities that are legislative requirements. These terms have been number-coded in the text where used, and the corresponding reference in the legislation can be found below.

1. Regulation 28 (1) of SI 2004/1031
2. Regulation 29 of SI 2004/1031
3. Schedule 1, Part 2 (4) of SI 2004/1031
4. Schedule 1, Part 2 (2) of SI 2004/1031
5. Schedule 1, Part 2 (9) of SI 2004/1031
6. Regulation 31A (4) of SI 2004/1031
7. Regulation 31A (7) of SI 2004/1031
8. Schedule 1, Part 2 (13) of SI 2004/1031

CHAPTER 14

Quality systems

Editor's note

All organisations involved in clinical trials must have a quality management system (QMS) in place to support the clinical trial activities they conduct. This ensures trial systems meet the requirements of the clinical trial legislation and associated guidelines and that processes are consistently applied. The extent and complexity of the QMS will depend on the size and nature of the organisation; however, essential features include clearly documented written procedures, adequate training of staff, and quality control and quality assurance procedures.

14.1 Quality system structure

An essential element of any clinical trial system is that there are clear written procedures in place to ensure that the system functions properly, that the roles, responsibilities and required tasks are clear to all parties involved and that there is provision for proper control, review and, when needed, change to the system. It is recommended that the standards to be followed in the quality system are also defined (for example, according to European Directives, UK legislation and ICH). It may also be relevant to refer to International Organization for Standardization (ISO) standards if these are used in the organisation.

Written procedures may take the form of policy documents, standard operating procedures (SOPs), working practices, guidelines or work instructions. The use and purpose of all written procedures used by an organisation should be clearly defined. The complexity of the quality system, and hence the written procedures, may depend on the type of organisation. In some organisations, for example, it may be appropriate to adopt a hierarchical approach to quality system documentation (see Figure 14.1). For others, a simpler system may be more appropriate, such as the use of only written procedures, forms and templates. Alternatively, there may be specific forms and procedures that are developed for each trial.

14.1.1   Different organisational models

14.1.1.1   Non-commercial organisations

In non-commercial organisations (for example, NHS Trusts), the quality system may be centralised, perhaps maintained by the research and development (R&D) office, and the procedures followed by all research teams. This model may be beneficial in terms of resources as it prevents different departments creating and maintaining a number of written procedures that are essentially very similar. It is also beneficial for an organisation to have one quality management system (QMS) for staff to follow, rather than individual sets of written procedures for different departments or funding streams. A common approach to quality will often make it easier for staff to comply with the system and for management to maintain oversight of it.

Alternatively, the quality system could be devolved with operational procedures being written by individual trial teams (for example, clinical trial facility/unit). In this case, the best use of resources and experience could be achieved by using an experienced trial team's procedures as the basis for creating new written procedures. Sometimes, the trial team may be following specific sets of written

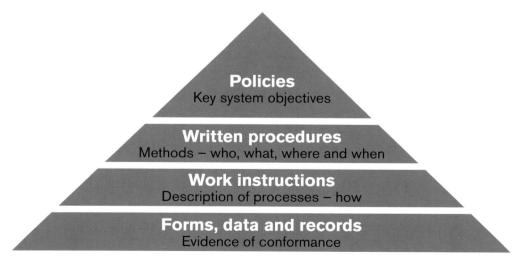

Figure 14.1 Example hierarchy of documentation in a quality system

procedures provided by outside organisations, such as the Medical Research Council (MRC) which applies a standard set of procedures across multiple sites. However this devolved quality system is approached, the sponsor should have assigned responsibility for ensuring that the localised procedures meet required standards and that sponsor oversight is maintained. Whatever type of system is used, centralised or devolved, the R&D office should ensure that it has procedures in place in order to maintain sponsor oversight.

In the case of a single investigator conducting a single trial, the quality system could be encompassed by the protocol containing all the trial-specific procedures that are to be followed, and therefore there will be no need to create a more complex quality system, where additional written procedures may not add value.

The research support services (RSS) of the National Institute for Health Research (NIHR) have developed a set of written procedures that can be used by R&D offices to ensure consistency across multiple organisations and sites running trials that are adopted into the NIHR portfolio. These procedures are available on the NIHR Clinical Research Network (CRN) website (www.crncc. nihr.ac.uk).

14.1.1.2 Commercial organisations

It is important that the procedures accurately reflect the functions that the organisation undertakes. For example, in some 'virtual' commercial sponsors (that is, those organisations that sponsor trials, but contract out all or the majority of their activities), it has been seen that their procedures cover activities that they are contracting out as though they are undertaking the activities themselves, which is inappropriate. Instead, the organisation's procedures should cover the function of overseeing the contractor performing the function. An example of this would be monitoring where the sponsor does not need a written procedure on how to undertake site monitoring visits, but does need a procedure to cover how it will assess and oversee the vendor undertaking the visit (for example, co-monitoring, review of reports). For these types of organisations, the quality system should include the contracting process, as this is a key activity. This is where the scope of work and roles and responsibilities are usually defined and therefore clear procedures surrounding this process will help to ensure there is appropriate delegation and oversight of a vendor by the sponsor.

Vendors, on the other hand, may have many written procedures which are very detailed as they may be carrying out a variety of activities for a number of sponsors. There may also be a subset of these written procedures if trial-specific or sponsor-specific procedures are warranted. The QMS of a vendor should clearly reflect the standards of the organisation. While it is recognised that procedures may vary from sponsor to sponsor, and the vendor will have flexibility in the quality system, the vendor should ensure that appropriate quality standards will always be met. Activities should be clearly defined as sponsors range from 'virtual' organisations to large global organisations.

Global pharmaceutical companies may have multiple layers of procedures in place, such as a quality manual, policies, written procedures, work instructions and technical guides, in order to manage multiple activities and functions. There may also be additional country-specific procedures in place in order to comply with differing regulatory and ethical requirements in relation to multinational clinical trials. In these more complex quality systems, written procedures, in particular global and local procedures, should not contradict each other.

Mergers and acquisitions can present a particular issue in relation to the QMS, where a sponsor can be conducting trials under more than one system, depending on which part of the new organisation the trial originated from. It is possible to manage more than one QMS while organisational changes are made; however, it should be clear which system is being followed and when changes occur to the system (particularly in relation to an ongoing trial), this must[1, 2] be documented. It is also recommended that there is a plan in place to manage the changes to the QMS.

As detailed above, it is recommended that an organisation has one QMS, but the complexity and size of an organisation may dictate that there may be a need for a number of systems or layers within its QMS.

14.1.1.3 General considerations

Any type of procedure that has been implemented to meet clinical trial legislation is recommended to be:

* reflective of the requirements in clinical trial legislation and applicable guidance (for example, EudraLex Volume 10)
* written and reviewed by adequately trained personnel (across different departments as required)
* approved by individuals within the organisation who have appropriate authority
* distributed and immediately available to all appropriate members of the organisation (and any other parties performing work on behalf of the organisation) once the procedures are effective (a period of time between

approval of the procedure and the procedure becoming effective would allow for training of relevant personnel)

- reviewed on a periodic basis to check that it still accurately reflects current practice.

It is also recommended that written procedures are user friendly and easily navigated to aid compliance; the length of a written procedure may need to be balanced against having a number of different procedures (that is, it may be more appropriate to produce a suite of written procedures rather than one written procedure that runs to hundreds of pages). The use of appropriate charts and diagrams within written procedures to explain activities can be very useful to the reader. While some organisations take the approach of having multiple written procedures to cover different functions, all activities should be covered without gaps in procedures that stretch across functions. It is recommended that organisations perform a gap analysis to ensure that their written procedures cover all activities.

Any significant deviations from procedures relating to clinical trial activities must[2] be documented. Information recorded, including the nature and impact of any deviations, may be important for trial reconstruction (for example, as illustrated in Figure 14.2, when revised written procedures are not implemented for a particular clinical trial in order to maintain continuity). It is recommended that the deviations are also captured centrally and taken into account during the next review of that

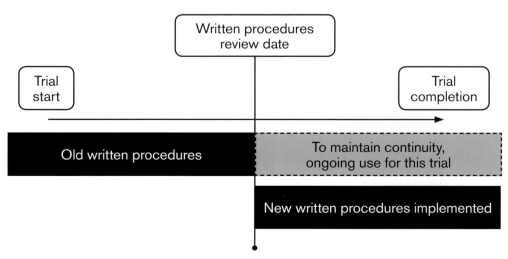

Figure 14.2 When revised written procedures are not implemented for a particular clinical trial in order to maintain continuity

procedure, as this may trigger a change to the system or may be used to identify any training needs. However, it may be necessary to implement some changes to the system prior to the next routine review – for example, if there is a significant change to the legislation, or if a significant gap or error in the procedures is identified that could affect safety or data integrity.

Where functions have been contracted out to a vendor, relevant procedures may be written and controlled by the vendor; the contract or work order may also define which written procedures will be followed. For example, Company X has subcontracted monitoring activities for a specific clinical trial to Company Y. It is acceptable for Company Y to perform these activities according to its own in-house written procedures; however, Company X (the contracting organisation) must[3] retain oversight which may be achieved by reviewing these procedures in order to ensure they are adequate, appropriate and compliant with applicable requirements and its own expectations. This review must[2] be retained as evidence of its assessment of the vendor (see section 1.3.2). Copies of these procedures, or a comprehensive list of the procedures being followed, must[1,2] be retained by the vendor, the contracting organisation or both. The contracting organisation should also have systems in place to ensure that it receives updates to the procedures used as they become available.

Alternatively, if the sponsor has requested that the vendor follow the sponsor's written procedures, then sponsors must[1,4] provide vendors with the written procedures and any subsequent updates. It is a common issue identified on inspection that vendors are not provided with adequate access to sponsor's written procedures, especially where there are updates during the course of the trial. This topic is also discussed in section 1.3.3.

A written procedure may cover one or more processes, or one process may have more than one procedure, depending on its complexity and the size and structure of the organisation.

Organisations running global clinical trials should ensure that they have procedures in place to meet local requirements. This is particularly important if the organisation does not have a local affiliate to help in the management of trials in that country. Any global written procedures should allow room for local affiliate procedures to be adapted to meet country-specific requirements. There have been examples seen on inspection where the local affiliate has not been involved in running a global trial, and only global written procedures are being used. This has led to the global team being unaware of specific local legislation and failing to comply with it – for example, failure to identify and report serious breaches in the

UK (see section 1.3.5 for further information on serious breaches). Other UK requirements that are sometimes not addressed in either global or local procedures include the requirement for urgent safety measures to be notified to the MHRA and the relevant research ethics committee (REC) within 3 days of action being taken (see section 2.3.7 for further information on urgent safety measures).

Organisations should control their procedural documents to ensure that staff are working to the current approved version of the procedure. Ways in which this can be achieved include version and date control of procedures, controlling the distribution of procedures and controlling access to them for updating purposes. For example, written procedures that are held electronically could be configured so that they display an expiry date when printed, or another watermark that reminds the user that only the electronic version is current. This practice will then minimise individuals referring to a paper version that may be out of date. Paper copies of written procedures may also be controlled by retrieving superseded versions when updates are issued. It is considered good practice for organisations to have a process in place that sets out how written procedures and other procedural documents are to be controlled. It is recommended that this document covers areas such as the maximum period for review of the different types of procedural document, the update and approval process, distribution of and training in new or updated procedural documents and the policy for retention of both current and superseded procedures.

It can be useful to employ tools to track the status of written procedures to ensure that they are reviewed and updated in a timely manner. Examples of such tools can range from a simple spreadsheet to register when written procedures are due for revision to a document control and approval system. If written procedures are reviewed, but it is determined that they are still current and no changes are required, this should also be documented. Details on the version control and preparation of written procedures are covered in Chapter 4.

Where there are a number of written procedures that cover the same or similar activities (usually where procedures cover activities that stretch across more than one department or function – for example, the regulatory green-light process (see section 1.5.2.3) may be covered in both clinical operations and clinical supplies written procedures), this can lead to an increased risk of contradiction if they are reviewed and updated at different times. It is therefore recommended that they are either updated at the same time (with input from both functions to ensure that they are consistent) or cross-refer to each other so that when one procedure is reviewed, it is checked against the other to ensure that one procedure does not contradict the other.

Written procedures and their use must[5] reflect the activities that are being performed and satisfy the principles of Good Clinical Practice (GCP). Examples of where poor management of written procedures may lead to issues are given below:

14

- Interactions between departments are not always taken into account when reviewing written procedures. This is important where a process involves more than one function. For example, gaps in the reconciliation of the pharmacovigilance database with the clinical database have been identified where neither the pharmacovigilance nor the data management function is clear about its responsibilities in this area.

- The R&D office developed a written procedure for IMP labelling, but the pharmacy department was unaware of this. The intention may have been to address a gap in the quality system, but by not involving other relevant departments this led to duplicate or contradictory procedures being produced.

- Where written procedures and forms are used jointly to detail procedures, these documents need to be managed appropriately. For example, in a Phase I unit there may be a written procedure to cover responsibilities and frequency of checks of the resuscitation trolley, but the required contents of the trolley may be covered in a form or checklist. If only the written procedure is reviewed and updated on a regular basis, important updates to the resuscitation trolley contents may be missed if the form is not controlled in the same way.

- Responsibilities are not always clearly defined in procedures. For example, sometimes when written procedures are designed to meet specific legislative requirements, the procedure paraphrases the legislation without detailing how that organisation can meet those requirements; that is, detailing that urgent safety measures or serious breaches must be reported to the MHRA within certain timeframes, but not specifying who is responsible for ensuring that this happens.

14.2   Training

Part 2 (2) of Schedule 1 to SI 2004/1031 requires that '*Each individual involved in conducting a trial shall be qualified by education, training and experience to perform his tasks.*'

In order to demonstrate that training has occurred, documentation must[2] be maintained and retained for all staff involved in the conduct of clinical trials and, where appropriate, for staff involved in supporting functions. The extent and content of this documentation is a business decision, but it typically includes:

- a current job description, dated and signed by the post holder and their line manager to demonstrate the date on which current roles and responsibilities have been agreed
- a curriculum vitae to demonstrate current and previous relevant education and experience, signed and dated to confirm the date of the document and ownership by the named individual
- confirmation that GCP training has taken place (including clear reference to the framework used in the training, such as UK Statutory Instruments and EU Directives)
- role-specific training relevant to the post holder's duties and clinical trial role(s) and responsibilities
- written procedures training records.

Additionally, for each trial an individual is involved with, there must[2, 4] be documentary evidence that they have received relevant trial-specific and (where required) therapeutic area training. These records must[2] be maintained as trial supporting documents (either centrally or with the individual trial site) for as long as they may be needed to support historical reconstruction of the trial.

In order to ensure that relevant staff have been appropriately trained, a process should be implemented so that the training requirements (in, for example, applicable written procedures, and for particular job roles and specific individuals in those roles) are formally documented. This could be in the form of a training matrix.

With regard to the training system, it is recommended that formal training plans are implemented that have been tailored to the individual needs of the clinical trial personnel (to ensure that they are, and remain, appropriately trained for their roles). The formal training plan may cover key training required to perform the designated tasks and be reviewed regularly by the individual and their line manager to ensure that training needs are being met.

In addition to formal training activities, organisations could consider making use of other methods of information sharing such as:

- posters in coffee points
- organisation's newsletters or bulletins
- intranet information sharing
- regular training or technical session at team meetings
- 'lunch and learn' style training events
- mentoring
- sharing good practice with other organisations or other internal departments.

A log of articles/journals reviewed could also be kept to demonstrate that an individual is keeping up to date with current thinking, as reading is also useful training.

14.2.1   GCP training

Regulation 28 of SI 2004/1031 states that no person shall conduct a trial otherwise than in accordance with the conditions and principles of GCP; it therefore follows that each person involved in a clinical trial must[4] receive some training in GCP commensurate with their roles and responsibilities. This training must[4] not be restricted to training in the UK Clinical Trials Regulations but should also include, as appropriate, training in other available guidance relating to clinical trials (for example, EudraLex Volume 10 or Annex 13 training if an individual is involved in reviewing/approving IMP labels). The frequency of GCP training is not specified in the regulations; however, it is recommended that training is given at intervals appropriate to ensure staff maintain awareness of the current UK regulations and applicable European guidelines. How often this training is repeated is a business decision for the organisation concerned. Systems should also be in place to allow for ad hoc training to be provided in the event that there are significant regulatory updates (for example, implementation of a new UK Statutory Instrument) between scheduled training events or to be provided as refresher training where, for example, staff have been on extended leave. Requirements for the frequency of GCP training should be documented in the organisation's procedures.

Training received can be tailored to the roles and responsibilities being undertaken by an individual. For example, it would not be considered necessary for an individual such as a ward nurse who is only responsible for obtaining blood samples from trial patients at an investigator site (which they would do as part of their normal clinical duties) to be trained in the full scope of GCP. Training/ awareness in the aspects of GCP relevant to that role would be considered acceptable (for example, recording of adverse events, documentation of activities in source notes or case report form (CRF), escalating any issues they identify as appropriate). Similarly, this would be the case if the management of the subject and administration of IMP was similar to the standard of care.

There may be staff involved in supporting activities who do not require specific GCP training (for example, phlebotomists or chemotherapy nurses where no trial-related activities are undertaken outside of their usual role). Where the administration of the investigational medicinal product (IMP) by chemotherapy nurses is routinely administered within the chemotherapy unit as standard treatment and all other protocol activities are undertaken by a member of the research team, then no protocol-specific or GCP training may be required; however, this should be reviewed as part of the risk assessment for the trial, with consideration given to GCP awareness training – for example, in the recording of adverse events (see Chapter 11).

It may be necessary for staff involved in trial activities to be aware of other regulatory requirements outside those of GCP. For example, healthcare professionals retaining tissue samples should be aware of the Human Tissue Act.

14.2.2   Training in written procedures

Training in an organisation's written procedures, or those of an external vendor, should be specific to the roles and responsibilities undertaken by particular staff members. The organisation should be able to demonstrate its expectations for training of staff in written procedures. Ways in which this can be achieved include listing training requirements for particular job roles in staff job descriptions and use of written procedure training grids and/or matrices to indicate what written procedure training is expected for each of the roles within the organisation. The complexity of the system used will depend on the type of organisation.

Consideration may also be given to the type of training required – for example, whether this is face-to-face training or a 'read and understand' approach. This will vary depending on the role and the procedure (that is, whether it is a new procedure, or the first time an individual has received training or whether it is an update). It is recommended that an appropriate and realistic time is allowed for written procedures to be 'read and understood' in order for this type of training to have any relevance. For example, it has been seen on inspection that a large number of written procedures (or, in some instances, all written procedures) have been recorded as 'read and understood' in one day. In this scenario, it is unlikely that all written procedures have been understood and that staff have been trained appropriately.

Some procedures cover particular 'hands-on' skills, such as laboratory procedures, clinical procedures or procedures carried out by an individual externally and unsupervised (such as monitoring and auditing). For these types of activities the organisation may wish to consider assessing the competency of the individual before they are allowed to perform that activity unsupervised or provide training on that task to another individual.

It is not a regulatory requirement to have a specific 'competency sign-off', indicating that the person is competent in a process. The organisation should, however, have processes in place to assure itself that its staff are indeed competent to perform their assigned functions. This is particularly relevant for complex tasks, where a simple 'read and understand' approach to procedures may not be appropriate. For example, at investigator sites, this could be complex dosing activities, venepuncture or interpretation of EEGs, while at the sponsor/ vendor site, this could be the use of data management systems or interactive response technologies (IRT) systems.

This assessment could be approached in several ways, including:

- ensuring that the training provided to staff for general and trial-specific activities is appropriate and effective (some organisations do have a competency assessment or check following training)
- ensuring that updates to training are provided as needed, particularly if trial or organisation processes or the protocol changes, or in the event of regulatory changes
- carrying out checks through audits or monitoring to ensure that on completion of training, staff are indeed carrying out their duties according to requirements and/or procedures; these checks should be documented in monitoring/audit reports and could take the form of a co-monitoring visit, or a peer review of interpretation of ECGs.

14.2.3 Trial-specific training

Trial-specific training must[4] be undertaken prior to commencement of any trial-specific activities (for example, activities such as reporting of serious adverse events (SAEs), or complex trial assessments or calculations, as listed in the trial protocol) and include any supporting trial manuals and guidance. All staff must[4] receive an appropriate level of training to allow them to perform their trial-related duties, taking into consideration training needs for staff who join a trial team after the trial has started.

With regard to trial-specific training, instances have been seen on inspection where a lack of training and understanding of protocol-specific requirements have had an impact on the outcome of the trial. For example, in a multinational trial, the protocol was ambiguous in relation to whether acute respiratory exacerbations required expedited reporting. The protocol-specific training did not adequately address this issue and this led to inconsistencies in how this information was collated and reported across sites and countries. Other examples seen include unclear instructions and training on how to conduct RECIST (Response Evaluation Criteria In Solid Tumours) calculations, which have led to incorrect results being documented. Also issues have been identified in relation to how creatinine clearance is calculated, which has led to incorrect data being collected and reported.

14.3 Quality control

Quality control (QC) is a fundamental approach to verify compliance with the Clinical Trials Regulations (Schedule 1, Part 2 (4) and (9) of SI 2004/1031) and should be implemented.

QC is an activity that involves the review of factors in a process as the process is occurring. This approach may be appropriate for some clinical trial activities as an 'in-process' assessment of performance and compliance. This real-time assessment of how systems are functioning can help build quality into processes rather than relying solely on an end-product assessment. The level and type of QC that should be undertaken is determined by the risk assessment of the clinical trial (if one is performed).

Any QC activities performed must[2] be documented and, where possible, performed by a second individual who is independent of initial activities. The documentation used to demonstrate that QC has taken place does not have to be particularly formal (that is, result in a report). Annotated sets of data could be acceptable, for example, if the provenance thereof could be determined.

Some examples where QC activities can be built into clinical trial systems and processes include:

- review and QC of trial documentation (for example, protocols, informed consent documentation, subject information sheets, clinical trial authorisation applications and contracts) – review of these documents prior to approval would help to identify errors, inconsistencies or non-compliances that would be more difficult to rectify once a document has been formally issued
- checks performed during monitoring on the quality and accuracy of data transcribed from source data into case report forms (that is, source data verification)
- checks on data entry for SAE information entered into safety databases
- system to verify accuracy of the clinical database (that is, data entry verification)
- accuracy of scanned documents (for example, into the electronic trial master file (eTMF) or electronic subject notes)
- review and QC of data used to make dose escalation decisions – these often form part of a safety report, but may bypass usual monitoring and data management processes due to the timelines associated with these trials
- review and QC of the analysis and incorporation of data in the clinical study report.

Written procedures detailing the requirements for QC activities should be in place and should include information relating to the expected scope and frequency of QC. In some (simple) trials, the QC procedures applied to the trial could be sufficiently outlined in the trial protocol. Expectations relating to acceptable standards of QC should be documented; this would usually define acceptable error rates and it is recommended that the process defines the actions to be taken where the QC checks show a failure to meet the acceptable predefined standard. For example, where source data verification of transcribed CRF data determines the error rate, a cut-off point can be identified to permit appropriate additional action to be taken. Such actions could be more frequent monitoring visits to a particular site, increased source data verification or additional site training in a particular area.

14.4 Quality assurance

Although the quality assurance (QA) function is not explicitly defined in the legislation, it is expected that the QA requirements[1] for a trial are assessed and the need for, and level of, QA determined.

14

There is a requirement[1, 5] to provide assurance that an organisation's clinical-trial activities are conducted in accordance with approved trial documentation and also to identify any deficiencies in supporting clinical trial processes and systems. A mechanism should therefore be in place to provide assurance that clinical trial activities are being performed in accordance with UK clinical trials legislation, guidelines, an organisation's procedures and GCP.

It is recommended that the frequency and approach to QA activities (for example, auditing) are proportionate to the nature and scope of clinical trial activities performed by the organisation. A risk-based approach may be appropriate providing that the organisation is able to provide a sound rationale. Audits must[4] be performed by individuals who have appropriate understanding of the clinical trial legislation to be able to assess whether the organisation is meeting the requirements of the legislation. Examples have been seen on inspection where poor QA activities (for example, audit findings are inappropriately collated, graded or they are repeated) have caused a trial (or site) to be inappropriately terminated or even reported as a serious breach to the MHRA, citing (incorrectly) GCP non-compliance.

Equally, it has been observed on inspection that an inexperienced QA or QC function missed important information such as missing subject records or compliance issues around subject recruitment, which were indicators of potential fraud. Obvious problems had not been detected or they had been detected but the auditor concluded that a trial was GCP compliant, therefore making an inappropriate assessment.

In addition, auditors should be independent of the activities being audited and, unless the size of the organisation does not allow, report into independent lines of management. In the non-commercial environment, independence of the QA function can be maintained by assigning QA functions across departments. For example, an oncology research nurse who is not a member of the trial team could conduct QA activities for a trial in a different department, such as the respiratory department, and vice versa. The support of senior management for the QA function is important to ensure that issues can be effectively and appropriately managed and escalated where necessary. Independence is therefore also key to the QA function for the same reasons.

In many organisations, QA activities are planned in advance on an annual or biennial basis. Audit schedules are recommended to be reviewed and approved by a member of staff with the appropriate authority. These audit schedules can be modified once implemented, as risks and priorities may change. However, these changes should be prospective and documented to indicate that they were performed in a controlled manner.

In addition to scheduled activities, unscheduled or 'for-cause' audits may be required in the event of serious non-compliance or other triggers. Planning for these types of audit will be different to those for scheduled audits, in that they cannot be allocated in advance and may therefore affect other planned QA activities.

Examples of the types of audits that may be performed by an organisation include:

- system audits – looking at the functionality of complete systems (for example, pharmacovigilance, data management)
- process audits – looking at the performance of specific processes within systems (for example, expectedness assessments, data query process)
- vendor audits – assessment of external service providers
- trial-specific audits – audit of all activities across a single trial
- investigator site audits – trial-specific assessment of trial activities in the clinical setting
- documentation audits – review of trial-specific or system documentation (for example, computer system validation package, protocols, interim reports or clinical trial report).

As previously indicated, the scope and frequency of audit activities will vary depending on the complexity of the organisation. Many organisations have implemented audit checklists and aides memoires to assist in conducting audit activities. These tools act as a prompt for auditors and are often customised depending on the type of audit being conducted. Also, these documents may form part of the quality system as controlled templates or forms associated with QA written procedures.

Records of audits that are planned and conducted should be distributed to the appropriate personnel (such as auditees and management). Following issue of the report there should be a system in place to ensure that appropriate corrective and preventative action to address the identified issues is proposed and agreed. Many organisations will not close audits until all actions have been completed. Where audits are closed and evidence of completed corrective and preventative actions has not been provided, follow-up action may be required in order to verify that proposed actions have been taken as indicated. This follow-up may be at the

14

next planned audit or sooner, depending on the severity and nature of the identified issue. The procedure should also allow for escalation of issues to appropriate personnel if, for example, there is a dispute over an audit finding or corrective and preventative action has not been taken. It is useful to implement a categorisation system so that issues can be graded according to significance/ impact on data, results or subject safety. 'Critical' or significant issues can then be identified using this system and actioned immediately and escalated appropriately. Records of audits that are planned and conducted must[2] be retained.

Many organisations use the output from audit activities to assist with generating metrics and to identify process improvements. In some situations, persistent and repeated non-compliance in certain areas can be indicative of flawed supporting systems rather than a problem with the particular area being audited. For example, where forms or templates are used to guide a particular process (such as drug accountability), repeated non-compliance when these forms/templates are completed could be associated with poor design of the forms rather than with how the activity is carried out.

In addition to audit activities, other techniques can be employed to assure the quality of work undertaken. Examples include:

- internal departmental assessments (for example, a local pharmacovigilance office reviewing their case-handling process)
- checklists – completed as processes are followed and used to identify gaps or flaws in those processes
- system tests – 'dummy runs' to ensure that processes function as intended (for example, 24-hour medical cover, emergency unblinding, recall processes).

14.5   Computer system validation

This section is not intended to cover all aspects of validation of computer systems as it is beyond the scope of this guide, but it is intended to give an overview of validation from a GCP compliance perspective. More detailed guidance on computer system validation is widely referenced and readily available:

- GAMP® 5: A Risk-Based Approach to Compliant GxP Computerized Systems, ISPE. www.ispe.org
- Computer Systems Validation in Clinical Research – A Practical Guide (Edition 2) ACDM. www.acdm.org.uk

- IC/S publication/recommendation: 'Good Practices for Computerised Systems in Regulated GxP Environments' (PI 011-3) Sept 2007. Secretariat of the Pharmaceutical Inspection Convention, c/o EFTA Secretariat 9–11, rue de Varembé, CH – 1211 Geneva 20, Switzerland. www.picscheme.org
- INS-GCP-3 Annex III to Procedure for conducting GCP inspection requested by the EMEA – Computerised Systems. www.emea.europa.eu

This section will therefore only provide an overview of the general principles to be applied when using a bespoke or a commercial off-the-shelf (COTS) product in clinical trial activities. There should be validation of the development or installation of the computer system itself, and also validation of any trial-specific builds/applications/programming undertaken subsequently using the validated system. These are undertaken together to demonstrate that the system and its use for a trial are 'fit for purpose'. All computer systems used in clinical trials, in particular those that impact on the quality of the trial data (and subject safety) should be validated. Computer systems in clinical trials are typically used to control a process, process data or store data. Examples of systems in the GCP environment are listed below:

- pharmacovigilance databases
- eCRF systems
- clinical trial databases
- electronic transfer of data (for example, laboratory data to the clinical database)
- IRT systems
- computer programming (for example, edit checks routines, statistical analysis)
- pharmacy electronic prescribing systems (for example, Chemocare)
- electronic diaries for subjects
- clinical trial management systems (CTMS)
- eTMF
- electronic health records.

14.5.1 Validation principles

Numerous definitions of computer system validation exist, but there are three key features:

- Appropriate controls of the system are in place throughout the system's lifetime.
- Documentation is available to support the application of the controls.
- The system is fit for purpose and performs reliably and consistently as intended.

The level of control and validation of the system to demonstrate its fitness for purpose is dependent upon whether it is an off-the-shelf package, an off-the-shelf package with a trial-specific configuration/build or a completely bespoke system. Also influential is the use and purpose of the system and how this relates to the two key GCP objectives of ensuring data/results integrity and the protection of the rights, well-being and safety of trial subjects. As such, a risk assessment and proportionate approach to the validation of the system would be considered acceptable by inspectors.

Off-the-shelf products (for example, MS Excel, SPSS, Oracle and SAS) are validated by the software developers before being released for sale, but may become unstable if they are incompatible with other software installed on the same operating system. However, in general, mainstream products tend to be used in the live environment within the same organisation for other activities, and the robustness and stability of the system is rarely a problem, so the risk of using these established systems is relatively low. When in doubt, installation, operational and performance qualifications should be undertaken and evidence must[2] be retained. Additionally, it may be appropriate to undertake vendor assessment to establish the aforementioned validation.

14.5.2 'Levels' of validation

Where a COTS package requires a trial-specific configuration (for example, MS Excel, eCRFs, eTMF, IRT), then some formal validation should be required to confirm that the system is fit for purpose for each particular trial. However, dependent upon the system, this could look very different yet still be acceptable (see examples below).

14.5.2.1 Example 1 (off-the-shelf package)

An investigator may use MS Excel to manage the trial data and undertake some simple analysis. There would be an expectation that there is a documented check on formatting of the cells (for example, numeric, dates) and any formulae that have been put into the system. This could simply be recording that the ranges of the cells have been checked, writing down formulae or confirming that the spreadsheet is consistent with the written 'specification' prior to use of the system.

Individual programs will require documentation to confirm fitness for purpose. This could be in the form of retained output from independent dual programming or input/output and logs to confirm that the program has performed as intended.

14.5.2.2 Example 2 (trial-specific configuration)

For the creation of a trial-specific application using a COTS package (for example, set-up of a trial in an IRT system or an eCRF system), the following validation documentation would be the minimum expected:

- approved specification
- testing documentation for developers and users
- signed validation report to confirm that all test failures have been resolved and specifications have been met)
- production of user instructions and training of users
- documented release (that is, the move to production environment from the testing environment).

It should be noted that the above documentation is descriptive of the purpose of the document, and the actual document itself could vary dependent upon its application. For example, the validation of a computer program could have the user requirements specified in a data management plan, statistical analysis plan or randomisation specification, and the functional specification and validation plan could be within a written procedure or guidance on programming practice.

14.5.2.3 Example 3 (bespoke system)

For bespoke application development, more comprehensive validation documentation would be required to demonstrate that the system was fit for purpose. This would typically include the following documentation:

- risk assessment
- user requirements specification
- functional specification
- validation plan
- code-testing documentation

- documentation of user acceptance testing (including retention of test scripts, failures and traceability matrix)
- validation report
- user manual
- training records
- records of release.

It has often been seen on inspection that not all the necessary records of validation have been generated or retained as required.[6] For example, there is no documentation to verify that the clinical database has been tested or a validation report has been approved after a system has already been released. Some systems inspected had not been validated at all.

14.5.3   Change control

There should be a mechanism in place for version control of the system/trial-specific build or application and a formal process to manage any changes to this to ensure the validated state is maintained. The version control may be based on minor incremental changes together with large-scale new releases. The change control documentation would typically include:

- request for a change and the reasons, details of requester
- risk assessment
- assessment and actions required (possible need for a validation plan)
- approval of planned change
- testing (and evidence of any corrective actions taken)
- validation report or similar
- evidence of release to production environment.

14.5.4   Other considerations

In addition to validation, there are other computer system requirements to consider and these include the following:

- system back-up (for accidental loss, disaster recovery)
- system security (that is, who has access and how this access is controlled)

- interaction of different systems (for example, direct electronic transfer of information/results from separate computer systems or merging of information between systems)
- audit trails (that is, the ability to verify who entered or changed data in the system, when this was done and what was changed)
- continued accessibility (clinical trial data are required to be stored for a lengthy period)
- training of staff, including investigator site staff.

The above considerations apply if the system is hosted on the server of the sponsor or of the vendor, or if it is hosted in a so-called 'cloud' space (that is, online storage of data generally hosted by third parties). Whatever the set-up used, it must[2, 6] meet the requirements for managing and storing data for clinical trials.

14.6   Chapter legislative references

Throughout this chapter, specific terminology – 'must', 'required' or 'requirement' – has been used to interpret activities that are legislative requirements. These terms have been number-coded in the text where used, and the corresponding reference in the legislation can be found below.

1. Schedule 1, Part 2 (4) of SI 2004/1031
2. Regulation 31A (4) of SI 2004/1031
3. Regulation 3 (12) of SI 2004/1031
4. Schedule 1, Part 2 (2) of SI 2004/1031
5. Regulation 28 (2) of SI 2004/1031
6. Schedule 1, Part 2 (9) of SI 2004/1031

Annexes

Introduction to GCP inspections

Editor's note

The MHRA Good Clinical Practice (GCP) Inspectorate is part of the Inspection, Enforcement and Standards Division of the MHRA. The function of the GCP Inspectorate is to assess the compliance of organisations with UK and EU legislation relating to the conduct of clinical trials in investigational medicinal products (IMPs) as part of the MHRA's mission to safeguard public health. This is achieved through carrying out inspections of sponsor organisations that hold clinical trial authorisations or organisations that provide services to clinical trial sponsors. These include pharmaceutical companies, contract research organisations (CROs), non-commercial organisations such as universities, NHS Trusts and charities, investigational trial sites, Phase I units, clinical laboratories, GCP archives, and other niche facilities, such as central ECG reading organisations, involved in clinical trial research. The MHRA Inspectorate initiated a voluntary GCP inspection programme in 1998 to develop the inspection methodology. A statutory GCP inspection programme has been in place since 1 May 2004.

Further information on the GCP Inspectorate, including details of the current level of fees for national GCP inspections, can be accessed via the Good Clinical Practice page of the MHRA website.

A.1.1 Legal basis for inspections

European legislation requires Member States to inspect organisations in relation to a clinical trial – Article 15 (1) of Directive 2001/20/EC states:

'To verify compliance with the provisions on good clinical and manufacturing practice, Member States shall appoint inspectors to inspect sites concerned by any clinical trial conducted, particularly the trial site or sites, the *manufacturing site of the investigational product, any laboratory used for analyses in the clinical trial and/or the sponsor's premises.'*

Article 23 (1) of Directive 2005/28/EC further defines that such inspections may take place on any of the following occasions:

'(a) before, during or after the conduct of clinical trials;

(b) as part of the verification of applications for marketing authorisation;

(c) as a follow-up to the granting of authorisation.'

UK inspectors have rights conferred under Regulations 325 and 327 of the Human Medicines Regulations 2012 (SI 2012/1916) as well as the Medicines for Human Use (Clinical Trials) Regulations 2004 (SI 2004/1031). These include the right to enter any premises involved in clinical trials of investigational medicinal products (IMPs) in the UK to carry out inspections, take samples, require the production of books and documents, and to take copies of, or copies of entries in, such books, and to document and seize and detain substances, articles and documents. It is a criminal offence under the Human Medicines Regulations 2012 to obstruct an inspector during the conduct of an inspection covered by these regulations. Inspectors carry cards of written authority as a means of identification and will produce them on request. Inspectors' rights are also stated on these cards.

A.1.2 MHRA GCP inspectors

All MHRA Good Clinical Practice (GCP) inspectors undergo a formal training programme and are educated, at a minimum, to relevant university graduate level or have equivalent experience in a relevant area (as required by Directive 2005/28/EC and the associated EudraLex Volume 10 guidance). New inspectors are trained through a combination of classroom training and accompanying accredited inspectors on inspections. The programme also includes training in the national and European guidelines for inspection, the systems needed to conduct clinical trials to GCP, and methods for evaluation and reporting of inspection findings. As well as national routine inspections, MHRA GCP inspectors also perform Committee for Medicinal Products for Human Use (CHMP) requested inspections on behalf of the European Medicines Agency (EMA) in the UK, EU and beyond. The MHRA GCP inspectors are regularly assessed according to internal procedures to ensure the standards of competence and consistency required are maintained, as well as undergoing external standards audits such as Benchmarking of European

Medicines Agencies (BEMA) and International Organization for Standardization (ISO) audits.

Outside of inspections, the inspectors are also involved in regular meetings with other agencies involved in clinical trials such as the Health Research Authority (HRA) and Human Tissue Authority (HTA), ensuring effective communication and streamlining of processes. The MHRA GCP Inspectorate also works closely internally with other MHRA divisions such as the Clinical Trials Unit (CTU) and Licensing Assessors. An example is the provision of advice on clinical trials, provided jointly with the MHRA CTU, either by telephone or via the Clinical Trial Helpline (clintrialhelpline@mhra.gsi.gov.uk).

MHRA GCP inspectors also attend the meetings of EU GCP inspectors, which are held on a quarterly basis at the EMA, to assist with harmonisation and the development of procedures for EU GCP inspections. The MHRA GCP Inspectorate (in addition to the MHRA CTU and HRA) also provides UK representation at the European Commission's ad-hoc group for the implementation of the Clinical Trials Directive 2001/20/EC, for the development of GCP legislation and guidance.

Interactions with external stakeholders include provision of speakers at requested training events and provision of symposia to the commercial and non-commercial sectors, input into the National Institute for Health Research (NIHR) training and research support services (RSS) standard operating procedures (SOPs), coordination of the MHRA GCP Consultative Committee, and developing internal and external guidance as new areas of regulation emerge. The MHRA GCP Inspectorate also launched the GCP Forum on the MHRA website in October 2011 to provide an opportunity for researchers and organisations to communicate with each other and discuss practical issues relating to clinical trials. The GCP Forum is moderated by the MHRA GCP inspectors to ensure that the discussions are in keeping with the legislation.

A.1.3 Types of GCP inspections

The types of inspections that may be conducted under the statutory programme are detailed below.

(i) *Routine national inspections*
These are scheduled inspections that organisations undergo on a periodic basis. Organisations are notified of these inspections in advance. These inspections are

A1

generally systems-based, meaning that inspectors examine the systems and procedures used to conduct clinical research in the UK by both commercial and non-commercial organisations, to comply with existing EU and national GCP regulations. The inspectors will select a number of clinical trials in order to get an overview of the work carried out by the sponsor and examine how the organisation's trial procedures are applied in practice. Inspections can also be trial-specific, in which case a particular trial which has been completed will be assessed. This trial is usually a pivotal or key decision-making trial, such as a trial to be submitted in support of a marketing authorisation application (MAA), or a trial that may significantly alter clinical practice.

(ii) 'Triggered' national inspections

These are ad hoc inspections that are triggered as a result of information received by the MHRA about suspected violations of legislation relating to the conduct of clinical trials (for example, information from a serious breach notification, a whistleblower, other MHRA departments or HRA). In rare circumstances, the organisation may receive little or no notification of these inspections in advance.

(iii) Requested inspections

These are MAA-related inspections. They may be performed at the request of the MHRA licensing division and conducted via national inspection procedures. Alternatively, they may be requested by the CHMP for applications via centralised procedures or by the Co-ordination Group for Mutual Recognition and Decentralised Procedures – Human (CMDh). The EMA coordinates these inspections, which are conducted by inspectors from the EU Member States. The general organisation and process for CHMP-requested GCP inspections is described in EudraLex Volume 10, Chapter IV.

A.1.4 Scope of GCP inspections

The inspection scope is limited to those trials that come under SI 2004/1031 (that is, it excludes non-interventional and laboratory studies that do not have a clinical component or contribute to trial end-points), and will cover work substantially performed after 1 May 2004.

In order to examine compliance of the procedures and systems used by the organisation for conducting trials in the UK, inspections may also include areas of the organisations that are partly or wholly located outside the UK.

A.1.5 Inspection schedule

The MHRA GCP Inspectorate has always used a risk-based inspection process for the routine statutory inspection programme; in May 2009 the compliance report system was launched to further inform the risk-based programme. This enables the Inspectorate to focus resources to improve the protection of public health where there is a potentially higher risk or where there would be a greater impact if compliance issues were to occur. This process uses the information provided by organisations in the compliance reports in conjunction with information and intelligence already held by the MHRA to determine an organisation's control of their risk. The resulting risk assessments are categorised into high, medium and low risk, and a proposed inspection frequency is assigned to a given organisation on the basis of this categorisation. In practice, this means that organisations with a higher risk rating will be inspected more frequently than those with a lower risk rating.

Factors that may affect inspection scheduling include:

- numbers of clinical trials sponsored, hosted or managed by a given organisation
- numbers of UK patients and the nature of trial subjects
- IMP characteristics, particularly regulatory status and IMP type
- outcome of previous inspections (including inspections from other competent authorities and GxP areas)
- non-compliance with reporting requirements (for example, safety reports, end-of-trial notifications, trial reports)
- organisations that have not previously been inspected.

Further details on the current risk-based inspection process can be found on the MHRA website.

A.1.6 Phases of the inspection process

There are three main phases of each GCP inspection (Figure A.1.1):

- planning
- conduct of the inspection
- reporting.

A1

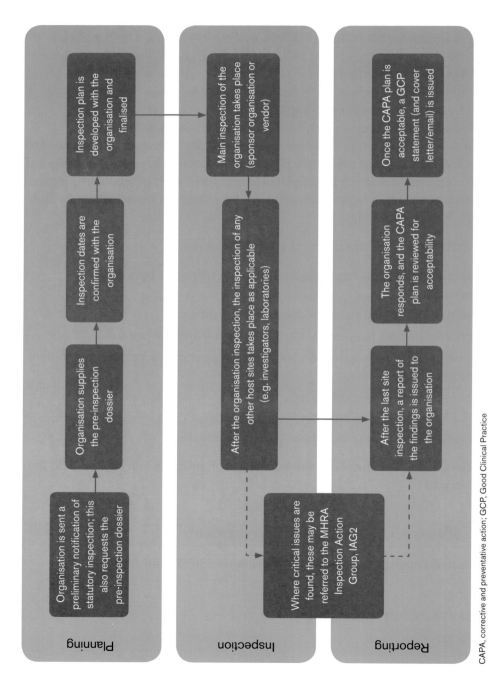

CAPA, corrective and preventative action; GCP, Good Clinical Practice

Figure A.1.1 MHRA GCP routine inspection process

A.1.6.1 Planning

For routine, national inspections, a preliminary notification is sent out to those organisations identified for statutory inspection. Each organisation will be requested to provide a GCP inspection dossier. This request for information includes a list of clinical trials, organisation charts, lists of written procedures and selected procedures (for example, safety reporting procedures), key contact details, overview of facilities, key service providers and clinical trial activities. This assists the Inspectorate in understanding who in the organisation performs clinical trial research, how this is generally conducted (management policy or procedures which direct the process) and where this research is performed. (Note: For non-commercial organisations this is in relation to those clinical trials of IMP where the organisation is the sponsor or co-sponsor and those trials that the organisation hosts on behalf of other non-commercial organisations.) The current version of the GCP inspection dossier template is available from the MHRA GCP website.

The lead inspector will review the dossier. If it is determined that an inspection of the organisation is not appropriate at this time (for example, if there has been little or no clinical trial activity since the previous inspection), the organisation will be informed. If the inspection is to go ahead, the inspector will contact the organisation to agree inspection dates and the agenda. Additional updated details may be requested nearer the date of the inspection. These usually relate to specific trials, such as recruitment and serious adverse event (SAE) numbers, but may also include specific written procedures. If there are any questions or concerns on the part of the organisation when compiling the dossier, these can be discussed by calling any of the MHRA offices where an inspector or administrator will help with any questions. A further confirmation letter (or email), issued once the inspection dates have been agreed, will provide further details on the logistics of the inspection, such as the inspection team, and also the fees applicable.

A draft inspection plan will usually be provided to the organisation for review and confirmation of personnel involved in interview sessions (see Table A.1.1 for activities that may be selected for review on inspection). A number of clinical trials are normally selected for detailed trial master file (TMF) review, although the inspection may not be limited to these. Any comments or clarification required in respect of this plan can be discussed with the inspectors. It is important that personnel who actually perform the activities are included in interview sessions, in order to gain most value from the inspection from both the Inspectorate's and

A1

Table A.1.1 Activities that may be selected for review on inspection

Organisation site inspection (commercial and non-commercial sponsors, vendors)		
Regulatory submissions	Monitoring	Medical advice
Contract management	Data management	Statistical analysis
Insurance	Quality assurance	Report writing
Project management	Training	Pharmacovigilance
Archives	Laboratories	Computer systems
Trial master file management for selected clinical trial(s)	Investigational medicinal product management	

Investigator site inspection		
Interviews	**Documentation**	**Tours**
Principal investigator	Case report forms	Pharmacy
Sub-investigator	Source data	Clinic
Pharmacists and pharmacy technicians	Investigator site file (plus support department files)	Support departments/sites (for example, pharmacy, laboratories, radiology)
Research nurses	Consents	Archives
	Investigational medicinal product accountability	Laboratory

Note: activities selected will depend upon the main areas of work carried out by the organisation and how much time is allocated to the inspection. Where time is limited, or where the inspection is triggered, only critical areas (either to the specific trials selected, or the specific queries raised) will be examined.

organisation's perspectives. Although face-to-face interviews are most effective, it is permissible to use teleconferences or videoconferences to overcome availability issues and to prevent personnel travelling unnecessarily long distances. If this is the case, time zones in different countries need to be considered. If there are any issues with timing of interviews because of clinical reasons – for example, when investigators are interviewed – inspectors can be flexible with timings to accommodate this. This should be resolved in the planning stage when the draft inspection plan is sent to the organisation.

Triggered and requested inspections differ from routine inspections, in that generally the objectives of the inspection are to answer specific questions raised (triggered inspections) or to satisfy the MHRA (or the CHMP) that a specific trial has been conducted in accordance with the legislation (MAA-related inspections). In addition, triggered inspections can be unannounced, in which case a detailed inspection plan might not be shared with the organisation.

Prior to the inspection, an organisation may be requested to make available additional documents, either prior to the site visit or for the first day of the inspection.

Requested documents may include:

- the TMF for a number of selected clinical trials
- CVs, job descriptions and training records for interviewees
- written procedural documents (for example, standard operating procedures (SOPs), working instructions)
- standard training material and presentations
- contracts and agreements templates
- evidence of corrective and preventative action (CAPA) taken in response to the previous inspection
- audit schedules
- serious adverse event (SAE) listings
- selected data listings from the clinical study report (usually for trial-specific inspections).

A.1.6.2 Conduct of the inspection

An opening meeting will be held on the first day of the inspection during which the scope and conduct of the inspection will be described.

The inspections themselves consist of site visits to the organisation (that is, commercial sponsors, non-commercial sponsors, contract research organisations (CROs)) and, if appropriate, one or two investigator sites (or other sites, such as a laboratory) involved in the organisation's current trials may also be inspected as an example of how the organisation's trial procedures were applied. (Note: Inspections of non-commercial investigator sites may take place at the same time as the inspection of the non-commercial sponsor organisations). Interviews with relevant personnel, generally as per the inspection plan, are conducted. Time is built into the inspection for the review of documentation, such as the TMF for the selected clinical trials or any other documents that have been requested during the inspection. The inspector may visit any facilities involved in clinical trials (for example, the pharmacovigilance department, data management unit, archives and pharmacy), and these visits may be pre-arranged by the inspector for logistical reasons or decided upon during the inspection. During the inspection, the inspection plan can and may be deviated from if the results of the inspection or unforeseen circumstances warrant this. Inspectors will also be flexible with the inspection plan in order to accommodate working patterns of individuals, wherever possible.

Inspectors do not hold a briefing at the end of every day to review deficiencies with the site. Issues will be raised at appropriate points throughout the inspection once associated document requests and written procedures have been reviewed. Instead, inspectors may discuss administrative or logistical issues (such as outstanding document requests or changes to the inspection plan) with the organisation at the end of each day.

In general, a closing meeting will be held on the last day of each inspection at each site, to provide oral feedback on any deficiencies identified and, if appropriate, information on any further sites to be inspected.

Points to consider in relation to the conduct of an inspection include the following:

- In general, the organisation is free to choose how many and which members of staff attend both the opening and closing meetings. Inspectors do not put restrictions on numbers attending, as long as space allows.
- Additional requests for documentation will be made throughout the inspection – these will be tracked via a form that the inspectors will maintain (an example document request form is shown in Table A.1.2). Copies of the forms may be taken at appropriate intervals to facilitate tracking. Most documents are used for reference only during the inspection. Therefore, to save time, provision of originals is acceptable (although do make the inspectors aware if documents are original so no notes are written on them). Any documents that the inspector wishes to retain will be clearly identified, in which case provision of a photocopy is usually acceptable.
- Any difficulties in obtaining documents during the inspection should be discussed with the inspection team at an early stage. Arrangements for providing documents post-inspection can be discussed.
- Note takers or observers are free to sit in on interview sessions as long as they do not interrupt the interview process.
- Organisations are free to take their own notes during the inspection, but recording of interviews or meetings is not permissible.

Table A.1.2 Example of a document request form used by MHRA GCP inspectors

Request no.	Document requested during inspection	Requester	Obtained	Reviewed	Retained
1	Written procedure for urgent safety measures	AB	✓	✓	
2	Training record for trial manager	AB	✓	✓	
3					
4					
5					

A1

- Post-interview clarification of responses is acceptable – inspectors understand the pressure a regulatory interview can impose, and that staff may be nervous.
- Internal audit reports will not routinely be reviewed, but may be requested in exceptional circumstances.

A.1.6.3 Reporting

Deficiencies found during MHRA GCP inspections are graded as follows:

(i) Critical

- Where evidence exists that significant and unjustified departure(s) from applicable legislative requirements has occurred with evidence that:
  - » the safety or well-being of trial subjects either has been or has significant potential to be jeopardised, and/or
  - » the clinical trial data are unreliable, and/or
  - » there are a number of major non-compliances (defined in (ii) below) across areas of responsibility, indicating a systematic quality assurance failure, and/or
- Where inappropriate, insufficient or untimely corrective action has taken place regarding previously reported major non-compliances (defined in (ii) below).

(ii) Major

- A non-critical finding where evidence exists that a significant and unjustified departure from applicable legislative requirements has occurred that may not have developed into a critical issue, but may have the potential to do so unless addressed, and/or

- Where evidence exists that a number of departures from applicable legislative requirements and/or established GCP guidelines have occurred within a single area of responsibility, indicating a systematic quality assurance failure.

(iii) Other

- Where evidence exists that a departure from applicable legislative requirements and/or established GCP guidelines and/or procedural requirement and/or Good Clinical Practice has occurred, but it is neither critical nor major.

Note: The grading of deficiencies as detailed above may be subject to change. Refer to the MHRA website for the most current information.

An inspection report is prepared by the lead inspector after the last site visit or on receipt of the last document requested, whichever is latest. It is reviewed internally to ensure consistency of classification of deficiencies prior to issue of the final report (grading of a deficiency may therefore change from what was initially communicated at the closing meeting). References to relevant sections in the regulations will appear in conjunction with those deficiencies classified as critical or major. The report is then sent to the inspected organisation (that is, commercial sponsors, non-commercial sponsors, CROs). Unless there are specific data or subject safety issues identified, a report will not be sent to the NHS Trust(s) associated with the selected investigator sites.

It should be noted that the factual matter contained in the inspection report relates only to those things that the inspection team sees and hears during the inspection process. The inspection report is not to be taken as implying a satisfactory state of affairs in documentation, premises, equipment, personnel or procedures not examined during the inspection.

A.1.7 Responding to findings

Following the issue of the inspection report, the organisation is requested to respond to any deficiencies identified and to provide the MHRA with an appropriate CAPA plan. The lead inspector will set the deadline for provision of responses. Note: During the inspection, the inspector may identify a deficiency that requires urgent action (for example, to safeguard the safety and well-being of trial subjects). In this circumstance, the inspected party may be requested to take immediate corrective action.

In relation to completing the responses:

- One person should assume overall responsibility for the responses. This individual should sign and date the document that includes the responses.
- Each inspection finding is numbered. A response should be produced for each inspection finding and the finding number should be referenced next to the response. Responses are not required in relation to recommendations or observations.
- Some of the findings in the report may be related to the systems/procedures of another party involved in the clinical trial. The inspector will expect the inspected organisation to supply responses for all findings by liaising with the other party.
- If the accuracy of information contained in the inspection report is challenged or if findings are disputed, then the respondent should enclose relevant documentary evidence supporting the responses. If a finding is not disputed, then documentary evidence is not required (unless specifically requested in the report).

When the deficiency is reviewed by the organisation, consideration should not only be given to correcting the specific examples cited in the inspection report, but also identification and correction of the root cause of the deficiency, where appropriate.

Other points to consider when responding to inspection findings are:

- The action must address the finding in terms of immediate corrective action and future preventative actions.
- Timelines should be clearly stated for each action.
- The organisation should not make promises it cannot deliver – that is, proposed timelines and actions should be realistic and achievable.
- Responses should be clear and succinct.

Following review of the responses, the inspector may contact the responsible individual to request additional information and/or to notify them that the responses do not adequately address the issues raised. It is routine practice for the responsible individual to be given one opportunity to provide additional information or clarification.

A1

A.1.8 Close-out of the inspection

Following review of the responses, the inspector will issue both a GCP inspection statement and a cover letter or email to formally close the inspection.

These documents may include a summary and evaluation of the findings or any further comment that the inspector wishes to make. For example, an organisation may also be required to provide quarterly reports on the progress of its CAPA in order to confirm that appropriate action is being taken.

GCP inspection statements are provided to the inspected organisation as a record of the inspection only; they are not intended as a statement of compliance. The statements are printed on headed paper and will include the number of findings in each critical and major category, and the topic area to which those findings related. Under certain circumstances, the issue of an inspection statement may be withheld. This may be warranted, for example, following referral to the MHRA Enforcement Group or where prompt follow-up inspection is directed by the MHRA Inspection Action Group (IAG) that considers issues related to GCP (IAG2).

A.1.9 Follow-up for serious inspection findings

Critical findings are routinely referred to IAG2, a non-statutory, multi-disciplinary group constituted to advise the Director of Inspection, Enforcement and Standards, the Director of Vigilance and Risk Management of Medicines and the Director of Licensing on any recommendation for referral or enforcement action appropriate to the divisions that arises from non-compliance detected during GCP and GPvP inspections (IAG1 covers issues from GMP and GDP inspections). IAG2 provides advice in cases where critical findings are identified during inspection and in other situations where serious non-compliance is identified that could affect the rights, safety or well-being of trial subjects or patients.

IAG2 meets regularly, usually monthly, to deal with ongoing business and to consider new referrals. Ad hoc meetings may be convened to address serious and urgent issues.

IAG2 recommendations for action may include:

* early re-inspection: this has been the most common recommendation to date. In most cases, on re-inspection adequate progress has been observed in

implementing the CAPA plan. In some cases, a further re-inspection has been required, and a minority of cases have been referred back to IAG2 for consideration of other actions

- request for provision of CAPA updates at periodic intervals
- recommendations for action in relation to pending or future clinical trial authorisation applications and/or recommendation for action in relation to existing clinical trials or existing clinical trial authorisations (for example, suspension or revocation)
- communication of the critical findings to external parties (for example, other competent authorities, other government departments, the EMA, the European Commission). Note: critical findings are routinely communicated to the National Research Ethics Service (NRES) under a memorandum of understanding
- meetings with senior representatives from the inspected organisations to review the implications of the critical findings, the organisation's proposed actions and the actions that may be taken if the non-compliances are not appropriately addressed
- issuance of an Infringement Notice (for example, to obtain a formal commitment for remedial action to be taken within a specified timeframe)
- referral to the MHRA Enforcement Group for investigation with a view to criminal prosecution.

A1

A.1.10 Re-inspections

Within the national inspection programme, there are a number of different reasons for re-inspection of an organisation:

- periodic national inspections performed as part of the routine statutory inspection programme (the frequency is dependent upon the risk-based inspection process)
- for inspections referred to IAG2, re-inspections to review corrective actions are normally required within 6–12 months
- UK and EU triggered inspections.

The focus of the inspection may be different from that of a routine, systems inspection depending on the reason for the re-inspection. One focus will be the improvement of the systems and processes resulting from the deficiencies identified in the previous inspection. A lack of action by the organisation will be taken into consideration when classifying inspection findings. Some areas may

A1

receive closer evaluation during re-inspection (for example, areas in which significant problems were previously identified; areas not looked at in detail on the first inspection; or areas of recent change). Some areas may not be evaluated to the same extent. For example, computer system validation may not be evaluated in depth if there have not been any upgrades or changes to the system.

A.1.11 Tips for preparing for a competent authority inspection

- Remember that inspections are a chance for the organisation to demonstrate regulatory compliance and an opportunity to improve its procedures and systems used for conducting trials in the UK.
- Be completely open and honest at all times.
- Communicate any issues or non-compliances that have already been identified by the organisation to the inspectors, at an early stage.
- Do not waste time and effort immediately prior to the inspection making quick fixes. These may often not be appropriate or may need to be changed after the inspection.
- Ensure all trial-related documentation is made available for selected trials – this should include the general TMF and UK country/site-specific sections, as well as any files that may be maintained separately (such as files for contracts, regulatory, pharmacovigilance, data management and statistics). Refer to section 10.6 for further information. European Guidance on the content of the TMF can be found in EudraLex Volume 10, Chapter V.
- Communicate promptly to the inspection team if there are any problems or difficulties in fulfilling inspection requests or if requests are unclear or ambiguous.
- The organisation may need to assign specific resource to assist with the coordination of the inspection. The individual or team assigned to do this must have good cooperation from other areas of the organisation.
- Ensure that everyone knows their role and responsibilities.
- Be prepared for deviations from the inspection plan at short notice.
- Ensure that interviewees and backroom staff are appropriate. Specific resources may need to be dedicated to address requests for documentation during the course of the inspection.
- Ensure that sufficient resources are made available to meet requests (for example, photocopiers, fax machines and adequate meeting rooms/offices).

- Ensure that the interview environment (for example, heating, lighting and ventilation) is suitable.
- Ensure that documentation is clearly labelled as per the inspector's request and that it is logged on the document request form.
- Implement a thorough communication strategy.
- Instigate a single contact point for coordination of requests coming from the inspection room.
- Ensure that relevant departments and sites are informed so that documents can be obtained from them if required.
- Ensure that there is a mechanism to obtain the relevant documentation, wherever it resides within the organisation, in a prompt manner.
- Ensure that teleconference or videoconference facilities are working and have been tested. Ensure that technical staff are available if problems arise.
- Check that the documents provided are complete and fulfil the request. Inadequate responses to requests may lead to additional requests and prolong the process.
- Finally, remember that the goals of the organisation and inspectors are the same – 'To protect public health'.

A1

Relevant legislation and guidance

A2

A.2.1 European legislation

Regulation (EC) No. 726/2004 of the European Parliament and of the Council of 31 March 2004 laying down Community procedures for the authorisation and supervision of medical products for human and veterinary use and establishing a European Medicines Agency.

Regulation (EC) No. 1394/2007 of the European Parliament and of the Council of 13 November 2007 on advanced therapy medicinal products and amending Directive 2001/83/EC and Regulation (EC) No. 726/2004.

Regulation (EC) No. 1901/2006 of the European Parliament and of the Council of 12 December 2006 on medicinal products for paediatric use and amending Regulation (EEC) No. 1768/92, Directive 2001/20/EC, Directive 2001/83/EC and Regulation (EC) No. 726/2004.

Regulation (EC) No. 1902/2006 of the European Parliament and of the Council of 20 December 2006 amending Regulation 1901/2006 on medicinal products for paediatric use.

Directive 2001/20/EC of the European Parliament and of the Council of 4 April 2001 on the approximation of the laws, regulations and administrative provisions of the Member States relating to the implementation of Good Clinical Practice in the conduct of clinical trials on medicinal products for human use.

Directive 2001/83/EC of the European Parliament and of the Council of 6 November 2001 on the Community Code relating to medicinal products for human use.

Commission Directive 2003/94/EC of October 2003 laying down principles and guidelines of Good Manufacturing Practice in respect of medicinal products for human use and investigational medicinal products for human use.

Commission Directive 2005/28/EC of 8 April 2005, laying down principles and detailed guidelines for Good Clinical Practice as regards investigational medical products for human use, as well as the requirements for authorisation of the manufacturing or importation of such products.

Directive 2011/62/EU of the European Parliament and of the Council of 8 June 2011, amending Directive 2001/83/EC on the Community Code relating to medicinal products for human use, as regards to prevention of the entry into the legal supply chain of falsified medicinal products.

Full text of the above can be accessed at: ec.europa.eu

A.2.2 UK legislation

The Human Medicines Regulations 2012, SI No. 1916 and the applicable Statutory Instruments, including:

* The Medicines for Human Use (Clinical Trials) Regulations 2004, SI No. 1031 and subsequent amendments, including:
  » The Medicines for Human Use (Clinical Trials) Amendment Regulations 2006, SI No. 1928
  » The Medicines for Human Use (Clinical Trials) Amendment (No. 2) Regulations 2006, SI No. 2984
* The Medicines for Human Use (Clinical Trials) and Blood Safety and Quality (Amendment) Regulations 2008, SI No. 941
* The Medicines (Products for Human Use) (Fees) Regulations 2012, SI No. 504 and subsequent amendments.

Full text of UK Statutory Instruments and Explanatory Memoranda can be accessed at www.legislation.gov.uk/.

A.2.3 Guidance documents and other useful reference texts

A.2.3.1 EudraLex documents

Relevant European guidance documents can be found in EudraLex Volume 10 (Clinical Trials), and also in Volume 4 (GMP guidance, in particular, Annex 13).

Key Volume 10 guidance includes:

- Detailed guidance on the request to the competent authorities for authorisation of a clinical trial on a medicinal product for human use, the notification of substantial amendments and the declaration of the end of the trial ('CT-1')
- Detailed guidance on the application format and documentation to be submitted in an application for an Ethics Committee opinion on the clinical trial on medicinal products for human use ('CT-2')
- Detailed guidance on the collection, verification and presentation of adverse event/reaction reports arising from clinical trials on medicinal products for human use ('CT-3')
- Annex 13 to the EU Guidelines to Good Manufacturing Practice, 'Manufacture of investigational medicinal products', July 2010
- 'Question & Answers' document
- Guidance on investigational medicinal products (IMPs) and non-investigational medicinal products (nIMPs)
- Detailed guidelines on Good Clinical Practice specific to advanced therapy medicinal products
- Recommendation on the content of the trial master file and archiving.

These documents (and others) can be accessed by searching on EudraLex at ec.europa.eu/health/documents/eudralex/index_en.htm

A.2.3.2 European Medicines Agency scientific guidance documents and reflection papers

There are also a number of scientific guidance documents and reflection papers published by the European Medicines Agency (EMA). These may be produced by a global group such as the International Conference on Harmonisation (ICH) and adopted by Committee for Medicinal Products for Human Use (CHMP), or produced by committees and working parties within Europe.

It is not practical to reproduce all guidance here; however, some useful documents, which are not included in EudraLex Volume 10, are highlighted as examples:

- European Commission Communication 2009/C28/01 ('Guidance on the information concerning paediatric clinical trials to be entered into the EU

Database on Clinical Trials (EudraCT) and on the information to be made public by the European Medicines Agency (EMEA), in accordance with Article 41 of Regulation (EC) No. 1901/2006')

- EMA GCP Inspectors Working Group, 'Reflection paper on expectations for electronic source data and data transcribed to electronic data collection tools in clinical trials' (EMA/INS/GCP/454280/2010)
- EMA, 'Reflection paper for laboratories that perform the analysis or evaluation of clinical trial samples' (EMA/INS/GCP/532137/2010)
- EMA, 'Reflection paper on expectations for electronic source data and data transcribed to electronic data collection tools in clinical trials'.

These documents (and others) can be accessed at the EMA website: www.ema.europa.eu/ema

A2

A.2.3.3 International Conference on Harmonisation (ICH) GCP documents

CPMP/ICH/135/95	E6	Guideline for Good Clinical Practice
CPMP/ICH/377/95	E2A	Clinical safety data management: definitions and standards for expedited reporting
CHMP/ICH/287/95	E2BM	Clinical safety data management: data elements for transmission of individual case safety reports
CHMP/ICH/166783/05	E2B (R3)	Data elements for transmission of individual case safety reports
EMEA/CHMP/ ICH/3943/03	E2B (R5)	Clinical safety data management: data elements for transmission of individual case safety reports: questions and answers
CPMP/ICH/381/95	Q2 (R1)	Validation of analytical procedures: text and methodology
CPMP/ICH/137/95	E3	Structure and content of clinical study reports
CPMP/ICH/363/96	E9	Statistical principles for clinical trials
CPMP/ICH/291/95	E8	General considerations for clinical trials
CPMP/ICH/286/95	M3 (R2)	Non-clinical safety studies for the conduct of human clinical trials and marketing authorization for pharmaceuticals
EMA/CHMP/ ICH/731268/1998	S6 (R1)	Preclinical safety evaluation of biotechnology-derived pharmaceuticals
EMEA/CHMP/ ICH/646107/2008	S9	Non-clinical evaluation for anticancer pharmaceuticals

Available from the ICH website: www.ich.org

ICH documents adopted by the CPMP/CHMP can be accessed at the EMA website: www.ema.europa.eu/ema

A.2.3.4 Committee for Medicinal Products for Human Use (CHMP) documents

CHMP/SWP/28367/07	Guideline on strategies to identify and mitigate risks for first in human clinical trials with investigational medicinal products
CHMP/EWP/2459/02	Reflection paper on methodological issues used in confirmatory clinical trials planned with an adaptive design
CHMP/QWP/185401/2004	Guideline on the requirements to the chemical and pharmaceutical quality documentation concerning investigational medicinal products in clinical trials
CHMP/BWP/534898/2008	Guideline on the requirements for quality documentation concerning biological investigational medicinal products in clinical trials
CPMP/EWP/QWP/1401/98 (Rev. 1)	Guideline on the investigation of bioequivalence
CPMP/ICH/381/95	Validation of analytical procedures
CHMP/EWP/5872/03	Guideline on data monitoring committees

These documents (and others) can be accessed by searching on EudraLex at: ec.europa.eu/health/documents/eudralex/index_en.htm

Advanced therapy investigational medicinal product trials

A3

> ### Editor's note
>
> An advanced therapy investigational medicinal product (ATIMP) is an advanced therapy medicinal product (ATMP) (as defined in Article 2 (1) of Regulation 1394/2007) which is tested or used in accordance with Article 2 (d) of Directive 2001/20/EC. The definition includes gene therapy, somatic cell therapy and tissue-engineered products.
>
> Clinical trials using ATIMPs are performed under the same clinical trials regulations as all other clinical trials; however, such trials also need to take into account the regulations specific to ATMPs. The regulation for ATMPs applied from 30 December 2008 (Regulation 1394/2007) and was incorporated into an amended Directive 2001/83/EC, together with Directive 2009/120/EC that amended Annex 1 of Directive 2001/83/EC. In December 2009, the 'Detailed guidelines on Good Clinical Practice specific to advanced therapy medicinal products' (hereinafter 'EU Guidance 2009') was published. The Medicines for Human Use (Advanced Therapy and Miscellaneous Amendments) Regulations 2010 (No. 1882) contain further detail on the implementation of the regulation into UK law.
>
> This annex covers some of the additional factors that should be taken into consideration by sponsors and research teams when planning and conducting ATIMP trials. Figure A.3.1 provides an overview of these considerations.

Archiving

- Systems in place to ensure trial documentation will be archived for the appropriate time period
- Appropriate contracts in place with concerned organisations (for example, tissue establishment(s) or manufacturer)
- If the trial is suspended or ended prematurely, or the sponsor ceases to exist as a legal entity, consideration will be needed to ensure archiving arrangements are in place for accountability/traceability records

Protocol

- Risk analysis to be conducted and documented
- Consideration for an ongoing risk analysis and communication of this to the investigator
- Training to be provided to all parties
- Considerations for devices in combined products
- Consider suitability of donated material, compliance with requirements and whether the donation is part of the trial process
- Will the sponsor expert be required at the application stage?

Informed consent

- Do the subject information sheet and consent form contain all of the specific information required by the ATIMP guidance?

Follow-up

- Systems in place for follow-up of subjects (both clinically and for data collection) to be defined in protocol
- Follow-up procedures for offspring and close contacts (considerations for consent)
- Training for investigators on requirements for follow-up
- A contingency plan for follow-up, in the event that the ATIMP development is halted, or the sponsor ceases to exist as a legal entity

ATIMP

- Clear traceability of the ATIMP at all sites involved (from manufacture through to application)
- Links from donor to recipient, and vice versa, which should be anonymised
- Contracts that include clear responsibilities with regard to traceability
- Traceability records to be kept for 30 years
- Regulation for procurement of human tissues must be considered
- Any precautions required in relation to viral shedding

Pharmacovigilance

- A pharmacovigilance process for ATIMPs that meets the additional requirements to expedite events related to the conduct of the trial
- Clear process for reporting adverse events in the protocol, to include events of concern (e.g. infection, lack of efficacy, events related to the application procedure, events related to mandatory concomitant medication)
- An alert card for each subject

ATIMP, advanced therapy investigational medicinal product

Figure A.3.1 Additional considerations for advanced therapy investigational medicinal product trials

A.3.1 Considerations for advanced therapy investigational medicinal product trials

The overarching principles in the ATIMP regulations and supporting guidance relevant to Good Clinical Practice (GCP) are as follows:

- The ATIMP must[1] be traceable from sourcing through to administration to the subject.

- If the product originates from a donor, records must[1] be sufficiently detailed to allow linking from donor to recipient and from recipient to donor; however, personal data should be protected by use of an anonymous coding system so that neither donors nor recipients remain identifiable.

- The protocol should specify the follow-up period for the subjects, and this must[2] be followed during and, if necessary, after the end of the trial, both for their own care and data collection as necessary.

- Medical care given to, and medical decisions made on behalf of, subjects must[3] always be the responsibility of a qualified medically qualified doctor or dentist, although there may be circumstances where a representative of the sponsor experienced in administration of the ATIMP also needs to be present during the application of the ATIMP to the subject. This expert may provide advice and information to the principal investigator or responsible medically qualified doctor, but the principal investigator remains responsible for any decision to halt or modify the application procedure.

A clinical trial involving an ATIMP must[4] comply with all of the standard requirements of GCP, as well as the additional requirements of the regulations and guidelines specific to ATMPs.

A.3.1.1 Traceability of an advanced therapy investigational medicinal product

Where an ATIMP contains human cells or tissues, it must[1] be possible to link the donor/source to the donation, to link the donation to the product and then to link the product to the subject. The traceability has to work in both directions from source to subject and from subject to source. It is the responsibility of the sponsor of the trial, the manufacturer and the investigator/institution where the product is used to ensure that a suitable traceability system is in place.

It is important to note that traceability is an area of overlap with Good Manufacturing Practice (GMP) since the traceability requirements also apply to manufacture and therefore must comply with GMP (in particular, Annex 2 and Annex 13 of EU GMP (EudraLex Volume 4). Traceability at the manufacturer is outside the remit of a MHRA GCP inspection, and would be covered by MHRA GMP inspectors. Traceability at blood establishments in the UK will be covered by the MHRA GMP inspections of these establishments. The Human Tissue Authority (HTA) assesses traceability systems for tissues and cells that may become ATIMPs further downstream when inspecting HTA-licensed establishments. There may also be other tissue establishments in the supply chain, some of which (for example, if embryonic stem cells are involved) may be inspected by other agencies depending on activities. For further details on the agencies involved and their inspection programmes, refer to the individual agencies' websites.

In practice, for GCP compliance, the standard investigational medicinal product (IMP) accountability contributes significantly to the traceability of the ATIMP from the manufacturer onwards. The manufacturer is responsible for traceability/accountability until the point of delivery to the trial site (assuming it is delivering the product) following which, the usual chains of accountability and associated documentation apply (that is, from pharmacy to trial team to subject).

Appropriate Qualified Person (QP) certification must[5] be in place prior to the release of the ATIMP. For short shelf-life products, GMP Annex 2 requires a two-stage QP certification, the first before administration (which will review the results and issues available at that time) and the other on receipt of the remaining test results, which may be after the subject has been dosed. Where the ATIMP is manufactured at a location that requires controlled storage temperature during transport prior to administration, there should be temperature monitor/log data and/or confirmation that such conditions have been met.

If the trial is suspended or prematurely ended (or the product development is discontinued), the sponsor retains its obligations to ensure that the traceability system is maintained (this includes where ATIMP ownership is transferred to another legal entity; the new owner should take responsibility for maintaining the traceability). If the organisation faces bankruptcy and the records cannot be transferred to another legal entity, then the traceability records (not all documents) should be transferred to the competent authority. This transfer of documents to the competent authority is only in relation to ATIMPs; there are no such arrangements in place for other types of trials.

Traceability procedures should either be described in the protocol or in an associated document (which should be sent to the competent authority for approval).

On inspection, the following examples have been seen where traceability and handling of the IMP was not appropriate:

- QP certification could not be traced through from vials manufactured to those dosed to subjects.
- ATIMP was dosed to a subject without evidence that appropriate temperature had been maintained during transport of IMP from the off-site freezer store to the hospital.
- Outputs from temperature data loggers were not retained in files for import of ATIMP that required cold-chain storage.

A.3.1.2 Contracts

Contracts should be put in place by the sponsor to guarantee the maintenance of traceability systems with the manufacturer, tissue establishment(s) or principal investigator/institution (which may include the surgeon who obtains the tissue or cells from a donor prior to manufacturing of the ATIMP), as applicable. These contracts will be key to ensuring the adequacy and duration of each party's responsibilities commensurate with the long-term nature of the follow-up, safety reporting and archiving requirements (for example, it has been seen that contracts in place with an ATIMP manufacturer only required retention of traceability records for 15 years, rather than the required 30 years). It is recommended that contracts encompass these obligations, including retention measures in the event of bankruptcy of one or more of the parties. Since there may be multiple parties involved that may not be routinely involved in clinical trials, it is important that responsibilities are clearly defined and documented for each party.

A.3.1.3 Risk analysis

It is the responsibility of the sponsor to ensure that an ongoing risk analysis of the ATIMP is performed and documented The risk analysis should be based on existing knowledge of the type of product and its intended use, including risks associated with the application method (for example, surgery, concomitant medication, associated devices). Among other aspects, the risk analysis will consider the need for, the duration and the nature of follow-up.

The risk analysis may be provided to investigators in the form of the investigator's brochure (IB). Maintenance of an IB for an ATIMP, including the requirement[6] for annual updates, is the same as that for an IMP and is covered in further detail in Chapter 4.

In practice, it is likely that the investigator/institution will additionally initiate their own safety management processes (for example, through risk assessments performed locally through the biological safety officer (or equivalent), as applicable). Where viral vectors are used, the sponsor would also usually perform an environmental risk assessment regarding viral shedding, and implement procedures as necessary to protect frontline healthcare professionals from potential risk of infection. Consideration would also be given to waste products and their potential effect on the public and environment.

A.3.1.4 Informed consent

As for any trial with an IMP, ATIMP consent material and procedures must[7] undergo an ethical review. However, there are specific elements for consent for ATIMPs that are included here for information. The investigator should inform the trial subject and, where applicable, their legal representative of the specific issues that arise for ATIMPs. In particular, both the informed consent form and any other written information to be provided to the subjects should include explanation of traceability arrangements, follow-up (before and after the end of the trial), the nature of the ATIMP (including risks to themselves and others), and the involvement of the sponsor (for example, the need, where applicable, for the presence of a representative of the sponsor for assistance during the administration of the ATIMP). Further details are available in section 11 (49h) of the EU Guidance 2009.

A.3.1.5 Pharmacovigilance

The EU Guidance 2009 states that new events likely to affect safety should be reported according to existing guidelines for expedited reporting and includes serious adverse events (SAEs) associated with trial procedures, lack of efficacy and events related to mandatory concomitant medication. The 'Detailed guidance on the collection, verification and presentation of adverse event/reaction reports arising from clinical trials on medicinal products for human use, June 2011' (hereinafter 'detailed guidance CT-3') states that these events do not need to be expedited; this requirement is therefore different for ATIMPs. The 'detailed guidance CT-3' also states that neither the sponsor nor investigator needs to actively monitor subjects for adverse events once the trial has ended; again this therefore differs for ATIMP trials as compared with clinical trials of medicinal products, and should be described in the protocol (or associated document).

The sponsor should consider any additional protocol- and/or product-specific requirements for adverse event reporting. In particular, the sponsor should consider issues that may be of concern such as adverse events related to the product application process, cases of infection, adverse events related to product failure or lack of efficacy, and adverse events related to mandatory concomitant medication. Adverse events may also occur that are related to medical devices that form part of the product or that are used for application of the product. Adverse incidents related to a medical device used in an ATIMP trial should be reported to the MHRA (see MHRA website for further details).

Causality assessment concerning the safety issues mentioned above should be described in the clinical trial protocol or associated document (and approved by the competent authority), and implemented in the adverse event reporting system. For example, the case report form (CRF) could be designed to capture differentiated causality (that is, suspected relationship to process, ATIMP, device or concomitant medication).

A.3.1.6 Follow-up

Clinical follow-up is defined in section 2 (4) of the EU Guidance 2009 as:

'a follow-up of individual subjects conducted by healthcare professionals. It includes prevention, screening, monitoring, diagnosis and treatment of diseases, injuries, complications, adverse reactions and medical errors'.

Safety follow-up is defined as:

'any systematic collection and collation of data that is designed in a way that enables learning about safety of a medicinal product. It may include passive or active surveillance, observational studies or clinical trials.'

Processes should be established to enable contact with subjects to be maintained throughout the required follow-up period. The need for, duration and nature of follow-up should be described in the protocol. This should be based on the nature of the ATIMP, the current state of knowledge and a risk analysis. Follow-up should be considered from the following aspects:

- for the protection of the subject – that is, clinical follow-up

- for the purpose of collection of specific data (that might not involve all subjects) – that is, safety and efficacy follow-up.

All subjects participating in a clinical trial with an ATIMP should receive from the investigator an alert card, which has been previously agreed by the sponsor and approved by the research ethics committee (REC), containing as a minimum:

- the name of the subject
- the investigator's contact number
- information regarding the medical treatment received.

Subject alert cards should inform medically qualified doctors treating the subject about the product used and any independent registries or other sources of data available in case of safety/efficacy issues, and of the need to inform the competent authority, the investigational sites and the sponsor in the event of certain serious adverse reactions.

The protocol should define the end of the trial and what follow-up should take place after the end of the trial. The safety and efficacy follow-up involving active data collection (for example, study visits) should form part of the clinical trial, whereas clinical follow-up and passive data collection may take place after the end of the trial.

Where follow-up after the end of the trial is required by the protocol, in particular when this occurs over the long term, the sponsor should ensure that there is a process in place for follow-up of the subjects treated with the product, even in cases where the product development is discontinued or the (former) sponsor ceases to exist as a legal entity. This process should be described in the protocol (as approved by the competent authority), which should be amended as needed. Where a subject is withdrawn from a trial at their own request or based on a decision of the investigator, the follow-up should be maintained, subject to the consent of the subject. Follow-up should also be considered for close contacts and offspring providing this has been approved by the REC and consent is in place for this. Where follow-up is via a third-party organisation, such as a government or health service registry, appropriate arrangements must be in place to cover, for example, the exchange of data.

A.3.1.7 Training

Those involved in the conduct of an ATIMP trial must[8] be aware of (and appropriately trained in) the regulations and guidance not only specific to these types of product, but also the GCP and GMP regulations. Findings seen on inspections of ATIMP trials can often be attributed to a lack of awareness of ATIMP guidance documents and content (by the sponsor or investigator, or both) or to ATMP organisations being new to regulated manufacture (GMP/GCP).

A.3.1.8 Essential documents and archiving

The requirements for essential documents for ATIMP trials follow the standards set out in SI 2004/1031, Directive 2001/20/EC and Directive 2005/28/EC. The EU Guidance 2009 defines the responsibilities for documentation for the sponsor, investigator, tissue establishment(s) and manufacturer(s) (as applicable), for the different trial stages (section 15 of EU Guidance 2009).

The sponsor of the trial, manufacturer, principal investigator/institution must[9] keep their records regarding ATIMP traceability for a minimum of 30 years after the expiry date of the product, or longer if required by the terms of the clinical trial authorisation. It is recommended that this includes the medical records of the trial subjects, and that these records clearly indicate that the subject was part of an ATIMP trial and as such should be kept for 30 years. Where archiving is contracted out, there should be appropriate arrangements in place that clearly state which documents relate to traceability and that these must[9] therefore be retained for the 30-year required period. These arrangements should also state the retention period for the other trial documents (that is, the usual archival period for clinical trials).

Examples of issues with essential documentation and archiving requirements for ATIMPs seen on inspection are:

- Gene therapy laboratory files did not form part of the trial master file (these omitted files contained key documents such as QP certification and IMP accountability).
- The archiving written procedure did not define those records that need to be retained by the sponsor for the 30-year retention period – that is, those records that form the ATIMP traceability audit trail.
- The contract with the NHS Trust archiving facility was not sufficiently detailed to ensure that the medical records would be retained for 30 years.

Further details on general essential documentation and archiving requirements can be found in Chapter 4.

A.3.1.9 Laboratory considerations

As most ATIMP studies will involve pioneering new techniques, it is likely that there will be new laboratory procedures and techniques developed alongside these. These techniques should be validated and records retained to ensure that processes are accurate, reproducible and can be interpreted and verified as required. (It is important to note that development and validation should be distinct.)

A.3.1.10 Considerations for medical devices

Where an ATIMP also incorporates a medical device (that is, a combined advanced therapy medicinal product), the protocol should contain a brief overview of:

- the characteristics, performance and purpose of the device
- confirmation that this product is in conformity with essential requirements of the regulations referred to in Article 6 of the Advanced Therapy 2008 Regulation (this regulation only applies to marketed devices; the MHRA Clinical Trials Unit would liaise with the MHRA Devices Division on this aspect, where necessary as part of the approval process)
- the rationale for the combination of ATIMP and medical device to aid understanding of the effect of each individually and in combination.

A.3.2 Annex legislative references

Throughout this annex, specific terminology – 'must', 'required' or 'requirement' – has been used to interpret activities that are legislative requirements. These terms have been number-coded in the text where used, and the corresponding reference in the legislation can be found below.

1. Section 4 (1) of SI 2010/1882
2. Regulation 29 of SI 2004/1031
3. Schedule 1, Part 2 (11) of SI 2004/1031
4. Regulation 28 of SI 2004/1031
5. Article 13 (3) of Directive 2001/20/EC
6. Regulation 3A of 2004/1031
7. Schedule 3, Part 1 (1) and (3) of SI 2004/1031
8. Schedule 1, Part 2 (2) of SI 2004/1031
9. Schedule 1 of SI 2010/1882

Considerations for use of electronic systems in clinical trial management

A4

Editor's note

Over the last two decades there has been increasing use of interactive voice response systems (IVRS) utilising telephones. Such systems have been developed further into interactive web-based response systems (IWRS) utilising the internet. For ease in this guide, these two terms will be combined into the general term 'interactive response technologies' (IRT) systems.

These systems were initially designed as a method for managing the medication supply chain in clinical trials and making the most efficient use of the drug supplies; this was particularly important where there was only a small quantity of product available, the investigational medicinal product (IMP) was particularly expensive or multiple sites were involved. In recent years, the use of these systems has expanded into other areas such as dose titration, unblinding and expiry-date updating. Also, in controlling randomisation and medication dispensing, the database of these systems can provide real-time project information and therefore act as a helpful trial management tool.

IRT systems may be bespoke in-house products designed by the sponsor or they may be managed by a vendor providing this service; the term 'provider' will be used in this annex to refer to either party.

A.4.1 What is an IRT system?

Essentially an IRT is a database that contains information on the subjects, the treatments and the sites which, after input from the site, advises the site which kit can be given to a particular subject. For this reason, an IRT consists of a number of databases, the main ones being a kit/treatment database and a subject database, with other ancillary databases completing the system.

Figure A.4.1 captures the links between the different databases involved in an IRT system. The subject database is where the subject randomisation numbers reside. This number should be unique to each subject on the trial and will include some demographic details, which can be used as a double check when entries are made into the IRT. The kit/treatment database is where the drug information resides. Each kit/treatment number is unique. The subject database is linked with the kit/treatment database. At a visit, the investigator (or delegate) will call the system or access it via the web to indicate that they need supplies for a particular subject. The system will then allocate a kit/treatment number based on the treatment to which the subject has been randomised. The randomisation database is where the treatment arms reside and will, of course, be linked directly to the subject database. The investigator site database is required for shipment details and the address of the site to be registered. It allows the provider to know what has been shipped to a site and to whom it was shipped. It will also have details of when the shipments were received at the site. Where a warehouse is used as a halfway house between the site of final release of IMP and the investigator site, details of the warehouse will be stored here, including the address and what medication is stored at that warehouse.

Often the IMP information is held outside the IRT system and the IRT system is manually updated by the sponsor (or delegate) responsible for the IMP. In these instances there can be a link from the sponsor drug supplies system directly or there can be a separate database within the IRT system. This holds details of the batch numbers of product and their expiry. This is particularly important when the IRT is used for the handling of expiry dates, rather than printing the expiry date on the label. This is deemed acceptable in Annex 13 of EU GMP (EudraLex Volume 4) which states that certain information can be omitted from the label if it is maintained by other means such as use of an IRT system.

It is recommended that IRTs are set up with various levels of access permission, usually provided via access codes assigned by the organisation responsible for managing the IRT. There should be a formal and documented mechanism for the granting of the correct level permission access code and revoking access (for example, when someone leaves an organisation or ceases to work on that clinical trial) to ensure adequate security and control of the system.

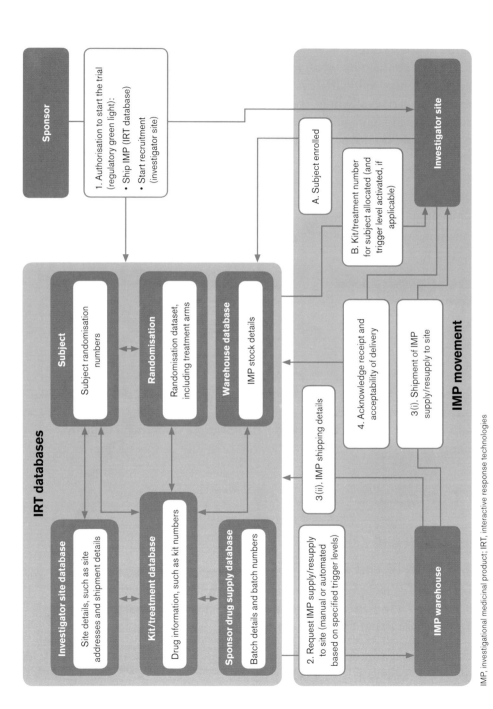

IMP, investigational medicinal product; IRT, interactive response technologies

Figure A.4.1 An example of the set-up and use of an IRT system

A4

Access is via the internet or the telephone. It is recommended that each member of the investigator site team with delegated authority from the principal investigator has a unique access code. The access permissions of different members of the team will differ depending on what they have been delegated to do and this should be represented in the IRT system. There should be an audit trail to demonstrate who did what when. This can be achieved in the IRT system through each individual having a unique access code; however, if this is not the case, then the audit trail should be documented elsewhere (for example, on paper).

The IRT system can accommodate a number of tasks, some of which may include:

- randomisation
- IMP dispensing
- stock control
- titration of doses
- blind breaking
- expiry date control
- site activation
- recall.

When setting up an IRT for a trial, it is recommended that early discussions take place between the relevant internal sponsor departments, contract manufacturing organisation (CMO) or the sponsor and IRT provider to determine what the requirements for the trial are and how they are best met by the system.

A.4.2 Setting up an IRT system

A.4.2.1 Design and validation

It is recommended that the protocol includes reference to the fact that an IRT will be utilised, even if at this point the provider (if not an internal system) is not known. The key to a robust IRT system for a trial is to ensure that the following is undertaken early on in the trial design process:

- Selection of most appropriate IRT provider, if not internal (see section 1.3.2 for information on selecting a vendor)
- Ensure sufficient time is allocated to set up and validate the system

- Identification of the manufacturing/assembly site(s)
- Inclusion of the manufacturing/assembly site(s) in the IRT set-up (It may be appropriate for the IMP contractor (if used) to have direct contact with the IRT provider to decrease the possibility for misunderstandings, but the sponsor must[1] maintain oversight)
- Ensure responsibilities between all the associated parties are documented clearly
- A thoroughly reviewed user requirements specification (URS) is advised as it may be difficult to make changes to the system at a later date. This can also include access permissions. For example:
  - » Who is responsible for activating sites (sponsor/provider)?
  - » Who can grant users access and permission settings for both the sponsor and site personnel?
  - » Who is able to unblind at the sponsor for expedited reporting?
  - » Who is able to unblind at the site for emergency unblinding?

Good communication between the sponsor and all the relevant parties can prevent many issues and avoid having to reprogramme the IRT system. For example, it has been seen on inspection that a lack of communication between two programming teams, one looking at bespoke code and the other at customisation of existing modules, resulted in several modules not being tested (as each group thought the other was doing it) and the system not being fully validated. In another instance, poor communication between the sponsor and provider project teams led to unblinded information being sent to the blinded project team at the sponsor.

The system will be designed based on the URS. Many providers will do this by way of a functional design specification (FDS), which gives the programmers something more technical to work from. Many systems are modular in nature, therefore it may be appropriate to validate only those bespoke programming elements and ensure that the overall system is operating as expected. Refer to section 14.5 for expectations on computer system validation.

The validation of the interfaces between the databases should form part of the testing of the system. Errors in the system can be catastrophic – for example, when the two treatment groups of a trial had been juxtaposed, subjects who should have been on the active arm were actually taking placebo. Issues such as this could invalidate a trial and necessitate a re-run. There are also many potential safety issues that could arise from the use of a poorly validated IRT system. For example, where calculations are undertaken within the system and the result is used to determine the next dose, if the calculation is incorrect or the algorithm linking it to the treatment is not accurate, then there is the potential for overdosing and/or underdosing subjects. Both outcomes could have serious consequences for the subjects.

The transfer of randomisation codes into the IRT should also be validated. Testing of this transfer is often performed using a dummy list. However, it has been seen on inspection that a dummy randomisation code was utilised during the testing phase, and this was the list that was then subsequently transferred into the live database, rather than the final version. This of course led to serious consequences for the trial.

A.4.2.2 User acceptance testing and 'go live'

Once the provider is satisfied with the system it will be open for sponsor (or delegate) user acceptance testing (UAT). Testing can take place either at the provider's premises or remotely. Issues can still be identified with the system, even when it has been released to the sponsor for testing. Hence, it is strongly recommended that the sponsor avails itself of the opportunity to conduct adequate UAT. A provider may offer to produce test scripts for UAT; however, it is strongly recommended that the sponsor produce its own. In this way, the sponsor has a better knowledge of the system and it has been seen that client UAT may uncover programming issues that may have been missed by the provider. The UAT also provides an opportunity to check that the system is consistent with the requirements of the protocol.

Once the sponsor has completed the UAT and any programming issues have been dealt with and retested, there will be a formal process at the provider for the system to 'go live' (that is, making the system available for use). Often this requires that the system is moved into the production area. Approval of the system should be formally documented and follow the activities described in section 14.5. There should have been some validation to ensure that the production area handles the IRT in the same manner that the test environment did. The system is then ready for use.

A.4.2.3 User access and training

Each individual accessing the system and their role should be documented in the delegation of authority log at the site and any project specification for the system.

It is advised that these individuals also each have their own unique access code. This is particularly important for an audit trail if different roles are given different access rights (for example, for unblinding or randomisation).

Prior to the use of the system at the site, training must[2] be undertaken, appropriate to the role of the individual. In many instances a user manual is provided to the site for the monitor to discuss at the initiation monitoring visit. Training must[2] also be provided to sponsor personnel who will be accessing the system. There have been a number of instances where changes in the system instigated by sponsor personnel have led to unblinding incidents. Training is equally important at the IRT provider, as inadvertent unblinding has occurred when unblinded data were sent to the sponsor's project manager.

A.4.3 Use of an IRT system

Figure A.4.1 provides an overview of the steps that generally take place when using an IRT system for a trial.

A.4.3.1 Activation within the system and initial drug shipment

It is recommended that each site is activated by a responsible individual at the sponsor or provider on an individual site basis once the authorisation to start the trial has been received for that site. The sponsor should be able to confirm that sites have been activated and that individuals at the site are able to access the system. It is important that this is done prior to IMP arriving at the site, particularly if the IRT will be used for breaking the blind in the event of a medical emergency.

As well as site activation, warehouse activations may also need to be considered. It is also possible that the QP has responsibility within the system; this could include verifying that supplies have been certified or that the expiry date has been updated in the system.

It is recommended that the sponsor define the stock levels to be sent to each site in the initial shipment. This will be based on anticipated recruitment rate, stratification of the randomisation and any past knowledge of the site. Site shipments from the warehouse should initially be triggered by the sponsor. The warehouse will receive a 'pick list' from the provider and will then send supplies to the site under the correct transport conditions. When the IRT is not used for breaking of the blind, randomisation code envelopes will be shipped along with trial drug. Some trials may have the supplies shipped on the basis of the randomisation of a subject within the IRT. This is also acceptable provided any

A4

risk with delays in shipping have been identified and mitigated. This may occur where there is some run-in period before IMP is administered to the subjects.

When supplies are received the site will acknowledge receipt; this may or may not occur via the IRT. This acknowledgement includes any confirmation that the integrity of the shipment was not compromised (for example, in the event of damaged containers or temperature excursions). Some sites may need to retrieve data from data loggers, which will mean that supplies will not be made available for dispensing at the site until the data have been analysed by the sponsor to ensure the integrity of the product. If there is no acknowledgement of receipt this may prohibit the use of those supplies, as the system will not recognise that they are available for use at the site. It is the responsibility of the investigator (or their delegate) to ensure that this task is completed. Temperature excursions should be managed as described in section 6.14.1. Quarantine procedures should be in place to ensure that the investigator and the IRT provider are made aware of any decision related to the use of quarantined stock.

A.4.3.2 Ongoing drug supply and other uses

Once activated at site and warehouse level, randomisation and dispensing can start at the site. As subjects enter the trial, the investigator or designee can contact the system to ascertain the treatment kit number to be assigned to that subject. The IRT will allocate the treatment kit based on the randomisation, visit and the expiry date of the stock. Additionally, the system can also determine what stock is at site and therefore when to re-supply sites (based on reaching re-supply trigger levels set by the sponsor). This can ensure that material is always available on site.

The site would usually receive a consignment report that would confirm the treatment kit number assigned to the subject number. Where the expiry date is controlled by the IRT (that is, the date is not printed on the label), the consignment report should also include the expiry date of the material. The checking of the expiry date should be inherent in the IRT system; however, it is good practice to double-check this at the site, as issues have occurred when the material supplied did not have a sufficient shelf life for the length of treatment. For example:

• IMP was assigned with the intention of the site being re-supplied and subjects returning prior to their next visit to receive new supplies and return the expiring

IMP. However, the subjects were never alerted to this, so they did not return for new supplies and took expired IMP.

- Expired IMP was not quarantined in the system, therefore allowing the expired IMP to be allocated to subjects.

To prevent such occurrences, two dates are often put into the system:

- A 'do not ship' date (that is, the date after which shipments should not be made from the warehouse to investigator sites after taking into account the length of time the IMP will be at site before it is allocated and the length of the treatment)
- A 'do not dispense' date (that is, the date after which the IMP should not be dispensed; this would include provision for the length of treatment and take into consideration the expiry date).

The IRT system can also be used for:

- **Dose titrations** Additional information may be entered into the system, such as haemoglobin levels or creatinine clearance rates, among other results. The IRT will then determine which kit/dose level will be administered to the subject.
- **Breaking of the blind** Procedures for breaking the blind via the IRT should be in place, for medical emergencies and expedited reporting. The procedures may include who is able to break the blind (and how this relates to access permissions) and the audit trail (electronic or paper) to demonstrate the procedure.
- **Product recall** This may be managed via the IRT where the system has access to all stock from the particular batches being recalled and is able to quarantine the stock electronically. This will ensure that this quarantined material is not inadvertently administered to subjects. It is important that the sponsor communicates this information quickly so that appropriate steps can be taken at the site.

A.4.3.3 Manual interventions

At times during the course of the trial, there may be a need for manual intervention (for example, if an incorrect kit has been dispensed to the subject or the electronic system is temporarily unavailable due to a fault). The IRT provider should therefore have procedures in place to manage such eventualities, such as an emergency contact number for the site to call. It is recommended that this helpdesk function is available on a 24-hour basis for global studies.

Where manual changes are made to the system, there should be a procedure in place to record these changes, including how the system would be updated to record the intervention. Where systems are updated in this way there should be quality control (QC) checks in place to ensure that the system is updated correctly. It has been seen on inspection that a lack of QC of manual changes has led to the system containing incorrect data such as expiry dates.

A.4.4 Maintenance of an IRT system

During the course of a trial there may be changes made to the system, such as those due to bug fixes or amendments in the protocol, which should be covered in a formal change control process (see section 14.5). The sponsor is responsible for updating the provider with any amendments to the protocol that could affect the IRT (for example, an extension of the trial, a change in treatment or a change in dosing). Issues have been seen on inspection when protocol amendments requiring a change to the IRT system have not been communicated to the provider, resulting in the system not being changed and IMP therefore not being administered as per the amended protocol.

A.4.5 What to do when the IRT system is unavailable

In the event that the system is not working (for example, because of technical difficulties at the site or at the provider, or because the server is being updated), there should be arrangements in place to allow the trial to continue at the site. This is particularly important when the subject has already started on the trial treatment, as it could affect the safety of the subject if they are unable to continue treatment, or it could affect the ability of the site to manage any emergency unblinding.

A usual method for ensuring continuity of the system is to have a facility to contact the IRT provider's helpdesk. Trained individuals, on the IRT provider's helpdesk, are recommended to have access to the randomisation scheme and be able to make a 'manual intervention' indicating which kit should be supplied to the subject. It is important that this is well documented, so that any of these interventions can be updated in the system as soon as the system is available. Issues have been seen where manual interventions have been made and there was a lack of documentation to demonstrate what randomisation had taken place while the system was down.

A.4.6 Close-down of an IRT system

When the trial is completed, the IRT system will need to be closed down to prevent further access to the system. It is the responsibility of the sponsor to let the provider know when this will occur. This will prevent investigators having the ability to randomise any further subjects. For example, it has been seen on inspection that, despite the target number of subjects having been reached, an IRT system had not been closed down as the provider had not been informed. This could have been avoided by programming a maximum number of subjects into the IRT system at the start of the trial. However, if subjects are still on treatment, the system should still allow access for any emergency unblinding, where applicable.

Any data residing with the IRT provider must[3] be reconciled with the clinical trial database and any queries must[3] be resolved before the closure of the clinical trial database. This must[4] all be clearly documented and retained (Chapter 10). Data may also be transferred to the clinical trial database from the IRT database as this may be the repository of information; this should be subject to the same data-transfer guidance as mentioned in Chapter 8.

A.4.7 Annex legislative references

Throughout this annex, specific terminology – 'must', 'required' or 'requirement' – has been used to interpret activities that are legislative requirements. These terms have been number-coded in the text where used, and the corresponding reference in the legislation can be found below.

1. Regulation 3 (12) of SI 2004/1031
2. Schedule 1, Part 2 (2) of SI 2004/1031
3. Schedule 1, Part 2 (9) of SI 2004/1031
4. Regulation 31A (4) of SI 2004/1031

Glossary

ADMINISTRATION OF RADIOACTIVE SUBSTANCES ADVISORY COMMITTEE

The committee established in line with the requirements of the Medicines (Administration of Radioactive Substances) Regulations responsible for issuing certificates for administration of radioactive medicinal products to humans.

ADVANCED THERAPY INVESTIGATIONAL MEDICINAL PRODUCT

Directive 2001/20/EC; EU Regulation 1394/2007: An advanced therapy medicinal product as defined in Article 2 (1) of EU Regulation 1394/2007 which is tested or used in accordance with Article 2 (d) of EU Clinical Trials Directive 2001/20/EC. This includes gene therapy, somatic cell therapy and tissue-engineered products.

ADVERSE EVENT

SI 2004/1031: Any untoward medical occurrence in a subject to whom a medicinal product has been administered, including occurrences that are not necessarily caused by or related to that product.

ADVERSE (DRUG) REACTION

SI 2004/1031: Any untoward and unintended response in a subject to an investigational medicinal product that is related to any dose administered to that subject.

ANNUAL SAFETY REPORT

SI 2004/1031: A report of all suspected adverse reactions that have occurred during that year in relation to any trials conducted (both inside and outside the UK) by the sponsor for that drug product.

ASSEMBLE/ASSEMBLY

SI 2004/1031: In relation to an investigational medicinal product, to enclose the product (with or without other medicinal products of the same description) in a container which is labelled before the product is sold or supplied or used in a clinical trial; or, where the product (with or without other medicinal products of the same description) is already contained in the container in which it is to be sold or supplied or used in a clinical trial, to label the container before the product is sold or supplied or used in a clinical trial in that container.

AUDIT

ICH E6: A systematic and independent examination of trial-related activities and documents to determine whether the evaluated trial-related activities were conducted, and the data were recorded, analysed and accurately reported according to the protocol, sponsor's written procedures, Good Clinical Practice, and the applicable regulatory requirement(s).

AUDIT TRAIL

ICH E6: Documentation that allows reconstruction of the course of events.

BENCHMARKING OF EUROPEAN MEDICINES AGENCIES

A cross-agency group established by the Heads of Medicines Agencies (HMA) for the purpose of identifying and sharing best practices across the European Union network of agencies.

BLINDING

Annex 13, EU Guidelines to Good Manufacturing Practice; ICH E6: A procedure in which one or more parties to the trial are kept unaware of the treatment assignment(s). Single-blinding usually refers to the subject(s) being unaware; double-blinding usually refers to the subject(s), investigator(s) and, in some cases, data analyst(s) being unaware of the treatment assignment(s). In relation to an investigational medicinal product, blinding shall mean the deliberate disguising of the identity of the product in accordance with the instructions of the sponsor. Unblinding shall mean the disclosure of the identity of blinded subjects or products.

CHIEF INVESTIGATOR

SI 2004/1031: In relation to a clinical trial conducted at a single trial site, the investigator for that site, or in relation to a clinical trial conducted at more than one trial site, the authorised health professional, whether or not they are an investigator at a particular site, who takes primary responsibility for the conduct of the trial.

This term is similar to the term 'coordinating investigator' in ICH E6 which denotes an investigator assigned the responsibility for the coordination of investigators at different centres participating in a multi-centre trial.

See also 'investigator'.

CLINICAL STUDY REPORT

ICH E6: A written description of a trial/study of any therapeutic, prophylactic or diagnostic agent conducted in human subjects, in which the clinical and statistical descriptions, presentations and analyses are fully integrated into a single report.

CLINICAL TRIAL

SI 2004/1031: Any investigation in human subjects, other than a non-interventional trial, intended to discover or verify the clinical, pharmacological and/or other pharmacodynamic effects of one or more medicinal products, and/or to identify any adverse reactions to one or more such products, and/or to study absorption, distribution, metabolism and excretion of one or more such products, with the object of ascertaining its (their) safety and/or efficacy.

CLINICAL TRIAL AUTHORISATION

SI 2004/1031: Authorisation to conduct a clinical trial granted by the competent authority.

CLINICAL TRIALS FACILITATION GROUP

The group established by the Heads of Medicines Agencies (HMA) in 2004 to coordinate implementation of the EU Clinical Trials Directive 2001/20/EC across the Member States. It acts as a forum for discussion to agree on common principles and processes to be applied throughout the European medicines regulatory network. It is composed of representatives from the competent authorities, the European Commission (EC) and the European Medicines Agency (EMA).

CLINICAL TRIAL SUMMARY REPORT

EudraLex Volume 10, Chapter I: Part of the end-of-trial notification, albeit usually submitted only subsequently to the end-of-trial notification. The sponsor should provide this summary report within one year of the end of the complete trial to facilitate entry of these details onto the EudraCT database.

COMPARATOR

ICH E6: An investigational or marketed product (that is, active control) used as a reference in a clinical trial.

(NATIONAL) COMPETENT AUTHORITY

A body with authority to act on behalf of the government of the Member State to perform a designated function; in the case of clinical trials, to ensure that the requirements of the Clinical Trials Directive are transposed into national law and are applied.

The Medicines and Healthcare products Regulatory Agency (MHRA) is the 'competent authority' in the UK.

See also 'Medicines and Healthcare products Regulatory Agency'.

CONTRACT RESEARCH ORGANISATION

ICH E6: A person or an organisation (commercial, academic or other) contracted by the sponsor to perform one or more of a sponsor's trial-related functions.

CIOMS I FORM

The CIOMS I form is the internationally recognised form for reporting of suspected unexpected serious adverse reactions (SUSARs). It was designed by the Council for International Organizations of Medical Sciences (CIOMS), an international, non-governmental, not-for-profit organisation.

DATA LOCK POINT

ICH E2F: The date (month and day) designated as the cut-off for data to be included in a development safety update report (DSUR). It is based on the development international birth date.

DATA SAFETY MONITORING BOARD

ICH E9: Also known as a data safety monitoring committee or data monitoring committee. An independent data monitoring committee that may be established by the sponsor to assess at intervals the progress of a clinical trial, the safety data and the critical efficacy end-points, and to recommend to the sponsor whether to continue, modify or stop a trial.

DEVELOPMENT INTERNATIONAL BIRTH DATE

ICH E2F: The date of the first authorisation to conduct a clinical trial in any country worldwide.

DEVELOPMENT SAFETY UPDATE REPORT

ICH E2F: A common standard for periodic reporting of drugs under development among the ICH regions. In the European Union, it replaces the annual safety report.

See also 'annual safety report'.

EUDRACT (EUROPEAN UNION DRUG REGULATING AUTHORITIES CLINICAL TRIALS)

The European database of clinical trials established in accordance with Directive 2001/20/EC.

EUROPEAN ECONOMIC AREA

SI 2004/1031: The European Economic Area (EEA) created by the EEA agreement, between the European Union (EU) and the European Free Trade Association. Includes Member States, Norway, Iceland and Liechtenstein.

EUROPEAN MEDICINES AGENCY

The European Agency established for the evaluation of medicinal products. It is a decentralised agency of the European Union, located in London. The Agency is responsible for the scientific evaluation of medicines developed by pharmaceutical companies for use in the European Union, using assessors and inspectors of the EU Member States.

(AUTHORISED) HEALTHCARE PROFESSIONAL

SI 2004/1031: An authorised healthcare professional is defined as a medically qualified doctor, a dentist, a nurse or a pharmacist.

HEALTH RESEARCH AUTHORITY

SI 2001/2323: An authority in England established on 1 December 2011. The authority exercises functions in connection with the facilitation and promotion of research and the establishment of research ethics committees.

HOSTING ORGANISATION

An organisation selected by the sponsor to undertake clinical trial activities, usually considered to be an investigator site, but may also be a vendor organisation.

HUMAN TISSUE AUTHORITY

A body with a remit to ensure that human tissue is used safely and ethically, and with proper consent. It regulates organisations that remove, store and use tissue for research, medical treatment, post-mortem examination, teaching and display in public. It also gives approval for organ and bone marrow donations from living people.

INSPECTION ACTION GROUP

A non-statutory, multi-disciplinary group constituted to advise the Director of the Inspection, Enforcement and Standards Division at the Medicines and Healthcare products Regulatory Agency (MHRA) on any recommendation for regulatory or adverse licensing action appropriate to the Division. IAG2 considers issues related to Good Clinical and Good Pharmacovigilance Practices.

INTEGRATED RESEARCH APPLICATION SYSTEM

The online Integrated Research Application System (IRAS) used to submit applications to research ethics committees in the United Kingdom for review and opinion.

INTENTION-TO-TREAT ANALYSIS

ICH E9: An analysis based on the intention to treat a subject (that is, the planned treatment regimen) rather than the actual treatment given.

INTERNATIONAL ORGANIZATION FOR STANDARDIZATION

Commercially developed international standards for quality, in a variety of different areas, developed to create industry-wide consensus.

INVESTIGATIONAL MEDICINAL PRODUCT

SI 2004/1031: A pharmaceutical form of an active substance or placebo being tested, or used, as a reference in a clinical trial, including products already with a marketing authorisation but, for the purposes of the trial, used or assembled (formulated or packaged) in a way different from the authorised form, or when used for an unauthorised indication, or when used to gain further information about the authorised form.

INVESTIGATIONAL MEDICINAL PRODUCT DOSSIER

SI 2004/1031: The dossier relating to an investigational medicinal product that accompanies a request for authorisation to conduct a trial in which that product is used.

INVESTIGATOR

SI 2004/1031; Directive 2001/20/EC: In relation to a clinical trial, the authorised healthcare professional responsible for the conduct of that trial at that site, and if the trial is conducted by a team of authorised health professionals at a trial site, the investigator is the leader responsible for that team and may be called the 'principal investigator'.

INVESTIGATOR'S BROCHURE

SI 2004/1031: A document containing a summary of the clinical and non-clinical data relating to an investigational medicinal product that is relevant to the study of the product in human subjects.

INVESTIGATOR (TRIAL) SITE

SI 2004/1031: A hospital, health centre, GP surgery or other establishment or facility at or from which a clinical trial, or any part of a clinical trial, is conducted.

MANUFACTURE

SI 2004/1031: In relation to an investigational medicinal product, any process carried out in the course of making the product, but not including dissolving or dispensing the product in, or diluting it or mixing it with, some other substance used as a vehicle for the purposes of administering it.

MEDICINAL PRODUCT

SI 2004/1031, Directive 2001/83/EC:

- Any substance or combination of substances presented as having properties for treating or preventing disease in human beings, or
- Any substance or combination of substances that may be used in or administered to human beings either with a view to restoring, correcting or modifying physiological functions by exerting a pharmacological, immunological or metabolic action, or to making a medical diagnosis.

MEDICINES AND HEALTHCARE PRODUCTS REGULATORY AGENCY

The Medicines and Healthcare products Regulatory Agency (MHRA) is the UK government agency responsible for ensuring that medicines and medical devices work, and are acceptably safe. The MHRA is an executive agency of the Department of Health and was established in April 2003 from a merger of the Medicines Control Agency and the Medical Devices Agency.

See also 'competent authority'.

MONITORING

ICH E6: The act of overseeing the progress of a clinical trial and of ensuring that it is conducted, recorded and reported in accordance with the protocol, written procedures, Good Clinical Practice and the applicable regulatory requirements.

NATIONAL RESEARCH ETHICS SERVICE

Part of the Health Research Authority (HRA); responsible for monitoring the performance of research ethics committees, and for providing advice and assistance to them as delegated by the United Kingdom Ethics Committee Authority (UKECA) to the HRA.

NHS TRUST/HEALTH BOARD

An appointed board that manages the National Health Service (NHS) through the four publicly funded healthcare systems in the UK. These are NHS (England), NHS Scotland (Scotland) and NHS Wales (Wales), and Health and Social Care (Northern Ireland). (Note: the term 'NHS Trust(s)', when used in the text of this guide, includes NHS Health Boards in Scotland, where applicable.)

NON-INTERVENTIONAL TRIAL

SI 2004/1031: A study of one or more medicinal products that are authorised, where the products are prescribed in accordance with the terms of that authorisation. The assignment of any subject involved in the study to a particular therapeutic strategy is not decided in advance by a protocol but falls within current practice, and the decision to prescribe a particular medicinal product is clearly separated from the decision to include the subject in the study. No trial-specific diagnostic or monitoring procedures are applied other than those which are ordinarily applied in the course of standard care, and epidemiological methods are used for the analysis of the data arising from the study.

NON-INVESTIGATIONAL MEDICINAL PRODUCTS

EudraLex Volume 10, Chapter I: Medicinal products used in the context of a clinical trial and not falling within the definition of an investigational medicinal product.

PATIENT (SUBJECT) IDENTIFICATION CENTRE

A site that is not performing any clinical trial activities (such that it is not a formal investigator site), however, may be used by an investigator site to help identify potential subjects and refer them to the investigator site for inclusion into a trial.

PER-PROTOCOL ANALYSIS

ICH E9: An analysis of the subset of subjects who complied with the protocol sufficiently to ensure that these data would be likely to exhibit the effects of treatment, according to the underlying scientific model. Compliance covers such considerations as exposure to treatment, availability of measurements and absence of major protocol non-compliances.

PERIODIC SAFETY UPDATE REPORT

Directive 2010/84/EU: Periodic safety update reports submitted by marketing authorisation holders containing summaries of data relevant to the benefits and risks of the medicinal product, including results of all studies with a consideration of their potential impact on the marketing authorisation; a scientific evaluation of the risk–benefit balance of the medicinal product; all data relating to the volume of sales of the medicinal product and any data in possession of the marketing authorisation holder relating to the volume of prescriptions, including an estimate of the population exposed to the medicinal product.

POST-AUTHORISATION STUDY

Directive 2010/84/EU: Any study relating to an authorised medicinal product conducted with the aim of identifying, characterising or quantifying a safety hazard, confirming the safety profile of the medicinal product, or of measuring the effectiveness of risk management measures.

PRINCIPAL INVESTIGATOR

See 'investigator'.

QUALITY ASSURANCE

ICH E6: All those planned and systematic actions that are established to ensure that the trial is performed and the data are generated, documented (recorded) and reported in compliance with Good Clinical Practice and the applicable regulatory requirements.

QUALITY CONTROL

ICH E6: Operational techniques and activities undertaken within the quality assurance system to verify that the requirements for quality of the trial-related activities have been fulfilled.

QUALITY MANAGEMENT

ISO 9000: Coordinated activities to direct and control an organisation with regard to quality.

QUALITY MANAGEMENT SYSTEM

ISO 9000: A management system to direct and control an organisation with regard to quality (for example, policies, written procedures, guidelines, templates).

REFERENCE SAFETY INFORMATION

EudraLex Volume 10, Chapter II: The information used for assessing the expectedness of an adverse reaction. It is contained in either the investigator's brochure or the summary of product characteristics.

RESEARCH AND DEVELOPMENT (R&D) OFFICE

The term R&D office in context of this guide is used for:

- R&D offices within an NHS Trust or Health Board
- business and innovation departments within a university
- any other terms used by non-commercial organisations for the group charged with sponsor's oversight of the clinical trial.

RESEARCH ETHICS COMMITTEE

Directive 2001/20/EC: An independent body in a Member State, consisting of healthcare professionals and non-medical members, whose responsibility it is to protect the rights, safety and well-being of human subjects involved in a trial and to provide public assurance of that protection, by, among other things, expressing an opinion on the trial protocol, the suitability of the investigators and the adequacy of facilities, and on the methods and documents to be used to inform trial subjects and obtain their informed consent.

RISK MANAGEMENT PLAN

Directive 2010/84/EU: A detailed description of the risk management system which comprises a set of pharmacovigilance activities and interventions designed to identify, characterise, prevent or minimise risks relating to a medicinal product, including the assessment of the effectiveness of those activities and interventions.

SERIOUS ADVERSE EVENT

SI 2004/1031: Any adverse event which results in death, is life-threatening, requires in-patient hospitalisation or prolongation of existing hospitalisation, results in persistent or significant disability or incapacity, or consists of a congenital anomaly or birth defect.

SERIOUS BREACH

SI 2004/1031: A breach which is likely to affect to a significant degree the safety, physical or mental integrity of the subjects of the trial, or the scientific value of the trial.

SPONSOR

SI 2004/1031: An individual, company, institution or organisation that takes responsibility for the initiation, management and/or financing of a clinical trial.

SUMMARY OF PRODUCT CHARACTERISTICS

Directive 2001/83/EC: The summary of product characteristics (SPC) describes the properties and conditions for use of a particular medicinal product, and is the basis of information for health professionals on how to use the medicinal product safely and effectively. It includes the composition, pharmaceutical form and strength, approved indications, side effects, warnings and precautions for use, shelf life, storage conditions and the name of the marketing authorisation holder.

SUSPECTED UNEXPECTED SERIOUS ADVERSE REACTION

SI 2004/1031: A serious adverse reaction, the nature and severity of which is not consistent with the information about the medicinal product in question, as defined in the summary of product characteristics for that product in the case of a product with an authorisation, or in the investigator's brochure relating to the trial in question in the case of any other investigational medicinal product.

See also 'serious adverse event'.

THE OVERVOLUNTEERING PREVENTION SERVICE (TOPS)

TOPS is a database that aims to prevent healthy volunteers from taking part too often in trials of new medicines.

THIRD COUNTRY

SI 2004/1031: A country or territory outside the European Economic Area.

See also 'European Economic Area'.

UNEXPECTED ADVERSE REACTION

SI 2004/1031: An adverse reaction, the nature and severity of which is not consistent with the information about the medicinal product in question, as defined in the summary of product characteristics for that product in the case of a product with an authorisation, or in the investigator's brochure relating to the trial in question in the case of any other investigational medicinal product.

UNITED KINGDOM ETHICS COMMITTEE AUTHORITY

A body consisting of the Secretary of State for Health (England), the National Assembly for Wales (Wales), Scottish Ministers (Scotland) and the Department for Health, Social Services and Public Safety (Northern Ireland); responsible for appointing research ethics committees, monitoring their performance and providing advice and assistance to them (this is delegated to the National Research Ethics Service via the Health Research Authority).

URGENT SAFETY MEASURE

SI 2004/1031: An urgent safety measure taken by the sponsor or investigator in order to protect the subjects of a clinical trial against any immediate hazard to their health or safety.

VENDOR/EXTERNAL VENDOR

All the various types of providers a sponsor may delegate their functions to (for example, CRO, laboratory, consultant, freelancer/contractor, niche provider).

VIRTUAL ORGANISATION

A small sponsor organisation comprising only a few key staff and which, as such, mainly contracts out all of its functions.

Index

contracting out *continued*
  of IMP activities 195–6
  of investigator site services 367–8
  of laboratory work 427
  of medical advice 169–70
  of monitoring 250
  of pharmacovigilance 138
  of QP certification 195–6
contract manufacturing organisations
    (CMOs) 4, 19, 36, 193, 194, 195,
    209, 231, 500
contract research organisation (CRO) 4,
    124, 138, 143, 176, 233
contracts/agreements
  for archiving 26, 356
  bespoke or non-standard 367
  between sponsor and vendor 186, 195
  with CMO 195
  for data management 289
  for documentation 231, 353
  investigator 367–8
  investigator sites 28
  for laboratory work 426–7
  model 28, 367
  for Phase I units 400
  preparation and oversight 27–8
  requirements 19
  with service providers 226
  for source data 388
  for traceability systems 491
  with vendors 19
coordinating investigator, definition 362
corrective and preventative action (CAPA)
    473, 476, 478, 479
correspondence
  organisation in TMF 339
  see also emails
co-sponsorship
  arrangements for DSURs 176
  see also sponsor, joint
cover letters 52, 63

data
  capture 264, 286–90
  coding 303
  completion of cleaning/validation
    process 305–6
  critical 247
  electronic transfer 287
  final, availability 322
  investigator's independent copy 278–9
  long-term access or backing up 278
  processing 265
  protection 420
  publication 90, 114, 264
  quality 303–4
  query process 299, 300–1
  recording in lab 430–1
  recording tools for trial subjects 280–2
  remote review 254
  self-evident corrections 299
  superfluous 274
  suspicious 324
  unavailability for inclusion in DSUR 177
  unresolved issues 305
  use in central monitoring 253–6
  verification 246–7, 286–7
data clarification form (DCF) 300–1
data collection
  for pharmacovigilance 172
  tools 268–9
data entry
  error detection and rectification 295
  by investigator site staff 391
  quality control 287, 288–9
  verification 453
data lock point (DLP) 174
data loggers 218, 219
data management
  documentation 267–8
  error rates, acceptable 453
  non-commercial operations 265
  overview of process 264–8
  personnel 265–7
  plan (DMP) 267
  quality control checks (QC) 265
  and statistical analysis 265
  statistical input 314–15
data management systems, competency
    sign-off 451
data manager, role at investigator site 365
data monitoring committee (DMC) 31,
    161, 163, 166–8, 236

investigational medicinal products (IMPs)
continued
expired 505
expiry date handling 498
from general stock 215
importation 186, 191–2, 407
labelling 39, 54, 185–7, 201–4
management by investigator 220–2
management in Phase I units 407–9
manufacture or reconstitution 204–5
manufacturing authorisation,
  requirements 185–7
monitoring 241, 245–6
off-label use 153, 155
oversight at investigator sites 39–40
packaging 185–6
prescribing 380–1
prescription requirements 228–9
product liability 30
QP declaration/certification 35–6,
  55–6, 189–94
quarantined shipment 37, 408
re-packaging for blinding 198
regulatory release 194–5
responsibility for quality 186
return 223, 380, 504–5
safety profile 139
self-administration by trial subjects
  226–7
shipment 217–18
site-to-site transfer 222–3
sponsor's responsibilities 1, 7, 35–40
starting dose 403–4, 414
storage and distribution 217–25
supplied to non-commercial sponsor
  165, 208
supplier as vendor 18
supply to subjects by post 223–5
unused, segregated 381
use after trial completion 227–8
see also medicines
investigator
adverse event reporting 32–3, 139–42,
  149–61, 381
adverse reaction reports to 437
chief *see* chief investigator

consent 373
definition 362, 363
duty of care to subjects 374
essential documents retention 352
independent copy of data 278–9
ongoing subject management 378
responsibilities 74, 362–3
  delegation to trial team 369
investigator site file (ISF)
archiving arrangements 26
electronic 346
indexing and organisation 333
in TMF 330–1
under investigator's control 355
investigator sites
agreements 28
approvals required 366
choice 361
closure 256–7
competency sign-off 451
decisions, documentation of 391–2
documentation 386
equipment and facilities 379–80
handling of laboratory samples 384–5
initial approach 364–6
oversight 21–2, 28
research team 361
resources required 361
role of trial coordinator 365
set-up 364–6
staff signature log 369
subcontracting of services 367–8
supply of IMP 40
team members 364–5
training requirements 368, 369–70
trial-specific documentation 388
investigator-initiated trials 170, 208
investigator's brochure (IB)
annual update 155
ATIMP 492
content and format 53
development and review 131
RSI 151, 155–6
specific guidance 118
sponsor's responsibilities 31–2
tabulation of adverse events 154–5